Applied Methods of Cost–Benefit Analysis in Health Care

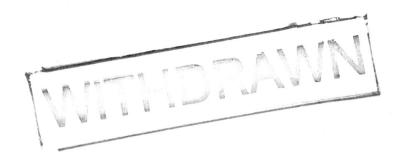

Handbooks in Health Economic Evaluation Series

Series editors: Alastair M. Gray and Andrew Briggs

Decision Modelling for Health Economic Evaluation
Andrew Briggs, Mark Sculpher, and Karl Claxton

Economic Evaluation in Clinical Trials
Henry A. Glick, Jalpa A. Doshi, Seema S. Sonnad, and Daniel Polsky

Applied Methods of Cost–Benefit Analysis in Health Care
Emma McIntosh, Philip M. Clarke, Emma J. Frew, and Jordan J. Louviere

Applied Methods of Cost-Effectiveness Analysis in Health Care
Alastair M. Gray, Philip M. Clarke, Jane Wolstenholme, and Sarah Wordsworth

Applied Methods of Cost–Benefit Analysis in Health Care

Edited by

Emma McIntosh
Philip M. Clarke
Emma J. Frew
Jordan J. Louviere

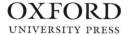

OXFORD
UNIVERSITY PRESS

Great Clarendon Street, Oxford OX2 6DP

Oxford University Press is a department of the University of Oxford.
It furthers the University's objective of excellence in research, scholarship,
and education by publishing worldwide in

Oxford New York

Auckland   Cape Town Dar es Salaam   Hong Kong   Karachi
Kuala Lumpur Madrid Melbourne Mexico City   Nairobi
New Delhi Shanghai Taipei Toronto
With offices in
Argentina Austria Brazil Chile Czech Republic France Greece
Guatemala Hungary Italy Japan South Korea Poland Portugal
Singapore Switzerland Thailand Turkey Ukraine Vietnam

ISBN 978-0-19-923712-8

Printed and bound in Great Britain by
CPI Antony Rowe, Chippenham and Eastbourne

Oxford University Press makes no representation, express or implied, that the drug dosages in
this book are correct. Readers must therefore always check the product information and clinical
procedures with the most up-to-date published product information and data sheets provided by
the manufacturers and the most recent codes of conduct and safety regulations. The authors
and the publishers do not accept responsibility or legal liability for any errors in the text or for
the misuse or misapplication of material in this work. Except where otherwise stated, drug

Series Preface

Economic evaluation in health care is a thriving international activity that is increasingly used to allocate scarce health resources, and within which applied and methodological research, teaching, and publication are flourishing. Several widely respected texts are already well established in the market, so what is the rationale for not just one more book, but for a series? We believe that the books in the series *Handbooks in Health Economic Evaluation* share a strong distinguishing feature, which is to cover as much as possible of this broad field with a much stronger practical flavour than existing texts, using plenty of illustrative material and worked examples. We hope that readers will use this series not only for authoritative views on the current practice of economic evaluation and likely future developments, but also for practical and detailed guidance on how to undertake an analysis. The books in the series are textbooks, but first and foremost they are handbooks.

Our conviction that there is a place for the series has been nurtured by the continuing success of two short courses that we helped develop – 'Advanced Methods of Cost-Effectiveness Analysis' and 'Advanced Modelling Methods for Economic Evaluation.' Advanced Methods was developed in Oxford in 1999 and has run several times a year ever since, in Oxford, Canberra, and Hong Kong. Advanced Modelling was developed in York and Oxford in 2002 and has also run several times a year ever since, in Oxford, York, Glasgow, and Toronto. Both courses were explicitly designed to provide a computer-based teaching that would take participants not only through the theory but also the methods and practical steps required to undertake a robust economic evaluation or construct a decision-analytic model to current standards. The proof-of-concept was the strong international demand for the courses – from academic researchers, government agencies, and the pharmaceutical industry – and the very positive feedback on their practical orientation.

So the original concept of the Handbooks series, as well as many of the specific ideas and illustrative material, can be traced to these courses. The Advanced Modelling course is in the phenotype of the first book in the series, *Decision Modelling for Health Economic Evaluation*, which focuses on the role and methods of decision analysis in economic evaluation. The Advanced Methods course has been an equally important influence on *Applied Methods of Cost-Effectiveness Analysis*, the fourth book in the series which sets out the key elements of analysing costs and outcomes, calculating cost-effectiveness, and reporting results. The concept was then extended to cover several other important topic areas. First, the design, conduct, and analysis of economic evaluations alongside clinical trials have become a specialized area of activity with distinctive methodological and practical issues, and its own debates and controversies. It seemed worthy of a dedicated volume, hence the second book in the series, *Economic Evaluation in Clinical Trials*. Next, while the use of cost–benefit analysis in health care has spawned a substantial literature, this is mostly theoretical, polemical, or focused on specific issues such as willingness to pay. In 2003 we ran a course entitled 'An Introduction to Stated Preference Discrete Choice Modelling in Health Care' in collaboration with Professor Jordan Louviere (CenSoC). Much of the material in this course focused on the valuation of benefits using stated preference discrete choice modelling, including the estimation of willingness to pay for use in cost–benefit analysis. The new material on discrete choice methods from this course along with existing work in the area of cost–benefit analysis from the authors provides the backbone for this third book in the series. We believe the third book in the series, *Applied Methods of Cost–Benefit Analysis in Health Care*, fills an important gap in the literature by providing not only a comprehensive guide to the theory but also the practical conduct of cost–benefit analysis, again with copious illustrative material and worked out examples. This book provides up-to-date practical guidance on using alternative methods of benefit assessment techniques such as stated preference discrete choice experiments within cost–benefit analysis.

Each book in the series is an integrated text prepared by several contributing authors, widely drawn from academic centres in the UK, the United States, Australia, and elsewhere. Part of our role as editors has been to foster a consistent style, but not to try to impose any particular line: that would have been unwelcome and also unwise amidst the diversity of an evolving field. News and information about the series, as well as supplementary material for each book, can be found at the series website: http://www.herc.ox.ac.uk/books.

Alastair Gray
Oxford
July 2006

Andrew Briggs
Glasgow

Web resources

In addition to worked examples in the text, readers of this book can download datasets, spreadsheets, formulas, and programs used in the relevant chapters.

Materials for this book are maintained at the following web address: http://www.herc.ox.ac.uk/books/cba

More information is available at the website. We anticipate that the web-based material will be expanded and updated over time.

Acknowledgements

I first became interested in cost–benefit analysis (CBA) in 1995 while working at the Health Economics Research Centre (HERU) at the University of Aberdeen. The health economic training obtained in those early days working with colleagues at HERU including Professor John Cairns, Professor Cam Donaldson, and Professor Mandy Ryan was enormously valuable and heavily influenced my areas of academic interest. These areas of interest continue today albeit diversified to accommodate for the increasing practical requirements of working in applied economic evaluation. My early interest in the use of stated preference discrete choice experiments (SPDCEs) in health economics also began at HERU and was inspired by the sound theoretical basis of the approach and the opportunities for the testing of economic axioms within health care. This interest was further developed by the intellectual generosity of Professor Jordan Louviere (Censoc, Sydney) and Professor Vic Adamowicz (University of Alberta) – both of whom have been hugely inspirational. Chapters 5, 10, 11, and 12 represent the development of such methods in health care.

Working with Professor Alastair Gray and Dr Philip M. Clarke at the Health Economics Research Centre (HERC) for the last ten years along with other HERC colleagues has further fuelled a more applied interest in CBA in health care. This has arisen through working in the development of stated preference techniques and applied methods of economic evaluation. I am hugely indebted to Professor Gray for his support and encouragement in all aspects of my work. Indeed, the work in Chapter 8, arguably one of the first identifiable CBAs in health care, arose from working with Professor Alastair Gray and clinical colleagues Professor Norbert Boos and Dr Mathias Haefeli in Switzerland and proved to be a most enjoyable collaboration. Working with Professor Tipu Aziz in Neurosurgery has also provided valuable opportunities to explore the strength of the CBA approach in health care. Indeed early work with the MRC hernia trials group arguably started this process. Dr Philip M. Clarke's novel work on the travel cost approach in Chapter 9 is an excellent example both in its theoretical grounding and the execution of the approach in health care. Chapters 6 and 7 produced by Dr Emma J. Frew provide a much overdue and valuable insight to the practical side of developing willingness to pay surveys in health care. I am grateful to Professor Andy Briggs for his editorial contribution to this book, particularly his assistance with appropriate methods of uncertainty in Chapter 12.

Finally, the support of my family, my husband Jeremy, and my three wonderful children, Angus, Archie, and Rebecca are acknowledged.

Emma McIntosh, PhD
Oxford, March 2010

Contents

Contributors

W.L. (Vic) Adamowicz
Department of Rural Economy,
University of Alberta,
Alberta, Canada

Norbert Boos
PRODORSO
Zentrum für Wirbelsäulenmedizin
Zurich, Switzerland

Richard T. Carson
Department of Economics
University of California
San Diego,
La Jolla, CA, USA

Philip M. Clarke
Sydney School of Public Health
Edward Ford Building,
The University of Sydney,
NSW, Australia

Achim Elfering
Institute of Psychology,
University of Bern,
Bern, Switzerland

Denzil G. Fiebig
School of Economics,
University of New South Wales
Sydney, Australia

Emma J. Frew
Health Economics Facility,
University of Birmingham,
Health Services Management Centre,
Birmingham, UK

Alastair Gray
Health Economics Research Centre,
Department of Public Health,
University of Oxford,
Oxford, UK

Mathias Haefeli
Centre for Spinal Surgery
University of Zurich
University Hospital Balgrist,
Zurich, Switzerland

F. Reed Johnson
RTI Health Solutions,
Research Triangle Institute,
North Carolina, USA

Jordan J. Louviere
UTS: CenSoC,
Centre for the Study of Choice
University of Technology,
Sydney, Australia

Emma McIntosh
Health Economics Research Centre,
Department of Public Health,
University of Oxford,
Oxford, UK

Atul Sukthankar
Centre for Spinal Surgery
University of Zurich
University Hospital Balgrist,
Zurich, Switzerland

Chapter 1

Introduction

Emma McIntosh

1.1 **Introduction**

In 1971, Mishan published the first comprehensive book on the subject of cost–benefit analysis (CBA) (1) and since then there have been a large number of texts in this field covering the theoretical basis of welfare economics (2–6;6–14) as well as books from a number of disciplines providing more specific technical guidance on the practice of CBA and valuing benefits in monetary terms (8;15–19) not forgetting the vast economic journal content for insights into methodological work in this area such as the *Journal of Health Economics, Health Economics, Social Science and Medicine,* and the *International Journal of Technology Assessment in health Care* to name but a few. Other than a recent general 'Handbook of Research on Cost–Benefit Analysis' by Brent (19) which has a limited section on health care, there is a distinct shortage of texts and journal articles offering practical, empirically-based advice on carrying out an applied CBA, least of all in health care. Indeed, it was noted by Pearce in 1971 (9) in reference to the theoretical and practical problems of CBA that there were 'serious problems' in actually applying the theory. The purpose of this handbook, therefore, is neither to provide an exhaustive treatment of the entire theoretical basis of CBA nor to debate the ongoing methodological work, but to supplement existing texts by providing key up-to-date methodological guidance in the specific area of applied CBA in health care while at the same time paying appropriate attention to their extensive theoretical basis where relevant. The aim of this book is therefore not to re-invent the theoretical wheel of CBA nor to condense it so much that it compromises the 'scientific foundations of the discipline in order to present the illusion of simplicity' (20), but to act as a handbook to assist researchers with up-to-date tools and practical suggestions for carrying out applied CBA in health care, and in doing so push forward this methodological area.

1.2 **Rationale for the book**

Given the failure of the market system in health care to allocate resources optimally, there is a requirement for economic measures of value to guide policy making in this area. This is similar to the situation in environmental economics as outlined by Freeman *et al.* (16). In the last 15 years, there has been a rapid rise in the number of methodological and applied contributions to the economics of health care. The majority of these contributions however have been in the area of cost-effectiveness and cost–utility analyses (17;21). This period has also seen a surge in the number of methodological applications in the area of contingent valuation and the measurement and valuation of monetary benefits. One notable development in the literature has been the increased use of both willingness to pay (WTP) and stated preference discrete choice experiments (SPDCEs) for estimating welfare values in health care as well as other areas including environmental and transport economics. Given this significant shift in the literature it is felt that a dedicated handbook to the practical application of CBA in light of these developments was timely. While the aim of the book is to provide guidance on the applied methods of CBA, this must be done within the realms of the rapidly developing literature in this area. It is for this reason that the book will focus on both the costing literature as well as methodological developments in the WTP literature and the fast evolving SPDCE literature. In doing so, the aim of this book is to provide guidance in carrying out applied CBA in health care that is as up-to-date as possible. While the distinguishing feature of this series of handbooks is its much stronger practical flavour than existing texts with plenty of illustrative material and worked examples, given the important theoretical basis of CBA, this book begins by introducing the basic theorems of welfare economics.

Since the purpose of this book is to act as a practical guide to applied CBA practitioners, much of the theoretical basis of welfare economics is assumed. Hence, the intended readers for this book are applied economic evaluation/CBA practitioners in health care and related areas such as environmental economists. However, for a more detailed introduction to the basic theories of 'normative' welfare economics including Pareto-improving criteria, theories underlying preferences and utility maximization, as well as the theory underlying the alternative types of welfare measures (compensating variation, equivalent variation, and consumer surplus), readers are referred to Boadway and Bruce (5), Layard and Walters (22), Layard and Glaister (23), and Mishan (1).

While CBA is a common form of economic evaluation across other sections of the economy such as the environment (see Chapter 5), other than methodological contributions in the area of benefit assessment such as WTP studies (see Chapters 6–8), the application of the CBA methodology in the health care sector has been notably limited with a widespread reluctance to use CBA for health care evaluations (2;24). As pointed out by Borghi (25) 'few WTP studies in the health sector have used their results within a CBA, an essential step to informing resource allocation decisions'. The main challenge of this handbook therefore is the compilation of evidence in the areas of benefit assessment and costing, and an attempt to produce some coherent guidance on applied methods of CBA in health care. As noted, this will require contributions from a number of developing literatures, most notably costing, WTP, and SPDCE. One immediate observation from these areas is the increasing reliance on statistical and econometric developments. While these developments have aided the 'accuracy' of such measures, these advances have been developed independently of one another and as a consequence little attention has been paid to the science of CBA as an entity (26). The aim of this handbook is to attempt to rectify this somewhat and not only pull these developments together in a coherent fashion but also to identify clear links between them with a view to providing some up-to-date guidance for carrying out applied CBA in health care.

1.3 What is cost–benefit analysis?

The basic idea of CBA is straightforward. To decide on the worth of a project involving public expenditure, it is necessary to weigh up the advantages and disadvantages. As Dasgupta and Pearce state, 'Cost–benefit analysis purports to be a way of deciding what society prefers. Where only one option can be chosen from a series of options, CBA should inform the decision maker as to which option is socially most preferred'(10). The key to this process is the unbiased and precise identification, measurement, and valuation of gains and losses (benefits and costs) arising from the project. Indeed, it is the search for unbiased and precise values of costs and benefits which is the root of much of the methodological work in the CBA area and is the main subject of this handbook.

1.4 Key concepts in welfare economics

At the very root of applied CBA methods is the theory of welfare economics. It follows that it is the purpose of any economic evaluation technique to assess the costs and consequences of a particular 'change in circumstances' e.g. a new bridge, clearing of a forest for recreational purposes, or indeed the introduction of a new drug for breast cancer patients. It is the reliance on the methods for measuring such *welfare change* for which applied economists have become known. Indeed Boadway and Bruce note that 'welfare economics can be viewed as an investigation of methods of obtaining a social ordering over alternative possible states of the world' (5). The reason economists require a social ordering is so they can compare all states of the world and rank each one as 'better than', 'worse than', 'or equally as good as' all the other states of the world. Ultimately, they are interested in 'ranking different *allocations of resources*, where this is used in its broadest sense to refer to the combinations of commodities produced and consumed by each decision maker in the economy and the combinations of factors used in the production of each commodity' (5).

In health care, resources are scarce. For this reason, choices have to be made regarding the best way to allocate resources amongst competing alternatives. Due to extensive market failure in health care, economists generally turn to neoclassical welfare economics as a framework within which to evaluate the costs and benefits of health care goods and services. Given this, the objectives of the remainder of this chapter are as follows:

◆ To briefly introduce the basic welfare economic theories including Pareto optimality

◆ To outline the key assumptions of normative economics and the basic theory of preferences

◆ To outline the main choices of benefit measure in CBA

◆ To discuss the concept of market failure in health care and the resulting requirement for economic evaluation methods

- To outline the main approaches to valuation of benefits in economic theory, namely revealed preference and stated preference methods
- To outline limitations with traditional neoclassical welfare economic theory and explore alternative theories
- To discuss the methodological challenges of measuring welfare change in 'hypothetical' health care markets using contingent valuation methods
- To introduce the concept of an alternative contingent valuation measure, namely stated preference discrete choice experiments (SPDCEs)

1.4.1 Basic theories

As noted by Groves: 'Utility is the subjective satisfaction of the household and cannot be observed directly. It must be inferred from observable attributes of household consumption behaviour and the hypothesis of utility maximization' (27). Such a basic, yet fundamental, statement is a useful starting point from which to explore the mechanisms of welfare economics. A distinction is usually made between analysing the consequences of a change and making judgements concerning the desirability of a particular change or policies. The former kind of analysis is called positive economics, while the latter is referred to as normative economics. Normative or *welfare economics* is concerned with evaluating the various consequences of a policy change and coming to a judgement concerning the desirability of the change. It is this type of economics and its role in applied health economic evaluation, with which this handbook is concerned.

Before getting into the details on the criteria used to measure welfare change, it is worth briefly outlining the concepts of 'welfare' and what a 'welfare measure' actually is.

1.4.2 The definition of welfare

Boadway and Bruce state that welfare economics can be 'viewed as an investigation of methods of obtaining a *social ordering* over alternative possible *states of the world*'. Such a view summarizes simply the basis of the practice of welfare economics. Such a social ordering then permits the comparison of states of the world and allows the ranking of each state in terms of 'better than', 'worse than', or 'equally as good as' (5;28). What exactly is welfare however? In the literature, this precise definition is skirted around, with texts referring to individuals 'well-being', resulting from consumption of goods, services, quantities, qualities, and so on. It follows from this, that in order to obtain a social ranking of states one must be able to find ways of measuring the impact of changes in resources upon human well-being. Therefore, if society wishes to make the most, in terms of individuals' well-being of its endowment of all health care resources, it must find a way of comparing the values of what its members receive from any health care change (i.e. the benefits) with the values of what its members give up by taking resources from other uses (i.e. the costs) (16). Finding an appropriate welfare measure therefore is a must. Standard economic theory for measuring changes in individuals' well-being was developed for the purpose of interpreting changes in the prices and quantities of goods purchased in markets. This theory became the basis for welfare measurement criteria when it was identified that the *trade-offs* people make as they choose less of one good and substitute more of some other good reveal something about the value people placed on these goods. Later sections in this chapter will explain how value measures based upon such substitutability can be expressed in a number of ways, not least willingness to pay (WTP) and willingness to accept (WTA) compensation for changes in quantity and quality of goods. The following section begins by introducing the concept of Pareto-improving criteria, a means by which social states can be ordered using some value judgement.

1.4.3 Pareto-improving criteria

The basic aim of welfare economics is to provide analysts with criteria according to which various policy proposals can be ranked such that we are able to assess the impact upon individuals' well-being. Much of the history of welfare economics has been dominated by the notion of a social welfare function (SWF) and the optimal output of an economy has been seen as determined by the point of tangency between the SWF and the production possibility frontier (PPF). The SWF remains frequently used for illustrative purposes in economics texts, but plays no role in *applied* welfare economics (29). An alternative, more applied approach which is also 'perhaps ethically more neutral' is the Pareto criterion (29), which states that policy changes which make at least one person better off without making anyone worse off are Pareto-improving and should be undertaken. Pareto improvements can occur from points in the interior of the PPF until the PPF is reached. Any point on the PPF is known as a Pareto optimal position.

The criterion used by welfare economics to judge a given policy is whether that policy is Pareto-improving. A Pareto-improving policy change is one which moves an economy to a position which is Pareto-superior (preferred) from a position which is Pareto-inferior (less preferred). Such a change is sometimes referred to as an increase in relative efficiency. Because in practice there are only very few, if any, policy changes which make no one worse off, the only way such a criterion can be implemented is to allow those who gain from a policy change to compensate the losers. According to the compensation test, the Pareto criterion is met if, after the gainers have compensated the losers, one agent is better off and no-one is worse off. In practice, however, compensation is rarely paid, and the strict compensation test (i.e. where compensation is paid) is not of great practical use (29).

John Hicks (1939) and Nicholas Kaldor (1939) proposed a welfare criterion which has been alternatively called the potential Pareto-improvement criterion (PPIC) or the potential compensation test (30;31). A potential Pareto improvement means that the gainers from the change could *hypothetically* compensate the losers from the change. The PPIC has been controversial because, without the *actual* payment of compensation, it is possible to make a very small group of people much better off while making the vast majority worse off. However, the PPIC has found wide acceptance and use among applied economists. Mitchell and Carson note that use of the PPIC has been justified on several grounds (29). The most common of these is the argument that projects should be decided on the basis of strict economic efficiency. In addition to this is the argument that the PPIC is only one piece of information available to

policy makers, who are free to reject policy changes with adverse distributional consequences if they wish (29).

CBA, often referred to as the applied side of modern welfare economics, operation-
alizes a variant of the Pareto criterion by placing monetary values on the gains
and losses to those affected by a change in the level of provision of a good for which
there is often no market, e.g. health care. This allows the calculation of net gain or
loss from a policy change, and determination of whether the change is potentially
Pareto-improving.

1.4.4 Preferences and utility maximization

It is important to outline two key assumptions of normative economics upon which
welfare economics theory is based. The first assumption is that economic agents
(patients, households, consumers, or firms) when confronted between a possible
choice between two (or more) bundles of goods, have preferences for one bundle
over another. The other main assumption is that through its actions and choices, an
economic agent attempts to *maximize* their overall level of utility or satisfaction.
When agents are given initial endowments of resources and allowed to trade, the
resulting actions and choices demonstrate a clear theory of value. It is exactly how
these 'values' are obtained which is the subject matter of much of this handbook.
Section 1.4.5 addresses the notion that people have preferences and the implications
of the axioms of such preferences.

1.4.5 Theory of preferences

Welfare theory starts with the premise that individuals[1] are the best judge of their
own welfare and that inferences about welfare can be drawn from each individual
by observing that individual's choices among alternative bundles of goods and services. If an individual prefers bundle **A** over bundle **B**, then bundle **B** must convey a
higher level of welfare. The individual chooses among available bundles on the basis of
their preferences and their budget set. Primarily it is assumed that the individual can
compare any two commodity bundles and declare that one is at least as good as the
other. In short, when x is at least as good as y, then xRy. If xRy and yRx, then the individual is said to be *indifferent* between x and y. It is assumed that the individual is
rational in the sense that their preference ordering is *reflexive* (xRy or x is at least as
good as itself), *transitive* (if xRy and yRz, then xRz) and *complete* (xRy or yRx or both
for any two commodity bundles x and y). If a further assumption about *continuity* of
preferences is made, then the individual's preferences can be represented by a real-
valued utility function $u(x)$. A utility function $u(x)$ will be a suitable representation of
the individual's preferences if $u(x) \geq u(y)$ whenever xRy for any pair of commodity
bundles x and y. As Freeman (1993) notes, the property of substitutability (continuity) is at the core of the economist's concept of value. This is because substitutability
establishes trade-off ratios between pairs of goods/attributes that matter to people.

---

[1] The term 'individual' is used here however often the term 'household' is used when discussing
these theories.

The importance of this observation will become apparent in later chapters on the use of WTP and SPDCEs to obtain measures of welfare, where substitutability is a crucial assumption for deriving welfare using such methodology.

This utility function $u(x)$ can be represented by a set of indifference curves, providing two further assumptions are made. The first is *non-satiation*, which states that utility is non-decreasing in any commodity and is increasing in at least one, i.e. more is preferred to less. This implies that the indifference curves have negative (or at least non-positive) slopes. The second is strict quasi-concavity which, in the two good cases, means decreasing marginal rates of substitution. In general, strict quasi-concavity implies a preference for diversity in consumption rather than specialization.

A further assumption about preferences that is useful is that of strong or *additive separability*. In this case, commodities or attributes of commodities can be partitioned into groups indexed $g = 1, \ldots, G$ and the utility function can be represented by

$$U = \sum_{g=1}^{G} \beta^g u^g(x_g),$$

where (β^g), $g = 1, \ldots, G$, are positive constants. That is, utility is the weighted sum of the utilities obtained from each commodity group x_g. The property of consumer preferences which gives rise to the additively separable form for the utility function is that the marginal rate of substitution between pairs of commodities in separate groups is independent of the level of consumption of any other commodity in any other group other than the two considered. (As Goldman and Uzawa have shown, this is a necessary and sufficient condition for additive separability (32)).

Section 1.4.6 outlines the possible measures of benefit which can be used within welfare economics.

1.4.6 Choices of benefit measure for estimating welfare change

The standard context in which to measure benefits is to evaluate price changes and hence changes in individual welfare. The basis for determining these values stems from the underlying preference structure of the individual and the assumptions made about how preferences should 'behave', as outlined earlier. Welfare measures are obtained by converting changes in utility to monetary values. There are three main methodologies to estimate welfare changes: consumer surplus (CS), equivalent variation (EV), and compensating variation (CV). CS is derived from ordinary, or Marshallian, demand curves. EV and CV, on the other hand, are derived from income-compensated, or Hicksian, demand functions.

Consumer surplus is often used as a welfare estimate because of the ease in estimation of Marshallian demand functions. The consumer's surplus on a good **y** is the difference between the maximum a consumer would be willing to pay for her current consumption of good **y** and the amount she actually pays for it. However, it has been noted that Marshallian welfare measures may be inappropriate because the underlying demand curves are not income compensated. Therefore, price effects are compounded by income effects (see Layard and Walters (22) for a more detailed description of such effects). Hence, welfare estimates based on CS are not unique if more than one price changes or if price and income change simultaneously. Thus, CV and EV, derived from Hicksian demand functions are more appropriate welfare measures in the context of policy decision making. CV is the amount of money we can take away from an individual after an economic change, while leaving her as well off as she was before it. For a welfare gain, it is the amount she would be willing to pay for a change. For a welfare loss, it is the amount she would need to accept as compensation for the change (22). For readers wishing to explore the differences between the Marshallian theory of consumption from the Hicksian theory in more depth please refer to Mishan (28) (Chapters 20 and 21).

Unlike CS, measures of CV and EV are not path dependant in cases of multiple price changes. According to Peters *et al.* (1995) both representations are equally valid, and it is difficult to discriminate between the two measures of welfare. Layard and Walters (1978;153) note, the ultimate problems of social choice can only be solved in principle by allowing for distributional judgements, and it is neither easier nor more difficult to make these in relation to EV or CV. But if the Kaldor criterion were used, this would be equal to the criterion that $\Sigma CV > 0$ provided that the act of hypothetical compensation, if actually undertaken, did not alter the structure of the relative prices (22). This equivalence arises because the *CV* (unlike the *EV*), is defined with reference to the *original level of utility*, as is the Kaldor criterion and for this reason it has been preferred by economists. This reasoning for using CV also fits in with the methods used for the economic evaluation of health care by estimating welfare gains and losses in a cost–benefit analysis (CBA). See Chapters 6–12 on estimating WTP and SPDCE in health care.

Examining the mechanisms by which CV is estimated, it is clear to see why this approach facilitates the valuations of goods and services, i.e. by the measurement of consumers' reactions to price changes. To see this and using Figure 1.1, suppose p_1 rises from p^0_1 to p^1_1, other prices remaining constant. We need to identify how much compensation is needed to make the consumer as well off as before (i.e. to hold u at u^0). This would be an amount equal to the change in the cost of securing u^0 (in health, this may be reflected in terms of the benefit from a successful hernia repair operation or seeing the GP of choice); this compensation is: $C(p^1_1, p^0_2, u^0) - C(p^0_1, p^0_2, u^0)$. This is a natural measure of welfare change, except that, since welfare has decreased, welfare is measured by the negative of this cost difference. This is CV. Thus, the CV and the compensated demand curve[2] are directly linked. The CV for a single price change (in p_1) is the *change in the area* (see shaded area in Figure 1.1) between the compensated demand curve for x_1 and the price line (p_1).

In Figure 1.1, if $p^1_1 > p^0_1$, the area above the price line is reduced, so the welfare change is negative.

---

[2] The compensated demand curve traces out the demand for goods (x) as price (p) varies, utility held constant.

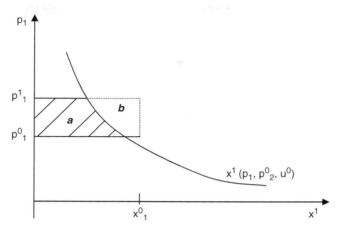

Fig. 1.1 The compensated demand curve.

1.5 **Requirement for economic evaluation in health care**

Section 1.4.6 outlined the standard measures of welfare in a competitive market where information on price and quantity is available. Section 1.5.1 introduces the concept of market failure and the resulting requirement for economic valuation in health care.

1.5.1 **Market failure**

In the case of a good or a commodity that is traded in a normal market, buyers and sellers reveal their preferences directly through their actions and price and quantity signals are observed, hence allowing CV to be estimated directly. This method of eliciting welfare change is called revealed preference (RP). However in health care, market failure often exists and as a result extensive government intervention is generally required. As a consequence of this market failure health care is often provided publicly. As outlined by Donaldson and Gerard (1993), the basic reasoning underlying extensive government intervention in health care is that the conditions required for perfect markets to operate are frequently violated. The characteristics of the health care market which cause failure are: risk and uncertainty associated with contracting illness, externalities, asymmetrical distribution of information about health care between providers and consumers and Oligopoly (including barriers to entry) (33).

As a result of market failure, the measure of 'value' usually obtained by measuring individuals' responses to price and quantity changes in the normal market is absent and preferences are not revealed in the normal manner. This is similar to the problem of preference revelation in environmental economics, as Freeman notes:

> The public good character of environmental services then leads to market failure. And without a market, there are no price and quantity data from which the demand relationships can be estimated (16).

As a consequence of this market failure, a number of practical methods that can be used to measure the WTP for non-marketed goods have been suggested in the literature. These include: stated preference (SP) survey techniques (see Chapters 6–8 and 10–12), the Clarke–Groves mechanism (34) (27), travel–cost methods (Hotelling 1947) (see Chapter 9), and hedonic approaches (35;36). In environmental economics, methods of valuing amenities have traditionally been categorized as direct and indirect. Indirect methods, such as the travel–cost approach, use actual choices made by consumers to develop models of choice. Direct methods ask consumers what they would be willing to pay/or accept for a change in a good or service. Direct methods are examples of contingent valuation stated preference techniques in that individuals do not actually make any behavioural changes, they only *state* that they would behave in this fashion.

Both direct and indirect methods have advantages and disadvantages. Direct methods are commonly criticized because of the hypothetical nature of the questions and the fact that actual behaviour is not observed (37). However, direct methods currently provide the main viable alternative to valuing goods and services where the consumer may have had little or no experience of the good being valued. This is the case in environmental economics, where direct methods are used for measuring 'non-use' values. In health economics, where consumers, i.e. potential patients, may have had little or no experience of the health care amenity requiring valuation and actual choices for treatments are often heavily influenced by professional advice (asymmetry of information) the direct methods are often the best option. Direct methods permit the valuation of a quality or quantity change involving a number of attribute level changes. The appropriate context in terms of information requirements and consumer sovereignty, etc. required for eliciting unbiased preferences can also be established within the direct methods and in doing so a hypothetical market framework is provided for decision making. In light of this, Section 1.5.2 briefly introduces the concept of economic evaluation in health care. For more details of these methods see Handbook 2 of this series.

1.5.2 Applied economic evaluation in health care

Economic evaluation is concerned with combining costs and benefits within an evaluative framework to provide information on the 'worthwhileness' of particular allocative decisions. Due to market failure, economic evaluation is commonly used as the workhorse for providing information for making resource allocation decisions in health care. The two principal economic evaluation techniques are: cost–benefit analysis (CBA) and cost-effectiveness analysis (CEA) (of which cost–utility analysis (CUA) is a form of). The techniques vary mainly in terms of how the benefits are valued however as will be shown in Chapter 4 there are specific costing issues relevant to CBA methods depending upon which measure of benefit is used.

Economic valuation of benefits refers to the assignment of values to non-marketed assets, goods, and services. Non-marketed goods and services refer to those which may not be directly bought and sold in the market place. Examples of non-marketed services in environmental economics would be clean air while in the National Health Service in the UK, health care is an example of a non-marketed good.

If a good or service contributes positively to human well-being, it has economic value. Whether something contributes to an individual's well-being is determined by whether or not it satisfies that individual's preferences. An individual's well-being is said to be higher in situation B than in situation A if the individual prefers B to A. The basic value judgement underlying economic valuation is that 'preferences count', although this does not imply that all decisions must be made on the basis of what people want. Other factors, such as what is morally appropriate, what is ethically acceptable, and what is reasonable and practical, must be taken into account, although such issues are less amenable to formal analysis.

As outlined earlier, there are two main ways of estimating the economic values attached to non-marketed goods and services: revealed preferences (indirect approach) and stated preferences (direct approach). Revealed preference approaches identify the ways in which a non-marketed good influences actual markets for some other good, i.e. value is revealed through a complementary (surrogate or proxy) market. An example of a revealed preference approach in health care would be the measurement of the travel costs incurred to attend a screening service (see Chapter 9) or assessing values for risk reduction in radon-induced lung cancer prevention (Kennedy (38)). Stated preference approaches or contingent valuation methods (direct methods), on the other hand are based on hypothetical or constructed markets, i.e. they ask people to state what economic value they attach to those goods and services. It is this approach which is the subject area of much of this handbook (see Chapters 6–8 and 10–12). In environmental economics, the National Oceanic and Atmospheric Administration (NOAA) panel undertook an investigation of the use of stated preference contingent valuation methodology for natural resource damage assessment (39). The NOAA panel concluded that contingent valuation studies 'can produce estimates reliable enough to be the starting point for a judicial or administrative determination of natural resource damages'. This handbook has made the assumption that this conclusion is transferable to health care assessment.

Finally, a third approach to economic valuation, more commonly used by environmental economists relies on the build-up of case studies from revealed and stated preference studies and then seeks to 'borrow' the resulting economic values and apply them to a new context. This is termed benefits transfer, see Bateman *et al.* (2002) for a comprehensive summary of this method (8).

Section 1.5.3 examines how estimates of contingent valuation have been derived in applied health economics with the use of hypothetical markets for health care goods and services. Chapters 6–8 provide applied examples of WTP studies in health care.

1.5.3 Eliciting WTP in the hypothetical health care market

In health economics, the most popular technique used to elicit monetary measures of benefit has been the use of direct stated preference (SP) contingent valuation methods to extract WTP for goods and attributes based on hypothetical markets. Contingent valuation methods use surveys to elicit people's preferences for goods by finding out what they would be willing to pay (accept) for specified improvements (downgradings) in them. Chapters 6–8 and 10–12 outline these applied methods in more depth.

The number of SP contingent valuation studies in health care is growing rapidly. In a review of the literature in health care contingent valuation studies, Diener *et al.* note that there is wide variation amongst health care contingent valuation studies in terms of the types of questions being posed and the elicitation formats being used (40). Much of the research into health care contingent valuation of recent years has in fact concentrated on these 'methodological' issues – the ultimate aim being to obtain the most valid, reliable, consistent, and meaningful measure of maximum WTP, derived through hypothetical means. Contingent valuation surveys typically aim to obtain an accurate estimate of the benefits of a change in the level of provision of a good, which can then be combined with the cost of producing the good, within a CBA. As Mitchell and Carson note 'In order to do this, the survey must simultaneously meet the methodological imperatives of survey research and the requirements of economic theory' (29). Mitchell and Carson go on to note that to meet the methodological imperatives requires that the scenario be understandable and meaningful to the respondents and free of incentives which might bias the results. Further, a survey must obtain the correct benefit measures for the good in the context of an appropriate hypothetical market setting. Section 1.5.4 provides a summary of the commonly used methods for eliciting WTP along with some of their key methodological issues.

Following on from the welfare economics concepts introduced earlier and the notion of 'value' required for benefit assessment, the technique of WTP as a benefit measurement tool is based on the premise that the maximum amount of money an individual is willing to pay (sacrifice) for a commodity is an indicator of the utility or satisfaction to them of that commodity. WTP has been used extensively in environmental, energy, and resource economics, where much methodological work has been carried out. Despite the theoretical merits of this approach, this literature has produced substantial criticism of the WTP approach (41;42). The majority of the criticisms are associated with the possible biases which are a threat to the validity of WTP results, such as 'yea-saying' (the tendency of some respondents to agree with an interviewer's request/value regardless of their true views), lack of association with real economic decisions and embedding/scope problems (this occurs when WTP values are the same, or not sufficiently differentiated, for commodities that differ from each other in their quantities or qualities) (43). Diener *et al.* (1998) explored the main elicitation methods for WTP in health economics, they were: open-ended questions, bidding games, payment cards, closed ended or 'take-it-or-leave-it' and closed ended with follow up (see Chapter 6 for details on these methods). The NOAA panel carried out an assessment of the various approaches to eliciting WTP (39). Their recommendations included promotion of the closed-ended format, face-to-face interviews instead of surveys, pilot surveying and pre-testing, and provision of accurate information on the goods being valued.

In terms of the WTP literature, evidence suggests that the different elicitation formats can yield significantly different results, although there exists no clear theoretical guidance as to which amongst them is 'correct' (44). Olsen and Smith (2001) review the extent to which the practice of WTP studies is consistent with the theory that underpins the approach. They conclude that WTP practice falls far short of the theoretical promise offered by the WTP method (45). Smith (2003) carried out a critical assessment of five key aspects in the use of WTP surveys in constructing the hypothetical health care market. Smith concluded that WTP studies in health care have performed poorly in the construction, specification, and presentation of the contingent market, and that there has been little, if any, improvement in this respect in the last 15 years (46). In summary, there remains no consensus on the 'best' approach and hence there is still a requirement for continued methodological work in the area of WTP surveys, and more generally contingent valuation methods in health care. See Chapters 5–11 for applied examples using these techniques.

Section 1.5.4 briefly introduces the methods of economic evaluation used in health care, concentrating specifically on the stated preference methods of benefit assessment used within CUA.

1.5.4 Non-monetary measures of benefit in health economics

There are three main types of economic evaluation commonly used in health economics: CBA, CEA, and CUA, although more recently CUA has been seen as a form of CEA. Until now, this chapter has concentrated on the valuation of benefits in monetary terms using standard welfare economic theory. Such benefits are used within a CBA framework. Such a conventional economics approach has been used to show that the amount people are willing to pay in terms of money is an indicator of their strength of preference for a good or characteristic of a good. As will be outlined in Chapters 6–12, WTP values are obtained by estimating the compensating variation measure of welfare, i.e. observing the reduction/increase in income levels people are prepared to accept for improvements/reductions in levels of attributes of a good. As a consequence, this handbook concentrates on the method of CBA as the main economic evaluation instrument. However, for a number of reasons, not least the fact that applied researchers often find valuing health related benefits in monetary terms objectionable, other economic evaluation techniques for combining costs with non-monetary benefits have been developed – these are CEA and CUA.

The subject of measuring health and measuring disease is the concern of many disciplines beyond health economics (47;48), including public health, epidemiology, and statistics. In health economics, it is widely accepted that it is theoretically possible to use numeraires, other than money, such as health state utility (49–52) in this measurement process. Culyer (1989) argued for an 'extra welfarist' approach to health; instead of attempting to devise measures of changes in utility, the task of measuring changes in 'health' was advocated, with the quality adjusted life year (QALY) as the instrument of choice (53;54). As a consequence, much of the health economics literature in recent years has concentrated on issues around measuring and valuing preferences for health care in non-monetary mediums, i.e. quality of life (55–58). This has led to the development of health state valuation measures including QALYs, and healthy years equivalents (HYEs). For more detailed descriptions of the traditional non-monetary approaches to benefit assessment within economic evaluation see Handbook 1 in this series.

1.6 **Structure of the book**

Following Chapter 1, Chapter 2 introduces the concept that it is important to be clear about what we are trying to value in health, in addressing this question it is noted that 'value' can be measured in two ways – in the preferences for health care goods and services or in the preferences for a change in health status. Chapter 2 then goes on to examine the valuation methods applied to both 'health' and 'health care' within the framework of the Household Production Model (HPM).

Following Chapter 2 on the classic HPM, Chapters 3 and 4 are dedicated to the costing side of a CBA. While there are a large number of useful costing chapters in economic evaluation texts (for example see Drummond *et al.* (59) these chapters aim to identify issues with costing specific to studies employing CBA methods. With inputs to production, namely costs, being more easily identified and valued, the main challenge for decision makers in health care is the valuation of benefits or 'output', however there remain a number of important costing issues pertinent to CBA which are outlined in Chapters 3 and 4. Chapter 3 introduces the concept of shadow pricing and outlines that due to a number of factors such as price and quantity constraints market prices are often inappropriate as measures of the marginal social costs of goods and services. Chapter 3 reveals that health and social care are no exceptions to this and summarizes the various ways in which shadow prices, or true opportunity costs are identified and measured in the health care market. The aim of Chapter 3 is to provide practical guidance as to the appropriate methods for shadow pricing in the health care setting. Up-to-date resources on the valuation of unpaid time are references including downloadable spreadsheets from www.statistics. gov.uk and the Centre for Time Use Research (CTUR) are utilized and recommendations made as to the most appropriate sources of values for health care economic evaluations.

Following directly on from Chapter 3, Chapter 4 entitled 'Costing methodology for applied health care evaluations' provides up-to-date practical guidance for costing in economic evaluations along with specific CBA-relevant costing issues. These considerations relate to the appropriate identification and measurement of costs specific to the timescale and context within which benefits are elicited. It is also important to align the cost units with the benefit data appropriately and matters such as divisibility of costs and their appropriate opportunity cost should also be considered. Since the use of SPDCE data alongside cost data within the formal CBA framework is a relatively new development in the literature, it is important that considerations for the costing within such CBA studies be examined. This chapter will provide a detailed and comprehensive summary of the identification, measurement, and valuation of the different types of costs arising in the health and social care setting. Methods such as annuitization, apportionment, discounting, and inflating will be introduced along with worked examples in health care. It is likely that some health care CBA studies will cross into many differing sectors of government and as such will require costing beyond the health sector hence these specific costing issues will be explored in this chapter. When CBA studies use welfare valuations derived from SPDCE studies, special considerations may be required for the costing side of the evaluation such as designing the SPDCE in line with available clinical trial attributes and levels and so on that reflect true shadow prices.

Before moving on to the more applied chapters of the book, Chapter 5 provides a comparison between health care evaluation methods and environmental methods. The resources devoted to high-profile contingent-valuation cases on environmental issues (such as the 1989 Exxon Valdez oil spill) resulted in distinguished economists, statisticians, and survey researchers applying their skills to valuation methods, including survey design, valuation theory, econometric analysis, and experimental economics and strategic behaviour. Natural Resource Damage Assessment (NRDA) cases have set high standards for acceptable practices involving survey design, information provision, treatment of strategic behaviour, and econometric analysis in contingent valuation applied to environmental issues. In doing so, health economic evaluation has benefited from this development and has the advantage of being able to draw upon on the environmental literature to develop and improve their health specific evaluation tools.

Chapters 6–8 focus on the use of the WTP method to estimate welfare in health care. The alternative elicitation techniques will be outlined and an introduction on how to design WTP surveys for use in a health care setting provided. Chapters 7 and 8 provide some detailed worked examples of the design and analysis of WTP studies in health care. Chapter 7 provides a methodological guide to carrying out a WTP survey in health care using applied examples in the area of screening for colorectal cancer. Chapter 8 provides another applied example of a CBA in spinal surgery. Chapter 9 follows on with an introduction to the theoretical basis of valuing time, this is then followed with an applied example of using revealed preference methods to value the benefits of health care using the travel cost approach.

In line with one of the key goals of this applied CBA book, Chapters 10–12 move into the realms of using SPDCEs to value the benefits for CBAs in health care. The use of SPDCEs within a CBA framework is a relatively recent development in the literature and to date there has been little applied guidance on how to use this approach in practice within CBAs with the exception of McIntosh *et al.* (26;60) and Lancsar and Louviere (61). Chapter 10 explores the specific issues around designing SPDCEs with particular attention to the use of experimental design theory and the random utility model and leading on from this Chapter 11 outlines the process of welfare estimation using SPDCE methodology.

Chapter 12 is entitled 'A practical guide to reporting and presenting stated preference discrete choice experiment results in cost–benefit analysis studies in health care'. The aim of this chapter is to provide some practical guidance for bringing costs and benefits together within health care CBAs using the specific methodology of SPDCE for the estimation of benefits. A further aim of this chapter is to outline ways of advancing the CBA methodology using SPDCEs by discussing methods currently used for cost-effectiveness analysis and highlighting how these same methods can be employed to enhance the usefulness of CBAs for health care policy makers. A checklist is also provided in this chapter which outlines the key areas of consideration when deriving a SPDCE-based CBA. Chapter 12 also provides a downloadable table containing SPDCE and conjoint studies carried out in health care – the table classifies the studies according to the following: country of study; respondents: category, e.g. health, non-health, process, and finally attributes included in the study. Finally, Chapter 13 concludes and summarizes the handbook.

1.7 **Conclusion**

The aim of this chapter was to provide a brief overview of the basic theories underlying welfare economics. In doing so, some theoretical context has been provided allowing the remainder of the content to be dedicated to applied methods of CBA in health care. As noted earlier, for more detailed introductions to the theories of normative welfare economics readers are referred to Boadway and Bruce (5), Layard and Walters (22), Layard and Glaister (23), and Mishan (1).

References

1. Mishan, E.J. 1971. *Cost-benefit analysis.* New York: Praeger.
2. Brent, R.J. 2003. *Cost-benefit analysis and health care evaluations.* Cheltenham: Edward Elgar.
3. Johannesson, M. 1996. *Theory and methods of economic evaluation in health care.* London: Kluwer Academic.
4. Layard, R. 2008. *Cost-benefit analysis.* 5th ed. Penguin Books.
5. Boadway, R.W. and Bruce, N. 1984. *Welfare economics.* 1st ed. Oxford: Oxford University Press.
6. Sugden, R. and Williams, A. 1978. *The principles of practical cost-benefit analysis.* New York: Oxford University Press.
7. Arrow, K.J., Cropper, M.L., Eads, G.C., Hahn, R.W., Lave, L.B., Noll, R.G., *et al.* 1996. Benefit-cost analysis in environmental, health, and safety regulation – a statement of principles. American Enterprise Institute for Public Policy Research.
8. Bateman, I.J., Carson, R.T., Day, B., Hanemann, M., Hanley, N., Hett, T., *et al.* 2002. *Economic valuation with stated preference: A manual.* 1st ed. Cheltenham: Edward Elgar.
9. Pearce, D.W. 1971. *Cost-benefit analysis.* 1st ed. London and Basingstoke: Macmillan Press.
10. Dasgupta, A.K. and Pearce, D.W. 1978. *Cost-benefit analysis: theory and practice.* 1st ed. London and Basingstoke: Macmillan Press.
11. Frost, M.J. 1975. *How to use cost benefit analysis in project appraisal.* 2nd ed. Westmead, UK: Gower.
12. Lesourne, J. 1975. *Cost-benefit analysis and economic theory.* 2nd ed. Oxford: North-Holland.
13. Warner, K.E and Luce, B.R. 1982. *Cost-benefit and cost-effectiveness in health care: principles, practice and potential.* 1st ed. Ann Arbor, MI: Health Administration Press, The University of Michigan.
14. Johansson, P.O. 1991. *An introduction to modern welfare economics.* Cambridge: Cambridge University Press.
15. H.M. Treasury, 2004. *The green book: appraisal and evaluation in central government.* 2nd ed. London: HMSO.
16. Freeman, A.M. 1993. *The measurement of environmental and resource values: theory and methods.* 3rd ed. Washington, DC: Resources for the Future.
17. Drummond, M.F., Sculpher, M.J., Torrance, G.W., O'Brien, B. and Stoddart, G.L. 2005. *Methods for the economic evaluation of health care programmes.* 3rd ed. Oxford: Oxford University Press.

18. Brent, R.J. 2006. *Applied cost-benefit analysis.* 2nd ed. Cheltenham: Edward Elgar.

19. Brent, R.J. 2009. *Handbook of research on cost-benefit analysis.* Cheltenham: Edward Elgar.

20. Birch, S. 2003. In: Brent, R.J., editor. *Book review: cost-benefit analysis and health care evaluations.* Cheltenham: Edward Elgar; Birch, S. 2004. *Social Science and Medicine* **59**: 885–887.

21. Gold, M.R., Siegel, J.E., Russell, L.B. and Weinstein, M.C. 1996. *Cost-effectiveness in health and medicine.* New York: Oxford University Press.

22. Layard, P.R.G. and Walters, A.A. 1978. *Microeconomic theory.* Singapore: McGraw-Hill.

23. Layard, R. and Glaister, S. 1994. *Cost-benefit analysis.* 2nd ed. Cambridge: Cambridge University Press.

24. Klose, T. 1999. The contingent valuation method in health care. *Health Policy* **47**: 97–123.

25. Borghi, J. 2008. Aggregation rules for cost-benefit analysis: A health economics perspective. *Health Economics* **17**(7): 863–875.

26. McIntosh, E., Donaldson, C. and Ryan, M. 1999. Recent advances in the methods of cost-benefit analysis in healthcare: Matching the art to the science. *Pharmacoeconomics* **15**: 357–367.

27. Groves, T. 1970. *The allocation of resources under uncertainty: the informal and incentive roles of prices and demands in a team.* Berkeley, CA: University of California.

28. Mishan, E.J. 1981. *Introduction to normative economics.* 1st ed. Oxford: Oxford University Press.

29. Mitchell, R.C. and Carson, R.T. 1989. *Using surveys to value public goods.* 3rd ed. Washington, DC: Resources for the Future.

30. Hicks, J.R. 1939. *Value and capital.* 1st ed. London: Oxford University Press.

31. Kaldor, N. 1939. Welfare propositions of economics and interpersonal comparisons of utility. *Economic Journal* **XLIX**: 549–552.

32. Goldman, S.M. and Uzawa, H. 1964. A note on seperability in demand analysis. *Econometrica* **32**: 387–398.

33. Donaldson, C. and Gerard, K. 1993. *Economics of health care financing: the visible hand.* 1st ed. London: Macmillan Press.

34. Clarke, E.H. 1971. Multipart pricing of public goods. *Public Choice* **11**: 17–33.

35. Griliches, Z. 1971. *Price indexes and quality change.* 1st ed. Cambridge, MA: Harvard University Press.

36. Rosen, S. 1974. Hedonic prices and implicit markets: product differentiation in pure competition. *Journal of Political Economy* **82**: 34–55.

37. Cummings, R.G., Brookshire, D.S. and Schulze, W.D. 1986. *Valuing environmental goods: a state of the arts assessment of the contingent method.* 1st ed. Totowa, NJ: Rowman and Allanheld.

38. Kennedy, C.A. 2002. Revealed preference valuation compared to contingent valuation: radon induced lung cancer prevention. *Health Economics* **11**: 585–598.

39. Arrow, K.J., Solow, R., Portney, P., Leamer, E.E., Radner, R. and Schuman, H. 1993. *Report of the NOAA Panel on contingent valuation.* Washington, DC: Resources for the Future. Report No.: 58.

40. Diener, A., O'Brien, B. and Gafni, A. 1998. Health care contingent valuation studies: a review and classification of the literature. *Health Economics* **7**(4): 313–326.

41. Kahneman, D. and Knetsch, J.L. 1992. Valuing public goods: The purchase of moral satisfaction. *Journal of Environmental Economics and Management* **22**: 57–70.

42. Diamond, P.A. and Hausman, J.A. 1994. Contingent valuation: Is some number better than no number? *Journal of Economic Perspectives* **8**: 45–64.

43. Svedsater, H. 2000. Contingent valuation of global environmental resources: Test of perfect and regular embedding. *Journal of Economic Psychology* **21**: 605–623.

44. O'Brien, B. and Gafni, A. 1996. When do the dollars make sense? Towards a conceptual framework for contingent valuation studies. *Medical Decision Making* **16**: 288–299.

45. Olsen, J.A. and Smith, R. 2001. Theory versus practice: a review of willingness to pay in health and health care. *Health Economics* **10**: 39–52.

46. Smith, R. 2003. Construction of the contingent valuation market in health care: a critical assessment. *Health Economics* **12**(8): 609–628.

47. Bowling, A. 1991. *Measuring health: a review of quality of life measurement scales.* 4th ed. Buckingham: Open University Press.

48. Bowling, A. 1995. *Measuring disease.* 1st ed. Buckingham: Open University Press.

49. Sackett, D.L. and Torrance, G.W. 1978. The utility of different health states as perceived by the general public. *Journal of Chronic Disorders* **31**(11): 697–704.

50. Torrance, G.W. and Sackett, D.L. 1972. A utility maximising model for evaluation of health care programmes. *Health Services Research* **7**(2): 118–133.

51. Torrance, G.W. 1976. Social preferences for health states: An empirical evaluation of three measurement techniques. *Socioeconomic Planning Sciences* **10**(3): 128–136.

52. Torrance, G.W., Boyle, M.H. and Horwood, S.P. 1982. Application of multiattribute utility theory to measure social preferences for health states. *Operations Research* **30**(6): 1043–1069.

53. Culyer, A.J. 1989. The normative economics of health care finance and provision. *Oxford Review of Economic Policy* **5**: 34–58.

54. Williams, A. 1985. Economics of coronary artery bypass grafting. *British Medical Journal* **291**: 326–329.

55. Buckingham, K. 1993. A note on HYE (Healthy Years Equivalents). *Journal of Health Economics* **12**: 301–309.

56. Buckingham, K. 1995. Economics, health and health economics – HYEs versus QALYs-a response. *Journal of Health Economics* **14**: 397–398.

57. Richardson, J. 1994. Cost utility analysis – what should be measured? *Social Science and Medicine* **39**: 7–21.

58. Drummond, M.F., Stoddard, G.L. and Torrance, W. 1987. *Methods for the economic evaluation of health care programmes.* 1st ed. Oxford: Oxford University Press.

59. Drummond, M.F., Sculpher, M.J., Torrance, G.W., O'Brien, B. and Stoddart, G.L. 2005. *Methods for the economic evaluation of health care programmes.* 3rd ed. Oxford University Press.

60. McIntosh, E. 2006. Using stated preference discrete choice experiments in cost-benefit analysis: some considerations. *Pharmacoeconomics* **24**(9): 855–869.

61. Lancsar, E. and Louviere, J.J. 2008. Conducting discrete choice experiments to inform healthcare decision making: A user's guide. *Pharmacoeconomics* **26**(8): 661–677.

Chapter 2

Methods for evaluating health and health care: Underlying theory and implications for practical application

Philip M. Clarke

There is however a special difficulty in estimating the whole of the utility of commodities some supply of which is necessary for life. If any attempt is made to do it, the best plan is perhaps to take that necessary supply for granted, and estimate the total utility only on that part of the commodity which is in excess of this amount. . .
*(Alfred Marshall 1920, p. 110)**

2.1 Introduction

Following on from the basic theory outlined in Chapter 1, one of the first questions that must be addressed is what are we trying to value? While this may appears a deceptively simple question, it is important to recognize that there are two domains in which value can be measured. It can be reflected either in the preferences for health care goods and services or in the preferences for a change in health status. Both domains are examined in this chapter within the framework of the Household Production Model (HPM). The main focus of this chapter is on *use* values, i.e. a consumer's preference for his or her own health or health care.

The remainder of this section provides background information on the origins of both these approaches. Section 2.3 outlines a two commodity HPM. In order to derive the results in this section, two simplifying assumptions about the nature of household production are made: (i) non-joint production of commodities and (ii) constant returns to scale. Section 2.4 shows how this model can be applied to value health and health care. The purpose of Section 2.5 is to clarify a point over which there has been some confusion in the literature – whether health can be represented as a single commodity. Section 2.6 then relaxes the two key assumptions invoked in Section 2.3. The implications for evaluation are then discussed in Section 2.7. We then consider other values for health with an emphasis on altruism in Section 2.8. The final section 2.9 contains a summary and some conclusions.

2.2 **Background**

Adopting a welfare economic framework to value changes in health dates back to 1968 (1), but it was Mishan (1971) (2) who had the greatest influence on the monetary valuation of health (3). The primary purpose of Mishan's work was to provide esti-mates of the costs and benefits arising from 'changes in the incidence of death, disable-ment, or disease caused by the operation of new projects or developments' (2, p. 687). His focus was very much on the valuation of life and limb (or changes in mortality and morbidity) and hence it lies within the domain of valuing health. Mishan's approach has largely been ignored by those health economists who prefer to value health in non-monetary terms by using measures such as QALYs.

Since the early 1990s, there has been renewed interest in valuing the benefits of health care in monetary terms. This has come from two different quarters. First, economists, who have applied Mishan's approach in other fields, e.g. environmental economics (see Chapter 5), have sought to apply these methods in the evaluation of health care. For example, the morbidity associated with a disease could be represented by different symptoms such as coughing or nausea. The benefits of relieving each symptom could then be measured. The value of a drug that cures the disease could be estimated by adding up the total value of the health benefits. A comprehensive over-view of this approach is contained in (3). More recent examples include, valuation of the benefits of relief from gastroesophageal reflux disease (4), symptom-free days of asthmatic children (5), and cure from a chronic illness such as gout (6).

The second approach involves the direct valuation of health care (see also Section 1.5.1 in Chapter 1) and, unlike the previous approach, it has been developed within the confines of health economics. Early examples of this approach include (7;8). More recently, this has been applied to value a wide variety of health care interventions (see Chapters 6–8). The valuation of health care goods and services, as opposed to measur-ing the benefits in terms of the health outcomes, represents a significant departure not only from the non-monetary valuation of health outcomes (i.e. QALYs) but also from the monetary valuation of health discussed earlier.

2.3 **A household production model of health care**

The household production approach developed by Becker (9) to model consumer choice provides a theoretical framework for valuing health and health care. Becker's approach to consumer theory draws a distinction between commodities and market goods. The household is viewed as combining market goods and their own time to produce commodities and it is these commodities that are the ultimate source of util-ity. The main advantage of this approach over traditional demand theory is that it separates the factors determining the process of production from those influencing consumer tastes.

The HPM has had great influence on health economics through the seminal work of Grossman (10). The 'Grossman model', as it has become known, regards health as: (i) a consumption commodity because good health is a direct source of utility and

(ii) an investment since improved health enables more market activities to be undertaken in the future. Grossman's full model will not be presented here, because the primary purpose of this chapter is to distinguish between the valuation of health and health care. For this reason, a simplified HPM is developed in the following sections.

2.3.1 A single period Household Production Model

It is assumed that an individual is endowed with a stock of health (H^s) which depreciates at a rate of δ. At the beginning of each period the individual must decide how much health to produce, but must always maintain their stock of health above a critical level (H^c) in order to survive. To abstract from intertemporal issues, we focus on a single time period in which the individual starts with an initial stock of health $H^s_t = H^s_{t-1} - \delta H^s_{t-1}$. The individual must then decide what quantity of health (H_t) and another commodity (Z_t) to produce during this period. At the end of period t, their stock of health depreciates by δH^s_t. The rate of depreciation is assumed to be exogenous and is known with certainty. Although this is a very simple model, it allows us to explore several important aspects of the HPM relevant to the measurement of welfare change.

The individual's decision over the optimum commodity bundle of H_t and Z_t can be divided into two stages: (i) a lower stage where market goods are combined with time to produce a feasible set of commodities and (ii) an upper stage where the commodity bundle that maximizes the individual's utility is chosen from this feasible set. The process of optimization involved in each stage is discussed in turn.

In the lower stage, the individual combines market and non-market goods to produce commodities. If there are n goods,[1] let x^H_j denote the quantity of the jth good used in the production of health and denote the corresponding input vector as: $X^H = (x^H_1,...,x^H_n)$. The input vector X^H will consist of any factor that influences health status (i.e. for goods that have no influence on health $x^H_j = 0$). Typically, this input vector includes health care and 'health creating' market goods (e.g. safety equipment) and non-market goods such as time. An individual's ability to produce health can also be affected by the environment in which they live. The health production function denoted by $H_t = f^H(X^H)$ is governed by the underlying technology available to the individual. We assume that this production function is strictly concave and is increasing in all its arguments. Similarly, denote an input vector $X^Z = (x^Z_1,...,x^Z_n)$ and define the production function for the other commodity to be $Z_t = f^Z(X^Z)$. The total quantity of each good consumed is represented by x_j (i.e. $x_j = x^H_j + x^Z_j$) and the vector of goods that the individual consumes by X, where $X = X^H + X^Z$.

Associated with every goods vector X is a feasible set of commodities, $G(X)$, that can be produced. A typical feasible set is depicted in Figure 2.1. Along the boundaries of this set is the 'production possibility frontier', which represents the maximum amount of Z_t and H_t produced for a given quantity of inputs. In order to maximize utility, the consumer must choose a point along this frontier. The exact point will be influenced by the relationship between the individual's current stock of health H^s_t, the rate of depreciation δ and the level of health that is critical for survival, H^c. In particular,

---

[1] Since all production is assumed to take place within a single period the subscript t has been suppressed on the input x_j.

if $H^s_{t+1} - H^c \leq \delta H^s_t$ then a minimum quantity of health (denoted by H^c_t) must be produced in the current period in order for the individual to survive. This level of health production is *essential* in the sense that the utility function is undefined for quantities of health below H^c_t. Alternatively, if $H^s_{t+1} - H^c > \delta H^s_t$, then the individual can choose not to produce health in the current period (i.e. $H_t = 0$) without affecting their survival. The exact quantity of health chosen beyond H^c_t is governed by the individual's preference for H_t relative to Z_t (i.e. the marginal rate of substitution between health and the other commodity) and the marginal rate of transformation between the two commodities.

In Figure 2.1, the consumer chooses the commodity bundle $(H_t{}^*, Z_t{}^*)$ since the highest available indifference curve (U^1_C) just touches the production possibility frontier at this point.

In order to operationalize the HPM, the input demand curves for goods and commodity outputs must be derived. Associated with X will be a vector of prices $P = (p_1, ..., p_n)$. In the first stage of the household production process we define a cost function, which represents the minimum cost of achieving a level of output for a given level of prices:

$$C(P,\ H_t,\ Z_t)\ =\ \min \sum_{j=1}^{n} p_j x_j \tag{2.1}$$

In general, the budget constraint in commodity space is non-linear. As a first step to deriving the commodity demand functions, the shadow prices $(s_H$ and $s_z)$ must be derived from the cost function:

$$s_H(P, H_t, Z_t) = \frac{\partial C(P, H_t, Z_t)}{\partial H_t}, \qquad s_Z(P, H_t, Z_t) = \frac{\partial C(P, H_t, Z_t)}{\partial Z_t}. \tag{2.2}$$

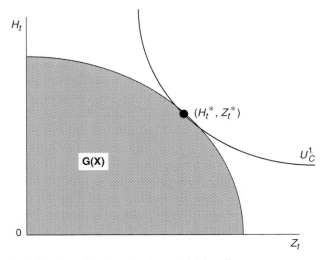

Fig. 2.1 Choice in the Household Production Model (HPM).

Unlike the standard utility maximization problem, s_H and s_Z are not exogenous to the consumer, but vary with the input prices and the chosen combination of commodities. In order for the problem to be tractable, it is normally assumed that *household technology exhibits constant returns to scale and no joint production*. Pollak and Wachter (11) demonstrate that under these conditions, the shadow prices are independent of the quantities of commodities chosen.

In order to complete the exposition of the basic model, we assume that both of these conditions hold, hence $s_H(P, H_t, Z_t) = s_H(P)$ and $s_Z(P, H_t, Z_t) = s_Z(P)$. The implications of relaxing these assumptions are discussed below.

At any point on the production possibility frontier, the marginal rate of transformation between the two commodities is the ratio of $s_Z(P)$ to $s_H(P)$. More formally, the commodity demands can be derived from the upper stage maximization problem:

$$\max U_C(H_t, Z_t) \tag{2.3}$$
$$s.t. s_H(P)H_t + s_Z(P)Z_t = y,$$

where y is the consumer's total income and $U_C(.)$ denotes utility in commodity space. To simplify the exposition, y is assumed to be exogenous. Equation (2.3) yields Marshallian commodity demand functions:

$$H_t^m = m^H(s_H, s_Z, y), \qquad Z_t^m = m^Z(s_H, s_Z, y). \tag{2.4}$$

These demand functions display all the properties of traditional demand functions. As Grossman (10, p. 225) notes the 'most fundamental law in economics is the law of the downward-sloping demand curve, the quantity of health demanded should be negatively correlated with its shadow price'.

The dual of the utility maximization problem in (2.3) is expenditure minimization subject to the attainment of minimum utility:

$$\min s_H(P)H_t + s_Z(P)Z_t \tag{2.5}$$
$$s.t. \ U_C(H_t, Z_t) \geq \bar{U}_C.$$

By differentiating the resulting expenditure function with respect to the shadow prices the Hicksian (compensated) demand curves can be derived for both commodities:

$$H_t^h = c^H(s_H, s_Z, \bar{U}_C), \qquad Z_t^h = c^H(s_H, s_Z, \bar{U}_C). \tag{2.6}$$

The demand functions for different inputs can also be derived since the utility function used to select the optimal commodity vector may also be defined over goods space. In Figure 2.1, the optimal bundle (H_t^*, Z_t^*) is produced by an input vector X. The Marshallian demand for goods can be derived by attaching the utility associated with the optimal commodity bundle with the input vector X (11). The Marshallian demand functions can be derived by

$$\max U_G(X) \tag{2.7}$$
$$s.t. \sum_{k=1}^{n} p_k x_k = y,$$

where $U_G(\cdot)$ is utility in goods space. This yields input demand functions for each good.

$$x_j^m = m^i(P, y). \tag{2.8}$$

Using the dual of (2.7), the Hicksian demand for goods can also be derived:

$$x_j^c = c^i(P, \bar{U}_G). \tag{2.9}$$

2.4 Valuing health and health care

The separation of health and health care in the HPM suggests that there are two different approaches that can be used to value a health care good or service. Either the benefits associated with its consumption can be quantified by valuing the health outcomes it produces (i.e. measuring the welfare change in commodity space), or it can be valued by directly observing the input demand function (i.e. measuring welfare change using the derived demand for the health creating good).

2.4.1 Valuing health

Health (H_t) is a non-market commodity which an individual cannot purchase directly. Instead it must be produced by consuming health creating inputs, like health care. Its valuation differs from the welfare measurement of price changes. Mishan (2, pp. 228–229) highlights this issue:

> In the market place, the price of the good... is fixed by the producer, and the buyer or seller determines the amount by reference to his subjective preferences. Where, however, the amount of a... good is fixed for each person—as may be the case with a change in risk—a person's subjective preference can only be determined by the price he will accept or offer for it; in short, his CV.

This suggests that the welfare change associated with an improvement or decline in health (which Mishan refers to above as a 'change in risk') must be defined in terms of a quantity change rather than a price change, because health is not a traded good.

The compensating variation (CV) associated with an improvement in health from H_t^1 to H_t^2 in period t can be defined using the expenditure function:

$$CV_q = e(s_H, H_t^1, U_C^1) - e(s_H, H_t^2, U_C^1) \tag{2.10}$$

In (2.10), CV_q represents the maximum amount of money that must be taken from the individual – that is, her willingness to pay (WTP), so that she remains at her initial level of utility (U_C^1). If the change in health was reversed (i.e. a decline from H_t^2 to H_t^1) then the CV is the minimum amount of compensation she requires to leave her as well off as before the reduction. Here, the CV measures the willingness to accept (WTA) compensation for a decline in health (12, p. 35). Alternatively, the equivalent variation (EV) for the same change in health can be defined using the final level of utility (rather than the initial level as in (2.10.)).

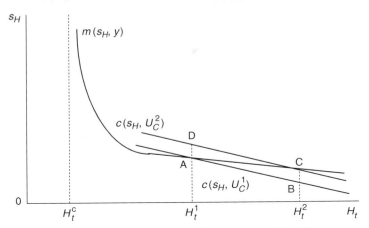

Fig. 2.2 The welfare benefits associated with an improvement in health.

The relationship between the various measures of welfare can be illustrated using the Hicksian and Marshallian commodity demand functions for health. Figure 2.2 illustrates three measures of welfare change associated with a change in health from H_t^1 to H_t^2. The ordinary Marshallian consumer surplus (CS) is the area under $m(s_H, y)$ between the two health states (i.e. $ACH_t^2 H_t^1$). The CV for the same change will be $ABH_t^2 H_t^1$ (i.e. the area under Hicksian demand curve $c(s_H, U_C^1)$. The EV for the same change in health will be the area under $c(s_H, U_C^2)$ or $DCH_t^2 H_t^1$.

The size of the benefit (or loss) associated with a change in H_t depends on the proximity of the change to H_t^c. If it is essential to produce a certain level of health in the current period to survive (i.e. $H_t^c > 0$) then the marginal valuation of health (represented by its shadow price s_H) will approach ∞ as the quantity of H_t approaches H_t^c. Welfare measures cannot be used to value a change that results in an individual's certain loss of life. Alternatively, if the individual can survive the current period without producing health, then $m(s_H, y)$ will intersect the vertical axis at a finite shadow price. In this case, any change in health (i.e. above $H_t = 0$) produces finite measures of welfare change, see (13) for a further discussion of this issue.

In practice, two techniques can be used to value changes in health status. The first involves observing the value of health implied by revealed preference (indirect methods) (see Chapter 9). This is often referred to as the defensive behaviour, or damage costs approach (14). The other method involves asking consumers to express preferences for a change in their health (direct methods) (see Chapters 6–8 and 10–12).

The revealed preference approach applies the HPM to derive the Marshallian demand function for H_t (2.5). The alternative approach is to use survey methods to value changes in health (direct methods). As outlined in Chapter 1, the most developed survey method is the contingent valuation approach, in which respondents are asked their 'willingness to pay' or 'willingness to accept' contingent on a market existing for the good or service. Typically, individuals are asked what they would be willing to pay to improve their health from H_t^1 to H_t^2 (i.e. a measure of the CV).

2.4.2 Valuing health care

Health care is normally combined with other market goods (e.g. a bus ticket to travel to the doctor, or an ambulance ride to hospital) and non-market goods (such as time) to produce health. All these goods represent inputs into the health production function. If health care is represented by x_1^H, the Marshallian demand (2.8) will be $x_1^m = m^1(p_1, \overline{P}, Y)$, where $\overline{P} = (p_2, p_3, \ldots, p_n)$. Similarly, the Hicksian demand (2.9) can also be defined as $x_1^c = c^1(p_1, \overline{P}, U_G)$. In the general case, x_1 may also produce Z_t, but health care goods – unlike some other inputs (such as the time) – cannot normally be divided between multiple uses. Consequently, in the following example we assume that $x_1^Z = 0$. The demand curves for x_1 can be used to calculate the welfare benefit (or loss) from a price change and in some instances it can be used to infer the value of change in health.

2.4.2.1 Welfare measurement of a price change

The effect of a change in the price of health care is graphically illustrated in Figure 2.3. In the first diagram (Figure 2.3i), the Marshallian demand for the good is $m^1(p_1, \overline{P}, y)$ and the Hicksian demand associated the initial utility (U_G^1) is $c^1(p_1, \overline{P}, U_G^1)$. The second (Figure 2.3ii), illustrates the health production function $f^H(x_1)$ and the third (Figure 2.3iii), represents commodity space (H_t, Z_t).

If the price of x_1 declines from p_1^0 to p_1^f, the individual will purchase a greater quantity of health care (i.e. increase consumption from x_1^0 to x_1^f). The effect that this has on H_t is illustrated in Figure 2.3ii. The increase in health care inputs from x_1^0 to x_1^f results in an increase in the production of health (i.e. H_t^1 to H_t^2). This in turn has an impact on the feasible production set $G(X)$ illustrated in Figure 2.3iii. Since x_1 only enters the health production function, the production possibility frontier shifts upward rather than outward. The combination of these factors results in a change in the optimal bundle of commodities from (H_t^1, Z_t^1) to (H_t^2, Z_t^2). As the commodity bundle (H_t^2, Z_t^2) is on a higher indifference curve (U_C^2), a decline in price leads to a welfare gain. Providing health is not a *giffen* good, the individual will increase their consumption of H_t following a decline in the price of a necessary input. The quantity of Z_t can rise or decline depending on whether it is a substitute or complement to H_t. The dotted line, **ab**, represents the marginal rate of transformation of H_t into Z_t and its slope is equal to $-s_H(P)/s_Z(P)$.

The Hicksian demand for x_1 can also be derived from this figure by removing income from the individual to bring them back to their original level of utility U_C^1 at the new lower shadow price. To do this, the dotted line **ab** is shifted back to the point at which it just touches U_C^1 (i.e. point **e** on the dotted line **cd**). At this lower level of utility, the consumer demands less health $(\overline{H}_1^f)$ and consequently less health care $(\overline{x}_1^f)$.

The CV associated with the decline in price is:

$$CV_p = e(p_1^0, U_G^1) - e(p_1^f, U_G^1) = \int_{p_1^0}^{p_1^f} x_1^c. \tag{2.11}$$

The area to the left of x_1^c between the initial and final price represents the welfare gain from the price fall (represented by the shaded area in Figure 2.3i). This area also

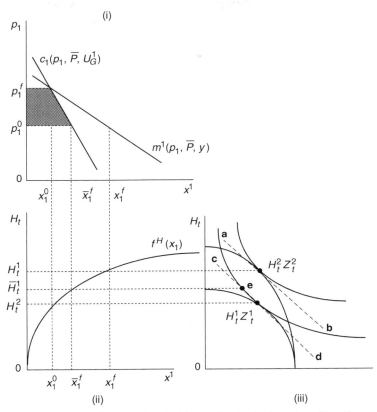

Fig. 2.3 The welfare benefits associated with a reduction in the price of health care.

represents the value of the change in health when the following three conditions are met: (i) x_1 is necessary[2] for the production of in H_t; (ii) x_1 does not produce Z_t; (iii) the change in health (H_t^1 to H_t^2) does not encompass H_t^c. Even if the first two conditions are not met, the input demands still represent the marginal value an individual places on different quantities of the health care goods x_1.

2.5 Measurement of output and welfare in the HPM

An important assumption underlying the valuation of health in Section 2.4.2.1 is that health can be represented by H_t. This notion that health is a single commodity 'output' has gained widespread acceptance, since it also ties in closely with the view that health

---

[2] A good is defined as necessary if it is impossible to produce an output without using a particular input. For example, if there were two goods (x_1, x_2) used in the production of H_t, then x_1 is necessary if $f^H(0, x_2)$ (15, p. 181).

status can be measured using QALYs, which is another one-dimensional measure of health. However, the use of such a broadly defined concept should be closely examined, since a commodity must represent the output of production processes and not a measure of utility (i.e. numbers representing preference ordering) (11, pp. 259–260). The measurement of the two most important health outputs – changes in mortality and changes in morbidity are considered below.

2.5.1 Mortality

An individual's risk of mortality is usually measured as the probability of dying over a fixed period of time (15). The effect that health care or other market goods, such as safety equipment has on mortality can be represented by changes in this probability (i.e. a change in risk). This is an objective measure in that it represents the individual's chance of survival and not the individual's preferences. It can therefore be regarded as a commodity 'output' within a household production framework.

2.5.2 Morbidity

Morbidity has been defined as 'a departure from a physical state of well-being, resulting from disease or injury, of which the individual is aware' (U.S. Public Health Service as cited in (15, p.168)). Morbidity, unlike mortality, has many dimensions. For example, a cancer patient's 'quality of life' will be governed by a range of factors including physical symptoms such as pain, body temperature, tenderness, discomfort, stiffness, and swelling in the treated area (16). Such patients might also experience psychological morbidity and anxiety stemming from a fear of death. It is difficult to measure many of these symptoms, even in physical terms. Although some symptoms can be measured on an objective cardinal scale (e.g. body temperature) other symptoms such as pain cannot be objectively measured. However, for illustrative purposes let us assume that morbidity can be represented by a series of symptom scores measured on different scales $(H_t^A, H_t^B, H_t^C, ..., \text{etc.})$. If health is to be represented by a single commodity, these scales must be combined into a single index (H_t). A vector of weights $(w_1, w_2, w_3, ...)$ can be used to represent the individual's *valuation* of different aspects of their health:

$$H_t = w_1 H_t^A + w_2 H_t^B + w_3 H_t^C. \tag{2.12}$$

However, it would appear that the resulting index is a measure of utility rather than a commodity, because the weights must represent preferences for different symptoms.

It is therefore not surprising that the focus of most quality of life research has been on developing *subjective* measures of health status, such as QALYs. These generally rely on techniques such as the *standard gamble method* to weight different health states. Responses to standard gamble questions depend not only on physical health but also on the utility gained from that health. Even the *visual analogue scale* involves a value judgement on the relative importance of one health state over another (17).

2.6 **Extensions to the Household Production Model**

The HPM introduced in Section 2.2 makes two important assumptions regarding the nature of production technology within the household: (i) there is no joint production; (ii) there are constant returns to scale. The implications of relaxing either of these assumptions is addressed below.

2.6.1 **Joint production and the Household Production Model**

Section 2.5.2 suggests that morbidity must be represented by a series of narrowly defined symptoms. This has important implications for the evaluation of health care because the existence of multiple health commodities increases the likelihood that household production involves one of the following forms of joint production:

(i) *Production indivisibility*: Arises when there are more commodities than goods. For example, if health care produces two and both commodities are produced in fixed proportions (i.e. $H_t^A = ax_1^H$ and $H_t^B = bx_1^H$, where a and b are the marginal rates of transformation. Indivisibilities in production occur if the input vector contains only one necessary good $X^H = (x_1^H, 0, ..., 0)$, because the feasible set is a ray from the origin in commodity space and a given quantity of x_1^H will produce fixed quantities of H_t^A and H_t^B. Points along the production possibility frontier will be consistent with an infinite variety of marginal rates of substitution since the consumer cannot choose to trade-off one commodity for another (18).

(ii) *Interdependent production functions*: Even if the number of goods is equal to the number of commodities, joint production can still occur if the different production functions are linearly dependent (19).

(iii) *Inputs confer utility*: If health care is a direct source of utility as well as producing other commodities. Mooney (20) terms this 'process utility'.

In Section 2.2, the derivation of commodity demand functions, represented by (2.4) and (2.6), depend on the shadow price (or marginal cost) being independent of the quantities of commodities chosen. However, if there is joint production, the marginal costs will also depend on the commodity bundle consumed (i.e. $s_H(P, H_t, Z_t)$ and $s_Z(P, H_t, Z_t)$). This has important implications for welfare measurement. Bockstael and McConnell (21) show that Marshallian commodity demands (2.4) do not exist, because it is impossible to uniquely define at each marginal cost a level of demand for which the income constraint holds. However, the presence of joint production does not preclude the derivation of Hicksian commodity demand functions (2.6), as the income constraint is not required to hold along the compensated demand curve. Even if the commodity outputs are jointly produced, the Marshallian input demand functions for goods can still be derived (2.8). Hence, revealed preference methods can be used to value health care treatments even if they cannot be used to value aspects of the individual's health (i.e. symptoms).

2.6.2 **Non-constant returns to scale**

In Section 2.2, the cost function is assumed to be linearly homogeneous in Z_t and H_t, which is predicated on the assumption of constant returns to scale.

This assumption should be relaxed because most health production processes are governed by biological relationships that are subject to decreasing returns and sometimes natural limits. The later can result in production having an upper bound; that is, increases in scale beyond a certain point result in no increases in output. In some instances, higher quantities of health care are harmful. For example, paracetamol, a common pain-relieving drug, is effective in small does (e.g. one or two tablets), but leads to kidney failure and even death if 20 or more tablets are consumed at one time. The difficulty of incorporating non-constant returns to scale into the HPM is that we face a similar problem to that of joint production, which means that the shadow prices are not only a function of input prices but also of the commodity bundle consumed. For this reason, only the Hicksian commodity demand functions can be estimated unless the entire cost function is known (21).

2.7 Implications for valuing the use benefits of health care

The discussion in Section 2.6.2 suggests that valuation of health using revealed preference methods faces formidable obstacles, because joint production and non-constant returns to scale are pervasive in the production of health. However, these features which are prevalent in commodity space do not affect the valuation of health care inputs in goods space. It is therefore quite possible to observe the demand for a health care good which reflects the combined value of all its outputs while being unable to observe the marginal value of a particular health commodity. However, all is not lost for those wanting to measure the value of health commodities, because Hicksian commodity demand functions still exist, and so it is still possible to apply stated preference methods.

Consider the case of indivisibility in production outlined above. What options are open to a researcher trying to evaluate a drug simultaneously impacts on two aspects of health H_t^A or H_t^B? One option is to use the contingent valuation method (CVM) to elicit preferences for the alleviation of each symptom by asking individuals their maximum WTP for a change in H_t^A or H_t^B (see Chapters 6–8). The benefits of the drug could be estimated by adding up the marginal benefit associated with the alleviation of each symptom. The other option is to use stated or revealed preference methods to directly value the drug. This involves observing the Marshallian demand for the drug. The merits of both these options are discussed below.

2.7.1 Valuing health care by valuing its outputs

The health outputs approach measures the benefits of a health care programme by valuing its outputs. This approach can be divided into a series of stages. In the first stage, all the relevant outputs of a programme need to be identified. In the second stage, the effects of treatment are quantified in terms of these outputs. In the third stage, the value of a change in each output must be elicited. Finally, the value of all outputs must be combined.

Up to this point, this chapter has been concerned with the technical issues surrounding the valuation of health and health care. There is a more fundamental question that also needs to be addressed. Namely, can an individual value changes in health commodities?

As Dolan (22) highlights, the valuation of health is predicated on the notion that an individual possesses a unique set of consistent preferences over health commodities. This assumption is not only germane to the monetary valuation of health but also to any method that requires an individual to express preferences for health outcomes such as QALYs or stated preference discrete choice experiments (SPDCEs).

A potential difficulty that arises when trying to value health is that most individuals are not familiar with the notion of expressing values directly for health-related commodities and so it may be difficult for them to form preferences even if they are able to value the good or service that produces these commodities. This problem is not unique to health, but arises whenever we attempt to disassemble a good into constituent commodity outputs. As Johansson (12, p. 77) notes we face the same problem when valuing a recreation trip:

> ... even if you know your WTP for a charter trip to the Bahamas, it may be difficult to specify the WTP for the weather, the WTP for the hotel, and so on; it is the package not a number of sub-components, that you buy.

Although it is possible to speculate on whether people have a consistent and complete set of preferences for health commodities, this issue ultimately can be resolved only through empirical testing.

2.7.2 Valuing health care directly

The alternative approach is to value health care directly either by observing the demand for health care inputs or by asking respondents what they would be willing to pay for a health care good. This is a much more holistic approach in that it requires respondents to weight up their preferences for the various commodities and transform them into a single value.

Unlike health symptoms, health care is exchanged in markets, but in many developed countries the government subsidizes care so that the user is charged a zero or nominal price. This generates its own problems, because a single point on the demand curve does not convey enough information to facilitate the calculation of the benefits associated with its consumption. This problem is quite different from that encountered when valuing health, because the cause is not an absence of (shadow) prices, but insufficient variation in the observed price to enable the researcher to value care (i.e. estimate the demand curve).

There are two approaches to overcome this problem. The first is to use other essential inputs in the HPM to derive values for a zero-priced health care good. The travel cost method discussed in Chapter 9 is a prime example of this approach. The second alternative is to construct a hypothetical market for health care using the CVM which is discussed in Chapters 6–8. The objective of both these approaches is to measure the consumer's WTP for health care. More recently, approaches using stated preference discrete choice experiments (SPDCEs) have also been used to measure consumer's WTP , see Chapters 10–12.

In Section 2.7.1, it was suggested that it is likely to be more difficult for an individual to form preferences for commodities than for goods. However, this does not mean that it is easy for the individual to value any type of good. There are some features of health care that make its valuation difficult. The rest of this section is devoted to examining this issue.

Underlying the direct valuation of health care is the assumption that the individual is aware of all the health commodities that are produced (e.g. H_t^A, H_t^B, etc.) and is able to weigh up the relative importance of each of these commodities using a one-dimensional metric that reflects their combined value (i.e. money). As Vatn and Bromley (23, p. 5) argue, an individual's ability to undertake such a task is likely to depend on her experience in valuing the good in question:

> ...this computational process is difficult for most goods. Long experience is required for it to work quickly – and well. Children sent to the bakery for their first bread purchase would not find the process simple. Adults are reminded of this when they undertake the purchase of an automobile.

The notion that preferences are not inherited, but instead are a learned behaviour is an interesting one. They are suggesting that the reason why adults can easily evaluate their preferences for common private goods such as bread is that they can ascertain its attributes (e.g. colour, freshness, texture) and have experience in measuring the relative importance of these attributes in monetary terms. Sloan (24) has referred to these as *experience* goods. Skills in purchasing experience goods are built up through a 'trial and error' learning process over a long period of time and cannot necessarily be transferred to goods with which they have less experience in purchasing (e.g. automobiles). This does not mean that adults cannot value such a good, but they must undertake 'preference research' by gathering information on the choices available to them before making a decision.

Why do people find it difficult to value unfamiliar goods? Vatn and Bromley (23) suggest that the process of determining preferences can break down for three reasons. Firstly, people find it cognitively difficult to observe and weigh up the attributes of unfamiliar goods. Secondly, health care contains potentially disparate attributes that cannot be mapped onto a single dimension. Finally, the value of one attribute may depend on another and so the value of the good may be different from the sum of its parts.

If this view of preference formation is correct, what implications does it have for the valuation of health care? It has long been recognized that health care is a good with special characteristics, as Arrow (25, p. 948) states in his seminal article on the welfare economics of medical care:

> The most obvious distinguishing characteristic of an individual's demand for medical services is that it is not steady in origin as, for example, food and clothing, but *irregular and unpredictable*. Medical services, *apart from preventative services*, afford satisfaction only in the event of illness, a departure from the normal state of affairs. *It is hard, indeed, to think of another commodity of significance in the average budget of which this is true.* {emphasis added}

These features suggest that it might be difficult for patients to determine preferences for many types of *curative* health care. It might be an even more difficult task than determining preferences for infrequently purchased private goods such as automobiles, because illness often denies an individual the opportunity to undertake preference research; this is especially true for acute conditions (24). Clearly, not all curative care falls into this category. For example, an individual might regularly suffer from migraines and therefore have a clearly defined set of preferences for different drug treatments even though the occurrence of this condition is unpredictable.

At the extreme are some health care goods where a one off decision to use must be made. An example is the decision to have a genetic test to see identify a disposition to a particular disease. As genetic tests are generally very accurate there is little value in retaking the same test. Sloan (24) refers to these as *credence goods* and argues that decisions about these goods must be based on the experience of others, reputation or trust in the doctor.

It is also important to note that Arrow in the above quote draws a clear distinction between demand for preventative and demand for curative heath care. The demand for the former is motivated by a desire to reduce the probability of experiencing deleterious health states in the future. Given that consumption of preventative services is not unpredictable, these may become experience goods, making it easier for individuals to form preferences – especially when a regular pattern of consumption is involved (e.g. taking anti-hypertensive tablets once a day or annual cancer screening tests).

Outlined in Chapter 1 (Section 1.5.1) were the characteristics of the health care market which cause market failure: risk and uncertainty associated with contracting illness, externalities, asymmetrical distribution of information about health care between providers and consumers and barriers to entry. As can be seen from the above discussion, it is not surprising given the complex nature of health and health care such assumptions often do not hold. A further complicating factor is altruism and the extent to which this fits with the assumptions of a competitive market is debatable. Further to this are the problems with quantifying welfare values which incorporate non-use altruistic values.

2.8 **Altruism**

Up until this point, the main focus of this chapter has been on quantifying use values for health and health care. It is also important to recognize that there are potential sources of value which may not be reflected in behaviour and these are often termed *non-use values*. An important source of non-use value is altruism, which arises whenever people are concerned about the well-being of others. Altruism within the family has been widely recognized since Becker (26), who argues that individuals not only maximize their monetary income but also a social income which includes the monetary value of the relevant characteristics of others who are part of their social group. It is also possible that altruism extends beyond the family, because individuals might be concerned about members of society outside their social group (see 27). Both forms of altruism can influence an individual's WTP for a health care programme that affects others.

In its most general form, altruism can be modelled as an interdependence between utility functions. Consider an individual who derives utility not only from the consumption of private goods (previously defined as x^i) and her health status (H^i), but who is also concerned about the well-being of another individual (r). This individual's utility function can be represented by:

$$U^i = U^i(x^i, H^i, U^r(x^r, H^r)). \tag{2.13}$$

Such an individual is often regarded as displaying *non-paternalistic* altruism, because any change that increases individual r's utility will in turn increase the utility of individual i.

This is not the only form of altruism that can exist. It has often been observed (e.g. 28–30) that in most societies there is a stronger support for increasing access to certain basic goods, such as health care, than increasing equality in the distribution of income per se. This may be due to individuals only being concerned about some aspects of the well-being of others. For example, the utility function of an individual that is only concerned about another individual's health can be represented by:

$$U^i = U^i(x^i, H^i, U^r(H^r)). \tag{2.14}$$

Equation (2.14) has been termed *health focused* altruism. It is theoretically possible that altruism may be *non-health focused*, in which case x^j rather than H^j would appear in the utility function.

There has been some debate on the importance of quantifying altruism when undertaking a CBA. This issue is highly relevant to the CVM since a respondent's WTP may in part reflect '*non-use*' values such as altruism. One side of this debate has argued that altruism should be given lesser (or no) weight when calculating the benefits of a programme. As Milgrom (31, p. 420) states:

> ...the part of willingness-to-pay (WTP) that arises on account of altruistic feelings must be excluded from the benefit-cost calculation in order to identify correctly the projects that are potential Pareto improvements.

Jones-Lee (32;33) offers some support for this view since he has shown that in a society where some or all individuals are *non-paternalistic*, the altruistic component of their WTP can be ignored since the marginal benefits and costs are scaled up by the same factor. However, the conditions under which this result holds are limited. Firstly, this only occurs for a marginal change and society must be at the *social welfare optimum* (i.e. the marginal social utility of income is equal across all individuals) (12, p. 132). Secondly, it only holds for non-paternalistic altruism, importantly if altruism focuses only on one aspect of well-being (e.g. health-focused altruism) then it should be taken into account (32).

The implications of each of these factors for health care contingent valuation studies have yet to be fully resolved as there are relatively few studies (e.g. 34;35) that have explicitly attempted to measure altruistic benefits. In these circumstances, Johansson (12) suggests collecting information on an individual's total WTP and the WTP for her own health.

2.9 Summary and conclusions

There is a fundamental difference between valuing health and health care. Health is not a traded good, and so we are restricted to valuing quantity changes. Whereas, when valuing changes in health care the situation is quite different, because health care goods are traded. Thus, we can potentially measure the welfare changes associated with either price or quantity changes. In practice, institutional restrictions mean that health care is often sold at a zero price, which creates difficulties for the measurement of value, but this problem is very different from that encountered when trying to value non-traded commodities such as health.

Under the HPM, the valuation of health and health care are linked, because health care is an input into the production of health. Under some conditions, the demand for health care or other health-enhancing products can be used to value health. However, these conditions are fairly restrictive. In particular, there must be constant returns to scale and no joint production. If these conditions are not met, the HPM breaks down and revealed preferences cannot be used to value changes in health. In contrast, there is no problem with using stated preference methods as these are not subject to the above conditions.

The penultimate section examines the processes by which individuals form preferences for health and health care. Although little empirical work has been conducted in this area it would seem likely that the more experience an individual has, in purchasing a good, the easier it is for them to form preferences. In this regard, individuals are likely to find it easier to value health care goods and services that are purchased on a regular basis, than to value changes in health commodities. This is particularly true when they have had experience in sacrificing the consumption of other market and non-market goods (e.g. time) in order to consume health care. The final section considers the valuation of altruism which is likely to be the main non-use benefit associated valuation of health, or health care.

References

* Marshall, A. 1920. *Principles of economics*. Vol 1. 8th ed. London: Macmillan.

1. Schelling, T.C. 1968. The life you save may be your own. In: Chase, Jr. S.B. editor. *Problems in public expenditure analysis*. Washington, DC: Brookings Institution.

2. Mishan, E.J. 1971. Evaluation of life and limb: A theoretical approach. *Journal of Political Economy* 79: 687–705 as reproduced in Layard, R. 1972. *Cost-benefit analysis*. Baltimore, MD: Penguin.

3. Tolley, G., Kenkel, D., and Fabian, R. 1994. Overview. In: Tolley, G., Kenkel, D.R., and Fabian, R., editors. *Valuing health for policy: an economic approach*. Chicago, IL: University of Chicago Press.

4. Kleinman, L., McIntosh, E., Ryan, M., Schmier, J., Crawley, J., Locke, G.R. 3rd, *et al.* 2002. Willingness to pay for complete symptom relief of gastroesophageal reflux disease. *Archives of International Medicine* 162(12): 1361–1366.

5. Walzer, S. and Zweifel, P. 2007. Willingness-to-pay for caregivers of children with asthma or wheezing conditions. *Therapeutics and Clinical Risk Management* 3(1): 157–165.

6. Khanna, D., Ahmed, M., Yontz, D., Ginsburg, S.S., and Tsevat, J. 2008. Willingness to pay for a cure in patients with chronic gout. *Medical Decision Making* 28(4): 606–613.

7. Johannesson, M., Jönsson, B., and Borgquist, L. 1991. Willingness to pay for anti-hypertensive therapy: results of a Swedish pilot study. *Journal of Health Economics* 10: 461–474.

8. Donaldson, C. 1990. Willingness to pay for publicly provided goods: A possible measure of benefit? *Journal of Health Economics* 9: 103–118.

9. Becker, G.S. 1965. A theory of the allocation of time. *The Economic Journal* **75**: 493–517.

10. Grossman, M. 1972. On the concept of health capital and the demand for health. *Journal of Political Economy* **80**: 223–255.

11. Pollak, R.A. and Wachter, M. 1975. The relevance of the household production function and its implications for the allocation of time. *Journal of Political Economy* **83**: 255–277.

12. Johansson, P-O. 1995. *Evaluating health risks: an economic approach.* Cambridge: Cambridge University Press.

13. Johannesson, M., Johansson, P-O., and Löfgren, K.G. 1997. On the value of changes in life expectancy: Blips versus parametric changes. *Working Paper No.152*, Stockholm School of Economics.

14. Dickie, M. 2003. Defensive behavior and damage cost methods. In: Champ, P.A., Boyle, K.J., and Brown, T.C. *A primer on nonmarket valuation.* Dordrecht: Kluwer, pp. 395–444.

15. Cropper, M.L. and Freeman, A.M. 1991. Environmental health effects. In: Braden, J.B. and Kolstad, C.D., editors. *Measuring the demand for environmental quality.* Amsterdam: Academic Publishers Elsevier/North-Holland.

16. Hall, J., Gerard, K., Salkeld, G., and Richardson, J. 1992. A cost-utility analysis of breast cancer screening in Australia. *Social Science and Medicine* **34**: 993–1004.

17. Mooney, G. 1986. *Economics, medicine and health care.* Brighton: Weatsheaf.

18. Hori, H. 1975. Revealed preference for public goods. *American Economic Review* **65**: 978–991.

19. Dickie, M. and Gerking, S. 1991. Valuing reduced morbidity: A household production approach. *Southern Economic Journal* **51**: 690–702.

20. Mooney, G. 1994. *Key issues in health economics.* London: Harvester Wheatsheaf.

21. Bockstael, N.E. and McConnell, K.E. 1983. Welfare measurement in the household production framework. *American Economic Review* **73**: 806–814.

22. Dolan, P. 1997. The nature of individual preferences: A prologue to Johannesson, Jönsson and Karlsson. *Health Economics* **6**: 91–93.

23. Vatn, A. and Bromley, D.W. 1995. Choice without prices without apologies. In: Bromley, D.W., editor. *The handbook of environmental economics.* Oxford: Blackwell.

24. Sloan, F.A. 2001. Arrow's concept of the health care consumer: A forty-year retrospective. *Journal of Health Politics, Policy and Law* **26**(5): 899–911.

25. Arrow, K.J. 1963. Uncertainty and the welfare economics of medical care. *American Economic Review* **53**: 941–973.

26. Becker, G.S. 1974. A theory of social interactions. *Journal of Political Economy* **82**: 1063–1093.

27. Culyer, A.J. 1971. The nature of the commodity 'Health care' and its efficient allocation. *Oxford Economic Papers* **23**: 189–211.

28. Tobin, J. 1970. On limiting the domain of inequality. *Journal of Law and Economics* **13**: 263–278.

29. Culyer, A.J. 1980. *The political economy of social policy.* Oxford: Martin Robertson.

30. Pauly, M.V. 1992. Fairness and feasibility in national health care systems. *Health Economics* **1**: 93–103.

31. Milgrom, P. 1993. Is sympathy an economic value? Philosophy, economics, and the contingent valuation method. In: Hausman, J.A., editor. *Contingent valuation: a critical assessment.* Amsterdam: North-Holland.

32. Jones-Lee, M.W. 1991. Altruism and the value of other people's safety. *Journal of risk and uncertainty* **4**: 213–219.

33. Jones-Lee, M.W. 1992. Paternalistic altruism and the value of a statistical life. *Economic Journal* **102**: 80–90.

34. Onwujekwe, O., Chimab, R., Shua, E., Nwagboc, D., Akpalac, C., and Okonkwoa, P. 2002. Altruistic willingness to pay in community-based sales of insecticide-treated nets exists in Nigeria. *Social Science & Medicine* 519–527.

35. Dickie, M. and Messman, V.L. 2004. Parental altruism and the value of avoiding acute illness: are kids worth more than parents? *Journal of Environmental Economics and Management* **48**: 1146–1174.

Chapter 3

Shadow pricing in health care cost–benefit analyses

Emma McIntosh

Whatever society's objective function is, there will be a sacrifice involved in applying resources to one use rather than another. The relevant price for cost-benefit purposes is therefore the price which reflects this opportunity cost. There exists, then, some set of prices called 'shadow' or 'accounting' prices, which reflect the true social opportunity costs of using resources in a particular project.
(Pearce 1971)

3.1 Introduction

The main reason for dedicating an entire chapter to shadow pricing is the practical relevance of shadow pricing within CBA studies. Indeed when the definition of shadow pricing is considered in Section 3.2, we could conclude that almost every chapter could fall under the heading of 'shadow pricing' the inputs or outputs of health care in one form or another. The CBA approach to economic evaluation permits a broad inclusion of costs and benefits due to the monetary benefit measure being all encompassing. While the CEA approach has often been criticized because of its narrow perspective, this has often been more about the decision makers stance as opposed to the methodology (Gold *et al.* recommend CEA from a societal perspective (1)) . The majority of CEAs in health care to date have generally considered quite narrow, often clinical measures of output. This has mainly been a function of the trial-based nature of many CEAs and the availability of relevant outcome measures. In addition to this, practical issues such as the limited availability of additional funding for the measurement and valuation of outcomes beyond the key clinical ones due to the extra costs involved. However, given the numerous possible inputs and outputs measurable within a broad societal perspective, shadow pricing is more likely to be required within a CBA, especially in areas such as mental health care and care of the elderly where often a large number of inputs such as 'informal' services beyond health are often utilized (2) for which market values may be more difficult to obtain.

Indeed, much of the applied component of this chapter will explore the shadow pricing of informal care provision in the health care market.

With the increasing popularity of CBA due to methodological developments in applied methods of benefit assessment methods such as WTP and SPDCE it is likely that the requirement for the shadow pricing of relevant inputs will increase. Further to this, as pointed out by Posnett and Jan (3), with health services becoming increasingly reliant on informal care and the associated shift in costs from the health care sector to the community, for instance through early discharge programmes, the substitution of inpatient care with ambulatory care and the move towards community care of the mentally ill – the greater the importance attached to recognizing and valuing the true cost of unpaid inputs. For all these reasons, this chapter aims to provide a brief practical guide to shadow pricing in health care. As pointed out by Macarthur (1997) (4) 'despite the huge literature on "efficiency" shadow pricing and the general consensus on methods and choice of numeraire, this method is infrequently practiced'. It is the contention that economists in health care do indeed practice shadow pricing, but are often not explicit about the nature of their costings and the shadow price nature of implicit costings. In order to avoid any confusion at the outset it should be noted that this chapter is dedicated to shadow pricing the *inputs* to health care, i.e. resources or 'costs' (as considered in the numerator of a CBA ratio) and not the shadow pricing of 'outputs' or outcomes of health care sometimes termed 'intangibles' (as considered in the denominator of a CBA ratio) in the more traditional economic textbooks (5). Such shadow pricing of 'outcomes' are explored within the chapters on WTP and SPDCE (Chapters 6–8 and 10–12).

3.2 **Definition of shadow pricing**

As Pearce outlines – the basic decision rule in CBA requires that benefits and costs be expressed in monetary units for each period of time over the economic life of the project (6). In order that this decision rule be consistent with the objective function of maximizing social welfare, it is necessary that the prices attached to the physical benefits and costs reflect society's valuations of the final good and resources involved. Pearce goes on to explain that whatever society's objective function is, there will be a sacrifice involved in applying resources to one use rather than another. The relevant price for CBA purposes is therefore the price which reflects this opportunity cost. The shadow price or 'accounting price' therefore reflects the true social opportunity cost of using resources in a particular project or good. In an undistorted economy, i.e. in a 'perfect market', prices are good reflections of opportunity costs partly because the perfect market is in equilibrium and the firms are price takers. Therefore, market prices can be used as reasonably good estimates of opportunity costs. In this case, market prices and 'shadow prices' will coincide. In a distorted economy, however, i.e. in an 'imperfect market', market distortions will cause shadow prices and market prices to differ. This makes CBA more complex to undertake, since 'shadow prices' or 'social values' cannot be directly observed and as a result, the true economic value of goods and services may not be known. The process of correcting distortions in market prices is called shadow pricing and it is used, often without formalizing as such, in most economic evaluations including the evaluation of health care interventions. In short, economists use shadow pricing to establish value in the presence of market failure, i.e. shadow pricing can be used in those cases where market prices need to be adjusted and/or no market price exists (7). Without using shadow prices to correct market distortions, cost estimates within CBA studies could be significantly biased. For a more detailed summary of the implications of market failure in health care, see (8).

3.3 Factors which can make market prices inappropriate as measures of marginal social costs

As noted, market distortions may cause market prices to be inappropriate as measures of marginal social costs (MSC), or marginal social values, of goods and services because the prices may not reflect the true economic value of goods and services, thus shadow prices and market prices may differ. MSC is defined as the total cost to society as a whole for producing one further unit, or taking one further action, in an economy. Therefore, the total cost of producing one extra unit of something is not only simply the direct cost borne by the producer but also the cost to the external environment, see Box 3.1.

With this definition in mind, and building on the section on market failure in health care in Chapter 1 (Section 1.5.1) possible causes of market distortions which would require researchers to undertake shadow pricing are outlined in Box 3.2.

3.3.1 Externalities

Externalities are spillovers from other people's production and consumption of commodities which affect an individual in either a negative or positive way, but which are out of the individuals' control. An example of a positive externality in health is vaccination against diseases such as measles, mumps, and rubella (MMR), these diseases have not only a direct effect on risks to one's own health but also on risks to others (9). For example, children who are vaccinated reduce the risk of contracting the relevant disease for all others around them, and at high levels of vaccination, society may receive large health and welfare benefits. When a factory emits pollution as a by product of its production process, this is a form of negative externality as pollution

Box 3.1 Components of marginal social cost (MSC)

MSC = MPC + MEC

Where:

MSC = Marginal Social Cost

MPC = Marginal Private Cost

MEC = Marginal External Cost

Box 3.2 Causes of market distortions

Externalities
Imperfect knowledge/information
Consumer surplus
Sales or price controls
Oligopoly
The existence of public goods
Monopoly
Property rights

can have a detrimental effect on the health and well-being of a population. The costs and benefit of such spillovers cannot be accounted for in market transactions because consumers and producers only consider costs and benefit to themselves. As a result, the market price will not measure the true MSC or benefit of vaccination or pollution.

3.3.2 Imperfect knowledge

In a perfectly competitive neoclassical model of the market, prices are set with the assumption that consumers and producers have perfect knowledge and information about all aspects of the economy relevant to their choices. This however is not always a realistic assumption. Indeed consumers, i.e. patients (those who are also not fully qualified medical personnel) are unlikely to have perfect knowledge about the costs and benefits of the health care they consume. For example, in attending the hospital for the birth of a first child the mother is not likely to have the full information on every alternative pain relief configuration or delivery option and resulting side effects, effects on baby, effects on recovery, long-term side effects, the costs of all of these options, and so on. In this situation, as with externalities, market prices may not reflect the true MSC or benefit.

3.3.3 Consumer surplus

Consumer surplus is the amount that consumers benefit by being able to purchase a product for a price that is less than they would be willing to pay. It is the difference between the price consumers are willing to pay and the actual price. If a consumer is willing to pay more for an extra unit of a good or service than they actually have to pay, failure to include his surplus may result in underestimation of the true value (marginal social benefit) of the good or service being purchased. Thus, the presence of consumer surplus not accounted for makes market prices an inappropriate measure of MSC.

3.3.4 Price control

The implementation of sales or price controls makes it difficult to know the true amount people are willing to pay for goods and services, hence difficult to access the true economic value of goods and services whose prices are controlled. For example, in the UK, the Pharmaceutical Price Regulation Scheme (PPRS) ensures the NHS has access to good quality branded medicines at reasonable prices, and promotes a healthy, competitive pharmaceutical industry. The PPRS sets the maximum price which may be charged by any manufacturer or supplier for the supply of a branded drug (10). Individual NHS trusts might be willing to pay more for a particular drug to be made available to their patients. As a result, the market price of the drug may not reflect how much a health care Trust is willing to pay for an additional unit of the drug to be made available to its patients, i.e. it will not reflect the true economic value (marginal social benefit).

3.3.5 **Oligopoly**

Oligopoly is a market structure characterized by the following: *few sellers* – a few firms that are so large relative to the total market that they can affect the market price; and *interdependence* – profit maximizing competitors set their strategies by paying close attention to how their rivals are likely to react. Because an oligopoly consists of a few firms, they are usually very much aware of each others' actions and are thus highly sensitive to changes in each others prices. This means that when price cuts do occur, the market tends to have to follow the lead of any one firm. Another characteristic of oligopoly is: *barriers to entry* – there are often high barriers to entry which can lead to a lack of price competition. This means that an oligopolist usually has little incentive to change its prices. It may cut prices where there are prospects of market share gains (i.e. when its rivals will not follow). It may increase prices if it feels sure that competitors will follow (or when the margin increase is sufficient to make up for the large loss in market share). Prices in an oligopoly therefore tend to be higher and change less than under perfect competition. These characteristics pose a problem from the point of view of consumers as the prices set are not determined by their willingness to pay as would be the case in a normal competitive market. Thus, the prices again do not represent the true MSC.

3.3.6 **Public good**

Public goods are goods and services whose use by one person doesn't reduce their availability to others. Public goods have the following characteristics: *non-excludable* – the goods cannot be confined to those who have paid for it; *non-rival* – the consumption of one individual does not reduce the availability of goods to others. The provision of information can be thought of as an economic good that has a high degree of publicness (11). For example, a patient obtaining information about the management of diabetes does not reduce the information available to another patient. Because public goods are usually provided free by the government, their market price is usually zero. If a public good has a beneficial impact to the people receiving them, most of them may be willing to pay for them. This is another case where the market price (which in this case is zero) of a good or service will not reflect its true cost or benefit to society.

3.3.7 **Monopoly**

Monopoly is a situation where there is only one buyer or seller. There are no competition or close substitutes and as a result, a monopolist is able to set prices. Many 'firms' in the health sector have some degree of monopoly power, for example, doctors have the power to influence their own prices (11). Prices within monopolies are usually higher than they would be in a competitive market, thus these prices would not reflect the true marginal social value of such service.

3.3.8 Property rights

Intellectual property rights (IPR), very broadly, are rights granted to creators and owners of works that are the result of human intellectual creativity. These works can be in the industrial, scientific, literary, or artistic domains (12). A patent is an example of an IPR. The marginal social benefit of a patent over time is the value of the incremental inventive activity generated by the patent in each time period and the MSC of a patent is the value of the incremental harm to society resulting from the patent in each time period.

3.4 Correcting market distortions

According to Macarthur (4), the operational function of shadow pricing is to go as far as possible in making corrections for the distortions outlined above so that a CBA can be carried out that is as complete as is required to allow a reasonably safe assessment. Based on this, it appears that shadow pricing is essentially an exercise in removing distortions in market prices. Dreze and Stern (13) have listed seven steps to correct such distortions alluded to above. Whilst not all will relate directly to health care, they provide a useful reference point for the practicalities of shadow pricing. The seven steps are outlined in Box 3.3.

Box 3.3 Dreze and Stern's seven steps to correct market distortions

1. Base the values of all traded goods on their border prices[1] (market value)

2. Remove the values of direct taxes and subsidies from the prices of all items

3. Make an adjustment to allow for the discontinuity between international and domestic values that is caused by the existence of taxes on international trade

4. Value non-traded inputs at their long-term marginal cost of supply

5. Make allowance where necessary for the fact that the wages of some kinds of labour – especially formal sector unskilled labour – may be higher than their opportunity cost at market value

6. Taking account of these basic shadow pricing requirements, calculate the border or market parity values of the goods and services used and produced by the project

7. Estimate the values of important consumer surpluses gained (and lost) in the project situation

[1] Border prices represent the values at which the economy can buy from and sell to the international economy. Where this option exists, it should be used at the basis for valuation (4).

3.5 **Shadow price numeraire**

From a practical standpoint and certainly for CBA studies, the appropriate numeraire for shadow pricing should be the value of a unit of currency used for some specific purpose in the domestic market. According to Macarthur (4), the most popular and certainly most frequently used is the unit of domestic currency that is converted into foreign exchange either in open markets or at the official exchange rate. This is known as the 'world prices' numeraire. For more technical descriptions of how to measure shadow prices of wage rates, foreign exchange, and public funds see Boadway and Bruce (14) as well as using Harberger's (1969) (31) weighted average shadow pricing formula. For the purposes of shadow pricing in CBA in health care economic evaluations, the unit of domestic currency is recommended.

3.6 **Shadow pricing in health care**

By far, the most literature on shadow pricing in health care is in valuing unpaid inputs in health care (3;15–17). One such unpaid input in health care is informal care, sometimes referred to as 'unpaid inputs' or 'unpaid time'. Section 3.6.1 explores this in more depth.

3.6.1 **Shadow pricing informal care**

Informal care can comprise a substantial part of long-term care and often substitutes formal home and nursing home care (18). Van Houtven and Norton show that informal care reduces formal health care use and delays nursing home entry (18). Informal care might thus contribute to the health-related quality of life of the care recipients and as such it has an intrinsic value which should be accounted for within any CBA where informal care occurs. In health care, unlike the available unit costs identifiable for formal care (see Chapter 4), market prices for such informal care services often do not exist. For example, the cost of informal care may not reflect the true societal value of resources attributed to this activity (19). The definition of informal care according to van den Berg is as follows: 'a non-market composite commodity consisting of heterogeneous parts produced (paid or unpaid) by one or more members of the care recipient as a result of the care demands of the care recipient' where 'heterogeneous parts' include: (a) home keeping, (b) personal care, (c) support with mobility, (d) administrative tasks, and (e) to some extent socializing.

Provision of informal care may also result in additional costs (although perhaps not direct financial costs within the health-care sector) which should also be incorporated into the value of the unpaid input. These additional costs are shown in Box 3.4.

Following in depth explorations as to how to calculate the shadow price of unpaid time and leisure, Posnett and Jan (3) outline a practical approach to the valuation of the opportunity cost of unpaid time inputs as a function of tying together the formal principles of shadow pricing and adapting them to the practice of evaluation. In order to do this however they relax some of the rigid assumptions underlying the theoretical basis of shadow pricing (for details of these models, see Posnett and Jan (3)). From these theoretical models, it is identified that several parameters are relevant to determining the value of unpaid time inputs which are listed in Box 3.5.

Box 3.4 Additional costs associated with informal care include the following

Additional 'costs'	Shadow price
Time spent travelling by patients, relatives, carers	Value of time
Time spent waiting for consultation, during consultation, treatment, and rehabilitation	Value of waiting time Opportunity cost of time
Leisure time lost (if time allocated to unpaid activity involves a displacement of non-working time)	Value of leisure activities forgone

Box 3.5 Parameters relevant to determining the value of unpaid time inputs

1. Whether the relevant time input involves working or non-working time
2. Whether lost output is likely to be replaced
3. The level of income tax
4. Sales tax
5. Deviation from competition in markets
6. Type of leisure activities forgone

From this identification of key questions, Posnett and Jan compiled a summary table identifying the opportunity cost of time based on working or non-working time. Table 3.1 reproduces this.

From Table 3.1, four main cases have been identified as follows:

(i) Where time inputs involve working time and where output is replaced, opportunity cost (Ω) is proxied by the net wage rate with any error likely to render this figure an overestimate

(ii) Where output is not replaced, the opportunity cost (the value of the marginal product) is best proxied by the full wage figure with any error causing this to be an underestimate

(iii) The opportunity cost (χ) of non-work time for those currently in employment may be proxied by the net wage rate although the real figure may be lower

(iv) For those not in paid employment and where unpaid household work is not replaced, a suitable proxy for opportunity cost is the market wage rate of a housekeeper

In the literature, two valuation methods are frequently recommended to value informal care, the opportunity costs and the proxy good method (20;21). Van den Berg *et al.* (17) applied both these methods to determine a monetary value for informal care in the Netherlands. As outlined by Van den Berg, the opportunity costs method values

Table 3.1 Opportunity cost of time

Current status?	Working		Not working	
Working time lost?	Yes		No	
Output/activities replaced?	Yes	No	Yes	No
Opportunity cost?	Ω	β	χ	**VMPh**
Proxy	w''	$w*$	w'' (employed) wa'' (not in paid work)	$wh*$

$\Omega = (uL' - uA')/\chi$

β = value of forgone consumption = VMP

χ = value of leisure = uL'/χ

VMPh = value of the marginal product of labour in household production

$(uL' - uA')$ = the marginal value of leisure less the marginal value of the marginal amenity derived from working

χ = marginal utility of money

w'' = net wage rate

$w*$ = full wage rate

wa'' = potential wage rate of the unemployed (average market wage for the relevant occupational group)

$wh*$ = full market wage of a housekeeper

Table replicated with kind permission from *Health Economics*, John Wiley and Sons Ltd (3).

the inputs of the production process. Van den Berg *et al.*, in line with Posnett and Jan (3) distinguish between different sources and amount of time foregone when valuing informal care using the opportunity costs method, this is shown in Box 3.6.

The proxy good method, also known as the 'market cost method' or 'replacement costs method' is an alternative to the opportunity costs method. As outlined by Van den Berg *et al.*, the proxy good method values time spent on caregiving at the (labour) market price of a close substitute, i.e. informal care time is thus valued at the wage rate of a professional caregiver. Importantly, the proxy values differ according to the task, e.g. housework valued at the market wage of a housekeeper and personal care valued at the market wage of a nurse. The two main methods of measurement for the proxy good approach are the diary and the recall method. Due to the time-consuming nature of the diary method the recall method is most often applied. With the recall method, respondents are asked retrospectively how much time they spent on different tasks during a certain time period. In summary, Van den Berg found that hourly values of informal care for stroke and rheumatoid arthritis patients ranged

Box 3.6 Value of informal care

Value of informal care = $n_i w_i + h_i s_i + l_i t_i$

Where t_i is the time spent on care tasks by caregiver i

w_i the net wage rate of i

n_i is the i's hours of forgone leisure

t_i the shadow price of leisure

from €10.64 to €20.24 using the opportunity cost and proxy good method. Following on from this, and the recommendation by Van den Berg that precise guidelines for the use of both methods is required, Section 3.7 takes a look at research into time use in the household. The values from such research could be used within the shadow pricing of unpaid inputs to informal care.

3.7 **UK specific values of unpaid time**

Recent research into the value of unpaid time is being carried out by the Centre for Time Use Research (CTUR) at the University of Oxford (http://www.timeuse.org). Placing money values on unpaid household production is of general interest for time use research insofar as activities move into and out of the economy. CTUR note that traditionally, this work has relied on identifying time devoted by households to the various categories of unpaid work, and valuing this by some appropriate wage rate. Recently, interest has focussed on an alternative approach in which household consumption events are counted, and then valued by market-equivalent prices, enabling, for example, the calculation of domestic productivity (i.e. the rate of domestic output per hour of unpaid labour) to be estimated in a non-circular manner. Work is currently underway to apply these methods to a number of datasets, to develop a view of international similarities and differences in the historical change in the money value of domestic production in the UK and elsewhere.

3.7.1 **Household Satellite Account**

The UK Office for National Statistics (ONS) is developing a Household Satellite Account (HHSA), which, for the first time, will measure and value the outputs produced by households in the UK. This unpaid work is not included in the UK National Accounts, and its measurement will provide a means by which the Government can monitor how the economy is affected by the way patterns of unpaid work are changing. The information will also be of use to policy makers where significant amounts of unpaid work need to be taken into account. The HHSA is part of the ONS series of experimental statistics. Estimates for the year 2000, complete with a detailed description of the methodology and assumptions used to produce the figures, are available from the website (http://www.statistics.gov.uk/hhsa/) and a guide to the methodology used is also available on the website (http://www.statistics.gov.uk/hhsa/hhsa/resources/fileattachments/hhsa.pdf).

The HHSA has been divided into a number of smaller projects covering the different areas of activity. The outputs relate to providing *housing, transport, nutrition, clothing and laundry services, childcare, adult care,* and *voluntary work.* The UK account component of HHSA brings together estimates of the output of housing, transport, nutrition, clothing and laundry services, childcare, adult care, and voluntary activity and shows the related inputs of intermediate consumption and household capital, and the calculation of gross and net value added. It also shows the adjustments that must be made to the National Accounts Gross Domestic Product estimates, if the HHSA estimates were to be combined with them.

While there are a great number of components of domestic unpaid work that may not initially appear relevant to health care, it is the case for many unpaid carers that these categories are indeed very relevant to them and many of these values can be used as shadow prices for informal care. Bonsang identified two types of formal home care, paid domestic help and nursing care, as being highly interacted with informal care (22). Hence, such HHSA values for informal adult care could indeed be relevant for health care shadow pricing. Values which could be used as shadow prices in economic evaluations of health care interventions are provided in Table 3.2.

Following on from these estimates, a number of more 'health specific' shadow prices for informal care could be obtained using relevant health care unit cost sources as proxies. In the UK, the publications 'Unit Costs of Community Care 2004' (23) and more recently, 'Unit Costs of Health and Social Care 2008' (24) have relevant sections containing unit costs and their breakdown of components. The schemas included in such detailed costing estimates are useful for identifying key components of cost often not included in unpaid care shadow prices.

Heitmueller and Inglis (25) explored the wage differentials and opportunity costs of informal carers using the British Household Panel Survey (BHPS). They reveal that on average an individual who experiences some informal care spells and does not work in these periods can expect to have lost between £41,000 and £52,000 of labour income between 1993 and 2002. Studies by the Scottish Executive Central Research Unit estimated the hourly market value of informal care to range from £7.50 to £9.24 (26;27).

Finally, Van den Berg *et al.* (16) recommend the use of the conjoint measurement method to identify values for informal caregiving (Chapters 10–12 provide details on the 'conjoint' stated preference methodology referred to here). Importantly in this work Van den Berg show that the conjoint method is probably better able to capture the heterogeneity of informal care and therefore the valuations provided will be more representative of the true shadow price. De Meijer *et al.* (28) further show that while contingent valuation methods are useful for valuing informal care for use in economic evaluations, non-response remains a matter of methodological concern.

Table 3.2 HHSA value of informal adult care by frequency and type of care

Type of help	Value used	Rate*
Practical	Care Assistant (hourly rate)	£5.58
Personal	Assistant nurse (hourly rate)	£6.02
Personal and practical	Assistant nurse (hourly rate)	£5.79
Continuous	Residential home fee (weekly)	£268

Source: HHSA estimate based on the Family Resources Survey 1999–2000 Residential care rates: Lang and Buisson Care of Elderly People Market Survey 2001. Assistant nurse and care assistant rates: New Earnings Survey

*Based on costs in the year 2000

Other shadow prices relevant to health care include the following:

◆ *Hospital beds* – the shadow price of inpatient stay may depend upon not only the specialty but the true cost of the hospital bed as a function of the bed-occupancy rate.

◆ *Ambulance service* – the shadow price of an ambulance journey may depend upon the true cost of running the ambulance service as a function of the call out rate.

◆ *Voluntary services* – the shadow price of the cost of voluntary service is a function of the opportunity cost of the volunteers own time as well as the value of their advice and information.

◆ *Consultation room costs* – it may be the case that appropriate consideration of the cost of the consultation room is required in which case it is important to account for throughput and true opportunity cost in estimation of the shadow price.

◆ *Land* – it is important to estimate the opportunity cost of the land which a health care project uses, i.e. the land were a new hospital is built. The economic price of the land is based on those areas where there will be a change in land use. The use of this land without the project (hospital building) provides the basis for its economic price. The opportunity cost (shadow price) of the land will be the net benefit that could have been achieved in its next best alternative use.

◆ *Donated health care equipment or medications* – during start up phases or clinical trial periods health care or drugs may be donated for which no market price exists but there is a clear value from its use, e.g. disposable laparoscopic surgical equipment donated during its introductory phase. For drugs provided at a discounted price, the shadow price is often assessed according to the price of another drug already on the market.

3.8 **The shadow price of labour in the health service**

Medical personnel working in private clinics and hospitals are generally better paid than those that work for Government-funded health services such as the NHS. Where NHS health professionals are paid below the market-clearing levels, this causes an artificial shortage. Where such shortages occur, wages may need to be adjusted upwards using shadow prices to reflect the true social cost of doctors and nurses in an economic evaluation. McGuire, Henderson, and Mooney (29) highlight two examples where the use of shadow pricing in health care is appropriate. The first example is that of the price of Doctors. The supply of doctors in most countries is limited through doctors' representative or governing bodies hence by acting as a cartel doctors may be able to price their labour more highly than in a competitive market. Thus, it may be necessary to derive shadow prices to value the *true opportunity cost* of such labour. Another situation is that of monopsony. Monopsony is a state in which demand comes from one source. If there is only one customer for a particular good that customer has a 'monopsony' in the market for that good, i.e. monopsony is equivalent to monopoly but on the demand side not the supply side. Hence, if a health service is a monopsonist in the purchase of 'nurse labour' they may be able to drive down the price of 'nurse labour' below its competitive level – again this implies the need for shadow pricing to value the true, higher, opportunity cost of such labour.

3.9 **Shadow pricing in health care: Limitations and cautions**

As outlined by Layard (30), shadow prices are 'imputed' prices. In light of this, in studies in health care as in any other area using such imputed prices they should always be subject to rigorous sensitivity analysis. The testing of the assumptions around the shadow prices used will allow the sensitivity of change to be explored appropriately. Further to this, as noted by Macarthur, while knowing the shadow price value will help in estimating the economic impact of a project it will give no help to understanding the distributional effects of what is known from a market price analysis.

3.10 **Summary**

The aim of this chapter was to outline the key definition of shadow pricing and, drawing on the available literature, provide some guidance on the process of shadow pricing as well as providing relevant examples in health care. The emphasis in this chapter was the valuation of informal care as it is recognized that health services are becoming increasingly reliant on informal care and the associated shift in costs from the health care sector to the community, for instance through early discharge programmes, the substitution of inpatient care with ambulatory care and the move towards community care of the mentally ill. In developing the shadow pricing of informal care and recognizing the heterogeneous nature of this commodity, the chapter outlined the recent research into the value of unpaid time as being carried out by the Centre for Time Use Research (CTUR) at the University of Oxford and the UK Office for National Statistics (ONS). The chapter then provided the reader with a number of 'health specific' shadow prices for informal care which could be used within economic evaluations in health care.

It is the contention that economists in health care frequently practice shadow pricing but are often not explicit about the process and see it as being part of a standard costing exercise. With the development of guidelines for costing and the call for increased accountability and transferability of costing methods, the shadow prices being used in health care economic evaluations will hopefully become more explicit.

References

1. Gold, M.R., Siegel, J.E., Russell, L.B. and Weinstein, M.C. 1996. *Cost-effectiveness in health and medicine.* New York: Oxford University Press.
2. Beecham, J. 1995. Collecting and estimating costs. In: Knapp, M., editor. *The economic evaluation of mental health care.* 1st ed. Aldershot: Arena, Ashgate, pp. 61–82.
3. Posnett, J. and Jan, S. 1996. Indirect cost in economic evaluation: The opportunity cost of unpaid inputs. *Health Economics* 5: 13–23.

4. Macarthur, J. 1997. Shadow pricing simplified: Estimating acceptably accurate economic rates of return using limited data. *Journal of International Development* **9**(3): 367–382.

5. Dasgupta, A.K. and Pearce, D.W. 1978. *Cost-benefit analysis: theory and practice*. 1st ed. London and Basingstoke: The Macmillan Press.

6. Pearce, D.W. 1971. *Cost-benefit analysis*. 1st ed. London and Basingstoke: The Macmillan Press.

7. Slothuus, U. 2000. *An evaluation of selected literature on the measurement of costs in health care evaluation*. Odense, Denmark: University of Southern Denmark. Report No.: Health Economics Papers 3.

8. Donaldson, C. and Gerard, K. 1993. *Economics of health care financing: the visible hand*. 1st ed. London: The Macmillan Press.

9. Donaldson, C and Gerard, K. 2004. *Economics of Health Care Financing: The Visible Hand*. 2nd Revised edition. Basingstoke: Palgrave Macmillan.

10. Department of Health. DOH, 2008. The Health Service Branded Medicines (Control of Prices and Supply of Information) Regulations 2008.

11. Folland, S., Goodman, A.C. and Stano, M. 2007. *The economics of health and health care*. 5th ed. Upper Saddle River, NJ: Pearson Prentice-Hall.

12. JISC Legal. Intellectual Property Rights. 2009.

13. Dreze, J. and Stern, N. 1994. Shadow prices and markets: policy reform, shadow prices and market prices. In: Layard, R. and Glaister, S., editors. *Cost-benefit analysis*. 2nd ed. Cambridge: Cambridge University Press.

14. Boadway, R.W. and Bruce, N. 1984. *Welfare economics*. 1st ed. Oxford: Oxford University Press.

15. van den Berg, B., Brouwer, W.B.F. and Koopmanschap, M.A. 2004. Economic evaluation of informal care: An overview of methods and application. *European Journal of Health Economics* **5**: 36–45.

16. van den Berg, B., Maiwenn, A., Brouwer, W.B.F., van Exel, J. and Koopmanschap, M.A. 2005. Economic valuation of informal care: The conjoint measurement method applied to informal caregiving. *Social Science and Medicine* **61**: 1342–1355.

17. van den Berg, B., Brouwer, W.B.F., van Exel, J., Koopmanschap, M.A., van den Bos, G.A. and Rutten, F. 2006. Economic valuation of informal care: Lessons from the application of the opportunity costs and proxy good methods. *Social Science and Medicine* **62**: 835–845.

18. Van Houtven, C.N. 2004. Informal care and health care use of older adults. *Journal of Health Economics* **23**: 1159–1180.

19. Drummond, M.F., Sculpher, M.J., Torrance, G.W., O'Brien, B. and Stoddart, G.L. 2005. *Methods for the economic evaluation of health care programmes*. 3rd ed. Oxford: Oxford University Press.

20. Russell, L.B., Siegel, J.E., Daniels, N., Gold, M.R., Luce, B.R., and Mandelblatt, J.S. 1996. Cost-effectiveness analysis as a guide to resource allocation in health: Roles and limitations. *Cost-effectiveness in health and medicine*. New York: Oxford University Press.

21. Drummond, M.F., Stoddard, G.L. and Torrance, W. 1987. *Methods for the economic evaluation of health care programmes*. 1st ed. Oxford: Oxford University Press.

22. Bonsang, E. 2009. Does informal care from children to their elderly parents substitute for formal care in Europe? *Journal of Health Economics* **28**: 143–154.

23. Netten, A. and Curtis, L. 2004. *Unit costs of health and social care*. Canterbury: Personla Social Services Research Unit, University of Kent at Canterbury.

24. Curtis, L. 2008. *Unit costs of health and social care*. Canterbury: University of Kent at Canterbury.

25. Heitmueller, A. and Inglis, K. 2007. The earnings of informal carers: Wage differentials and opportunity costs. *Journal of Health Economics* **26**: 821–841.

26. Scottish Executive Central Research Unit. 2001. Providing free personal carer for older people: research commissioned to inform the work of the Care Development Group. Edinburgh: Scottish Executive Central Research Unit.

27. Scottish Executive Central Research Unit. 2002. *Over the threshold? An exploration of intensive domicilliary support for older people*. Edinburgh.

28. De Meijer, C., Brouwer, W., Koopmanschap, M., van den Berg, B. and van Exel, J. 2010. The value of informal care – A further investigation of the feasibility of contingent valuation in informal caregivers. *Health Economics*. Forthcoming; Published online 23rd June 2009.

29. McGuire, A., Henderson, J. and Mooney, G. 1992. *The Economics of Health Care*. 2nd ed. London: Routledge.

30. Layard, R. 2008. *Cost-benefit analysis*. 5th ed. Penguin Books.

31. Harberger, A.C. (1969). Professor Arrow on the social discount rate. In: Somers, G.G. and Wood, W.D. (eds). *Cost-benefit analysis of manpower policies*. Proceedings of a North American Conference. Kingston, ON: Industrial relations Centre, Queen's University.

Chapter 4

Costing methodology for applied cost–benefit analysis in health care

Emma McIntosh

4.1 Introduction

Following Chapter 3 on shadow pricing the inputs of health care, the aim of this chapter is to outline key applied costing methodology for economic evaluation and more specifically to outline those specific costing issues which have particular relevance to CBA studies. It is also the purpose of this chapter to act as a reference source for health care costs or 'price weights' for use in economic evaluations.

It is generally accepted that the costing approach should be the same no matter which economic evaluation technique is being used: cost-effectiveness, cost–utility or cost–benefit analysis. Indeed, in clinical trials it may be the case that prior specification of the economic evaluation technique is not possible until data on the costs and effects become available (1). However, with new developments in benefit-assessment methodology in CBA such as Stated Preference Discrete Choice Experiments (SPDCE) there are a number of considerations when costing specifically for a CBA study. These considerations relate to the appropriate identification and measurement of costs specific to the timescale and context within which benefits are elicited. It is also important to align the cost units with the benefit data, and to consider matters such as divisibility of costs and their appropriate opportunity cost. Since the use of SPDCE data alongside cost data within a formal CBA framework is a relatively new development in the literature, it is important that considerations for the costing within such CBA studies be examined. Chapters 10–12 explore benefit assessment for CBA studies in health care using SPDCEs. Specifically, Chapter 12 provides practical examples of development of a CBA plane akin to a cost-effectiveness plane. This chapter will outline key costing methods, provide sources of health care unit cost data and provide guidance on the appropriate types of costs to be included within CBAs. Downloadable excel spreadsheets are provided for the purposes of annuitization and discounting cost data for a CBA. Guidance will be provided on costing for a CBA study in health care as well as checklists provided for those carrying out applied CBAs. Further, with the methodology of CBA being recommended for the economic evaluation of public health interventions, this chapter contains a worked example of a costing exercise for such an intervention and explores the specific issues it raises such as the importance of accounting for multi-sector costing across the differing government sectors and the challenges with estimating the long-term costs and benefits of such interventions.

It should be noted that beyond this chapter there are a large number of useful costing methodology references including Chapter 3 'Valuing Medical Service Use' in the second book of this series of handbooks by Glick et al. (2). Other references include Gold et al. (3), Johnson et al. (4), Drummond et al. (5), and the National Institute for Health and Clinical Excellence (NICE) Appraisal Methods Guidance (6).

4.2 Identification, measurement, and valuation of resource use data

There are three key components to a costing exercise: identification, measurement, and valuation of relevant resources. This section will outline the main types of resources to be identified within an economic evaluation.

4.2.1 Identification of resource use for inclusion in an economic evaluation – the relevant perspective

As outlined in Drummond et al. (5), the use of the terms direct, indirect, and intangible costs are no longer recommended due to inconsistent use of terminology across studies giving rise to confusion regarding whether an item is a cost or a benefit as well as confusion with definitions used in other disciplines such as accountancy. Further, it is more useful to think about 'resource use' rather than 'cost' at the outset. These resource-use items can then be combined with unit costs or 'price weights'(2) to produce a 'cost' item for use within an economic evaluation. The relevant identification of resources is also a function of the perspective to be adopted within the CBA. The UK NICE guidance for the assessment of health technologies used the concept of a reference case which 'specifies the methods considered by the Institute to be … consistent with an NHS objective of maximizing health gain from limited resources'. In relation to this, the NICE guidance reference case recommends that costs should relate to resources that are under the control of the NHS and Personal Social Service (PSS). Whilst this is a useful starting point and indeed it may be the case that for many cost-effectiveness studies this perspective is suitable, it will be the case that for many CBA studies this perspective may be somewhat narrow and will not fit well with economic welfare theory to which CBA adheres, which implies that all costs, apart from non-resource costs, be included. In CBAs, in health care the concern is with *public choices*, according to Sugden (7) for most public decisions, a broader, social objective is more appropriate than a narrow financial objective. In health economic CBA studies, this relates to the use of a broader perspective than health care. A recent study by Basu et al. explored the social costs of crime reduction, specifically armed robbery and the cost-effectiveness of substance abuse treatment (8). Whilst not reported as a CBA, this framework would have been ideal for such broad categories of resources spanning government sectors such as health care, employment, and justice. Table 4.1 classifies possible resources for inclusion in a health care CBA into broad categories.

Table 4.1 Examples of types of resource use for inclusion within cost–benefit analyses in health care

Health sector resources	Community health and Personal Social Service resources	Patient and family resources	Other government sector costs	Productivity gains/losses
• Hospital ward stay • Outpatient hospital attendances	Community-based social care, e.g. social worker and local authority occupational therapist	Travel time and expenses Out-of-pocket costs	Housing Employment	Value of changes in productivity (patient or carer)
• Staff time • Drugs • Consumables • Theatre time • Equipment • Capital items • Overheads • Community-based health care, e.g. GP attendances	Nursing home Community-based health care staff Residential care Local authority day care	Over-the-counter medications Opportunity cost of leisure time Childcare costs Herbal remedies	Education Home affairs and justice Social welfare	Transfer payments (tax receipts and sickness benefit payments)
• Paramedic and emergency ambulance services	Foster care services	Domestic resources, e.g. *cleaning and gardening costs due to ill health*	Transport	

Whilst it may also be the case that the CBA framework can be used for a narrowly defined clinical economic evaluation, due to its 'all encompassing' outcome measure it is ideally placed to be used in areas such as the evaluation of complex public health evaluations.

4.2.2 Measurement of resource use for inclusion in an economic evaluation

Once items of resource use have been identified as being relevant to the economic evaluation at hand, the *measurement* of resource use is a practical step within any CBA or economic evaluation more broadly. If the economic evaluation is being carried out wthin a prospectively designed study such as a randomized controlled trial (RCT), then this process often consists of designing relevant 'data capture' questionnaires to be sent to patients at various timescales throughout the economic evaluation period for retrospective recall of resource use over a particular period of time. Such detailed patient-specific costing is often termed 'micro-costing', 'bottom-up' costing, or 'activity-based costing'. With microcosting, very detailed patient-specific resource use is measured for each facet of a patient's care. Given this level of detail, hence accuracy, such costing is often considered the 'gold standard' in economic evaluation.

Indeed, Wordsworth *et al.* in their comparison of micro- and macro-costing methods for multicentre studies showed that micro- or bottom-up costing methods should be considered for technologies with a large component of staff input or overheads, significant sharing of staff or facilities between technologies or patient groups and health care costing systems which do not routinely allocate costs to the intervention level (9).

In addition to such micro-costing, to aid recall 'resource use' diaries may be designed to be held by the patient for 'real time' documentation of resource use. If the economic evaluation is being carried out alongside an RCT, then it is usually appropriate to collect the resource use data for the time period within which outcomes, preferences, or welfare measures are also being collected – this allows costs and benefits to be matched up within the analytical process. There is a small but emerging literature on patient resource use recall producing evidence that patient memory is unreliable after a three-month period and declines in a linear fashion between 3 and 12 months (10). Further evidence from the available literature suggests that there is a tendency to underreport community service utilization, which appears to be exacerbated when the recall period is extended (11). Van den Berg and Spauwen (12) show that when using recall of resource use in an informal care giving setting respondents tend to overestimate the time spent on providing informal care to patients. Resource use data can also be collected from a number of secondary sources including health records and primary and secondary care information systems. Examples of data capture instruments including questionnaires and resource use diaries in the area of Parkinson's Disease surgery and a broader public health, parenting intervention can be downloaded from the website: www.herc.ox.ac.uk/books/cba/support.

An alternative approach to the detailed micro-costing methods are 'gross costing', 'macro-level', or 'top-down' costing methods. Such macro approaches use readily available costs such as Diagnosis Related Groups (DRGs) to cost health care episodes. A practical solution for health economists, and recommended by a number of researchers as well as being used in accountancy practice for hospital costing systems (13–16), is to use both micro- and macro-level costing methods. It is argued that the use of both methods may be advantageous because different methods can serve different purposes. For instance, a top-down or 'macro-costing' approach can be used to assess long-run average costs, while a bottom-up or 'micro-costing' approach can be used to assess local cost variation. Each economic evaluation however will be different and the researcher needs to weigh up the research advantages involved in labour-intensive micro costing versus the readily available macro costing and the extent to which key cost drivers are influenced by either method. It may be the case that a 'reduced list' of resources predict a large proportion of costs and that detailed micro-costing beyond this reduced list may not be worth the research effort (17).

For further statistical guidance on analysing cost data such as dealing with missing cost data, censored cost data, sample size considerations, and handling uncertainty in trial-based economic evaluations please refer to the second and fourth books of this series of handbook (2). However, it should be noted that whilst the results of economic evaluations should always be reported in a statistically meaningful way no amount of statistical analysis can compensate for poor quality cost data (18).

4.2.3 **Valuation of resources**

Once resource use has been identified and measured, it is then appropriate to value it. The recent increase in economic evaluation studies has fuelled considerable advances in the provision and accessibility of cost data both at the level of the trust and at the national level including data such as Health Care Resource Groups (HRGs), the online National Schedule of Reference costs (19) and the Scottish Health Service Costs Book (www.isd.org). The development and implementation of such a national tariff of reference costs came about due to the demand for reliable, robust costing information. Further, since such cost data is being used more proactively by such bodies as the Audit Commission, HM Treasury, the Office for National Statistics (ONS), private, voluntary, and academic organizations, the need for comparable, high-quality data is reinforced (20). These references are often accompanied by useful technical manuals on how the costs have been compiled (20). Information Services Division (ISD), Scotland's national organization for health information, statistics, and IT services, produce the Scottish Health Service Costs Book. Scotland has some of the best health service data in the world. Few other countries have information which combines high-quality data, consistency, national coverage, and the ability to link data to allow patient-based analysis and follow up. The UK Personal Social Services Research Unit (PSSRU) compiles an invaluable source of cost data in the form of its annual compendium of 'Unit Costs of Health and Social Care'(21) along with schemas of how the unit costs were devised. Such detailed costing schemas are also useful for identifying appropriate ranges for sensitivity analyses. As a consequence of such readily available unit cost data, the valuation of resources is less onerous than was historically the case. James and Stokes also provide a useful reference source for identifying UK primary and secondary health economic data more generally (22). Box 4.1 outlines some frequently referenced sources of UK health care unit cost data.

A further consideration for cost data are the differing *types* of cost which affect how resources are measured and valued. Box 4.2 outlines the differing types of cost.

Economists often emphasize the importance of the distinction between average cost and marginal cost with the use of the example provided by a study exploring the

Box 4.1 Sources of UK unit cost data for economic evaluations in health care

Type of resource	Source
Healthcare Resource Groups HRGs and national reference costs	www.dh.gov.uk (search for 'reference costs')
Scottish health service costs	http://www.isdscotland.org (search for 'costs book')
Unit costs of health and social care	Unit costs of Health and Social Care (21) and online at www.pssru.ac.uk (search for 'unit costs')
Drug dosage and price	BNF www.bnf.org MIMS www.mims.co.uk

Box 4.2 Types of cost

Definition	Description
Total cost (TC)	Sum of all the costs of producing a particular quantity of output
Fixed cost (FC)	Costs which do not vary with the quantity of output in the short run (usually about 1 year), e.g. rent, equipment lease payments, some wages and salaries
Variable cost (VC)	Costs which vary with the level of output, e.g. medical consumables such as sutures, patient meals
Average cost (AC)	Total cost/quantity
Marginal cost (MC)	The *extra* cost of producing one *extra* unit of output

cost-effectiveness of the six stool guaiac (23). Indeed, in an economic evaluation most types of cost outlined in Box 4.3 are likely to be used in one manner or another however when it comes to reporting the final cost-effectiveness ratio it is the marginal cost per marginal unit of health benefit which is the important one. In CBA studies, it is also the case that all types of costs may be relevant however when it comes to reporting the final result with the marginal cost and the marginal benefit being the same unit it is recommended that net benefit (monetary benefit minus monetary cost) be the figure reported.

4.3 Costing methodology in economic evaluations

A recent study by Clement *et al.* show that different costing methodologies can produce markedly different cost estimates (24). In the UK, NICE issues guidance on around 20 technologies per year and economic evaluation plays a major role in the decisions made by NICE. To aid this process and to improve the comparability both within and between submissions, NICE has devised the concept of a reference case which was developed by experts in the methodological aspects of economic evaluation. The reference case, based on that published by Gold *et al.* (3) 'specifies the methods considered by the institute to be the most appropriate for the Appraisal Committee's purpose and consistent with an NHS objective of maximizing health gain from limited resources'. As discussed earlier, while the appropriate perspective for an economic evaluation in health care may go beyond that of the NHS, this reference case is a useful starting point for cost (and benefit) methodology. Box 4.3 provides a summary of the UK's NICE reference case requirements.

As outlined in Box 4.3, the NICE reference case states that costs to the NHS and PSS are the most relevant. However, its guidance states that non NHS/PSS costs *can* be included but *outside* the reference case. This is important for the development of the CBA framework in health care evaluation. NICE accepts that some technologies may have a substantial impact on the costs (or cost savings) to other government bodies hence their recommendation in these circumstances is that 'costs to other government bodies may be included if this has been specifically agreed with the Department

Box 4.3 The UK's NICE reference case

Element	Reference case
Defining the decision problem	Consistent with NICE's scope
Comparator	Routine therapies in the NHS
Perspective on costs	NHS and PSS
Perspective on outcomes	All health effects on individuals
Type of study	Cost-effectiveness analysis
Synthesis of outcome evidence	Systematic review
Measure of health benefits	Quality Adjusted Life Years (QALYs)
Health state descriptions	Validated generic measure
Method of preference elicitation	Choice-based
Source of preference data	Sample of public
Discount rate	Annual rate of 3.5%* for costs and benefits
Equity	QALY given same weight for all recipients
Dealing with parameter uncertainty	Probabilistic methods

* Current recommendations in 2010.

of Health'. When non-reference-case analyses include these broader costs, explicit methods of valuation are required. NICE states that in all cases such broader costs should be reported separately from NHS/PSS costs and that these costs should not be combined into an incremental cost-effectiveness ratio (ICER; where the QALY is the outcome measure of interest). Further, NICE states that costs borne by patients may be included when they are reimbursed by the NHS or PSS and when the rate of reimbursement varies between patients or geographical regions, such costs should be averaged across all patients. Productivity costs and costs borne by patients that are not reimbursed by the NHS and PSS should be excluded. The guidance also states that NHS reference costs should be the source of resource use valuation (see Box 4.1) and that prices should be public list prices to NHS with no VAT costs. For more information on the NICE reference case, see www.nice.org.

4.4 Discounting and annuitization of costs

A crucial element of costing methodology is the methods used to account for the differential timing of costs and consequences. As pointed out by Drummond *et al.* (25) even in a world with zero inflation and no bank interest, it would be an advantage to receive a benefit earlier and to incur costs later. This is termed 'time preference'. This section of the chapter summarizes a number of formulae, technical appendices, and provides details of downloadable material to be used for costing exercises available from the website: www.herc.ox.ac.uk/books/cba/support. Further to this, for a comprehensive technical guide to economic appraisal in Central Government see 'The Green Book',

HM Treasury (26) as well as online calculators for estimating net present costs in public sector economic appraisals: http://eag.dfpni.gov.uk/npc-calculator.xls.

Section 4.4.1 outlines the concept of discounting.

4.4.1 Discounting

As noted above, it is an advantage to receive a benefit earlier and to incur costs later – this is termed *positive time preference*. Some reasons for positive preference include a shortsightedness or an impatience for the future, i.e. myopia; due to future uncertainty, people may prefer to have all the benefits now and incur costs later and finally individuals are hopeful that economic growth will mean that we will be wealthier in the future so that having an extra Pound (£) today is of higher value to us than having an extra £ in the future. While the practice of discounting costs in health care is regarded as being fairly uncontroversial, this is not the case for the discounting of health benefits, for a review of this see Smith and Gravelle (27) as well as Van der Pol and Cairns (28), and Cairns (29). The NICE reference case currently recommends a discount rate of 3.5% for both costs and benefits (see Box 4.3). The use of a discount rate has the effect of reducing the value of future costs and benefits in present day terms. The key terms are 'present value' and 'discount factor'. Using the NICE recommended rate of 3.5%, this essentially implies that society values £1 today equally with the certainty of £1.035 in a year's time. Another way of putting this is to say that £1 in a year's time is worth only 96.62 pence now (£1/1.035 = 0.9662). Hence, 96.62 pence represents the 'Present Value' (PV) of £1 and the figure 0.9662 represents the relevant 'discount factor'. The example in Box 4.4 shows how the present value

Box 4.4 Example of present value as a function of differing discount rates

Year of payment (mid year)	Present value Discount rate -3.5% (At middle of year)	Present value Discount rate -6% (At middle of year)	Present value Discount rate -10% (At middle of year)
0	£1.0000	£1.0000	£1.000
1	£0.9662 $(£1 \times 1/1.035^1)$	£0.9434 $(£1 \times 1/1.06^1)$	£0.9091 $(£1 \times 1/1.10^1)$
2	£0.9335 $(£1 \times 1/1.035^2)$	£0.8900 $(£1 \times 1/1.06^2)$	£0.8265 $(£1 \times 1/1.10^2)$
3	£0.9019 $(£1 \times 1/1.035^3)$	£0.8396 $(£1 \times 1/1.06^3)$	£0.7513 $(£1 \times 1/1.10^3)$
4	£0.8714 $(£1 \times 1/1.035^4)$	£0.7921 $(£1 \times 1/1.06^4)$	£0.6830 $(£1 \times 1/1.10^4)$
5	£0.8420 $(£1 \times 1/1.035^5)$	£0.7473 $(£1 \times 1/1.06^5)$	£0.6209 $(£1 \times 1/1.10^5)$
10	£0.7089 $(£1 \times 1/1.035^{10})$	£0.5584 $(£1 \times 1/1.06^{10})$	£0.3855 $(£1 \times 1/1.10^{10})$

of £1 declines in future years when the rate of discount is 3.5% per annum, 6% per annum, and 10% per annum. In showing the differing discount rates and the impact over time hopefully the concept of positive time preference will be made clear.

From Box 4.4, it can be shown that with no discount rate all values are £1 in year 0; however as we progress into future years the impact of discounting on the present value becomes apparent. In addition, the higher the discount rate, i.e. the more positive the time preference, the less the present value of £1. We can see that £1 in 10 years' time using a discount rate of 3.5% is worth £0.7089 now as compared to £1 in 10 years' using a discount rate of 10% – worth only £0.3855. In most economic evaluations, it is sufficient to carry out discounting on costs and benefits identified at annual intervals. For access to a downloadable spreadsheet containing discount factors for all discount rates in all years, please refer to: www.herc.ox.ac.uk/books/cba/support.

4.4.2 Equivalent annual cost

Capital costs tend to occur at a single point in time however, capital assets are used over time and can be sold at any time therefore the opportunity cost of capital is spread over time. As a consequence of this, the appropriate costing of capital items requires the calculation of an equivalent annual cost (EAC). This EAC is therefore the capital cost apportioned into EAC as a function of its expected lifespan and appropriate discount rate. In addition to this, however, to obtain a 'unit cost per use' items of capital generally also require the inclusion of annual servicing and replacement part costs and these 'annual costs' should then be divided by the annual throughput of patients using the equipment to obtain a unit cost per use.

Example: A stereotactic frame for performing neurological surgery may cost £82,250 but in order to obtain a 'cost per use', i.e. 'cost per patient' we need to account for both the lifespan of the equipment as well as the estimated 'number of uses'. To do this, we must firstly identify the EAC of the equipment based upon its true retail cost, express this as a function of its lifespan and the appropriate discount rate, add in the annual costs of servicing and maintenance, and finally divide by throughput. An example of this is provided in Box 4.5.

Box 4.5 Annuitization and per patient costing of equipment

Cost (£)	Lifespan	EAC of £1 per annum for 3 years @ 3.5% p/a	EAC of equipment	Annual cost of servicing, maintenance and replacement parts	Annual through-put (no. of patients)	Cost per use (£)
£82,250	3 years	0.3569	£82,250 × 0.3569 = £29,355.03	£1,736	40	(£29,355.03 + £1,736) ÷ 40 = £777.28

4.4.3 Handling uncertainty in cost data

The example provided in Box 4.5 also affords the opportunity of showing the importance of allowing for uncertainty in the estimates of cost (and outcome) data. Briggs distinguishes among a number of different types of uncertainty depending upon whether the data are patient level or from decision analytic models. In stochastic analyses, such as individual patient data from clinical trials they identified four main types of uncertainty: methodological; sampling variation; extrapolation; and generalizability/transferability. For all types of uncertainty apart from extrapolation, where modelling methods are recommended, sensitivity analysis is the recommended approach to handling uncertainty. Sensitivity analysis is a method whereby various parameters in the analysis are varied in order to test the impact on the overall result. The main types of sensitivity analysis are one way; multi-way; scenario analysis, threshold analysis, and probabilistic sensitivity analysis (PSA). See Briggs (30), Drummond *et al.* (25), and Glick *et al.* (2) for fuller expositions of these methods.

Obvious parameters influencing cost and which may make the total cost variable 'sensitive' to change and therefore impact the overall result of the study include the following: source of unit costs; cost perspective; lifespan of capital items; patient throughput; discount rate; and annual service and maintenance costs. Box 4.6 outlines the impact on the cost per use of £777.28 from the example in Box 4.5 based on changing the key assumptions regarding lifespan, throughput and annual service and maintenance costs.

Box 4.6 shows that in this example, the cost per use of £777.28 based on the baseline assumptions outlined in Box 4.5 is sensitive to changes in the lifespan and throughput of such a costly piece of equipment but less sensitive to changes in the annual service and maintenance costs.

4.4.4 Allocating overhead costs

Hospital running costs are usually apportioned across specialty and patient type and these costs are partly 'direct hospital costs' such as medical and nursing staff, but there are also resources which are shared between many different departments or programmes, these 'joint resources' are termed 'allocated costs' or 'overhead costs'. If individual projects in a CBA are to be costed, then some consideration needs to be taken of relevant overhead costs. Examples of overheads in a hospital are shown in Box 4.7.

Box 4.6 Sensitivity analysis of cost data (from Box 4.5)

Assumption	Cost per use (£)
Lifespan of **5** years	£498.86
Annual throughput of **60** patients	£518.18
Reducing the annual service and maintenance costs by **50%**	£755.58

Box 4.7 Examples of overhead costs in a hospital

Administration	Portering
Catering	Waste disposal
Bedding and linen	Laundry
Heating	Property maintenance
Cleaning	Depreciation
Rent and rates	Uniforms

As noted by Drummond *et al.*, there is no *right* way to apportion such costs. The obvious approach to use for economists is the use of marginal analysis, that is to simply see which resources would be impacted by the addition, expansion, removal, or reduction of a programme. However, with CBA it may be the case that two completely separate programmes, in differing specialties are being compared for 'value for money' in which case an alternative method for allocating overheads is required. Drummond *et al.* (25) go into detail on the technicalities of overhead allocation including the following methods: 1. Direct allocation; 2. Step-down allocation; 3. Step-down allocation with iterations; and 4. Simultaneous allocation. However, they also provide a simple, crude approach as shown in Box 4.8.

In developing their simple approach to the allocation of overheads, Drummond *et al.* note that the effort one would put into overhead costing depends on the likely importance of overhead costs. This is an important point as Tan *et al.* (31) showed that overhead costs were the second most important cost component in their micro-costing of dental fillings in Europe. Their study showed that overheads covered 24% of the total costs, ranging from 7% in England to 41% in Germany. In this study, overhead costs

Box 4.8 Simple approach to allocating overheads

1   Identify those hospital costs unambiguously attributable to the treatment of programme in question. Allocate these to the programme.

2   Deduct, from hospital operating expenses, the cost of departments already allocated above and departments known not to service the programme being costed.

3   Allocate the remainder of hospital operating expenses on the basis of number of patient days, for example,

Hospital cost of the programme	=	Directly allocatable costs	+	Net Hospital *Expenditure* Total number of hospital patient-days	x	Hospital patient days attributable to the programme

4   Finally, undertake a sensitivity analysis.

Adapted from Drummond *et al.* (25), p. 70.

were allocated on the basis of 'average treatment time', 'total overhead costs per year', and either the number of workable hours or the number of hours dedicated to direct patient care only.

From the ISD online data referred to above the overheads for Scottish hospitals can be directly accessed from downloadable Excel spreadsheets, along with their method of allocation (www.isdscotland.org). For example, the overhead expenditure on catering and cleaning from April 2007 to March 2008 at Glasgow Royal Infirmary was £1,740,000 and with 40,016 patient consumer weeks this gives rise to a cost per patient consumer week of £43. This can be compared to the equivalent overhead cost per patient consumer week at Ninewells Hospital, Dundee of £77.

4.4.5 Productivity costs

This section explores the methods used to incorporate productivity 'costs' often termed 'indirect costs' into CBA studies. As well as exploring traditional methods such as the human capital approach, the friction–cost approach and the US Panel approach this section explores the use of a new approach based upon the theory of equality of opportunity developed by Roemer (32).

Productivity costs as defined by the Washington Panel are: '…costs associated with lost or impaired ability to work or engage in leisure activities due to morbidity and lost economic productivity due to death' (3). Brouwer *et al.* propose an alternative definition of productivity costs as 'Costs associated with production loss and replacement costs due to illness, disability and death of productive persons, both paid and unpaid' (33). There are three main methods for estimating production costs, the human capital method, the friction cost method, and the US Panel approach. These approaches are described briefly.

The human capital method documented by Rice and Cooper (34) estimates 'production costs' based on the present value of the additional stream of income for a patient/carer as a result of a given healthy care programme. The friction cost method, proposed by Koopmanschap *et al.* (35) is a relatively newer approach which estimates the cost of lost production as a function of the time-span organizations require to restore the initial production level. There are a number of concerns arising with both approaches. The human capital approach is criticized for providing an estimate of *potential* lost production as opposed to *actual* lost production, adopting the unrealistic assumption of 'full employment' and discriminating in favour of the economically active. On the other hand, the main objections to the friction cost approach by critics such as Johannesson and Karlsson (36) and Liljas (37) is that the absence of productivity costs after the friction period implies that the opportunity cost of labour is set at close to zero after the friction period. Both critics argue that in order to be consistent in the analysis, the same approach would have to be taken towards direct health care costs including labour costs. If a value close to zero was applied to labour costs, this would substantially reduce the costs of health care interventions. It is this flaw which, they suggest, illustrates the main limitation of the friction cost approach.

Unlike the human capital approach and the friction cost approach which recommend that production costs enter the cost side of the CEA or CBA equation the US panel approach (Gold *et al.* (3)) recommends that production costs enter the cost–benefit equation in the *benefit* side and this has caused much debate. In short, the panel recommends that researchers use health state values which implicitly incorporate the impact of illness on ability to work and financial loss. This approach originates from the guidelines for the CEA of health care interventions generated by a multidisciplinary panel designated by the US Public Health Service. For a comprehensive guide to all three methods both theoretically and practically as well as a direct comparison of the methods see Pritchard and Sculpher (38).

More recently, Herrero and Moreno-Ternero (32) have proposed a method for calculating the production costs of an intervention in a manner that accounts for differences in 'productive effort'. In the human capital approach, Herrero and Moreno-Ternero deem that a key feature is missing. This feature is that of disentangling the effect of circumstances (aspects that are beyond the control of a person but that affect her pursuit of welfare) and effort (to be understood as those aspects that also influence a person's welfare but over which a person has at least some responsibility) in the outcomes of individual earnings. Herrero and Moreno-Ternero's position is that the earnings gap due to a disease, illness, or impairment is well computed only if we compare the earnings of an impaired person with the earnings of a healthy person who has the same remaining circumstances and has expended the same relative degree of effort. To develop this model, Herrero and Moreno-Ternero rely upon the recent theory of *Equality of Opportunity* developed by Roemer (39) who builds on key earlier contributions by political philosophers such as Richard Arneson, G.A Cohen, Ronald Dworkin, John Rawls, and Amartya Sen.

4.5 Special costing considerations for CBA studies

Moving on from the fundamental tools of costing, and in line with the main focus of this book, there are some specific costing issues within a CBA in health care when using SPDCE and WTP methods to derive welfare measures. These issues are related to: units of benefits and units of costs; aligning costs with preference data; and beyond discounting to 'appropriate lifespan' of preferences. Chapter 12 provides some further guidance for combining costs and SPDCE-derived benefits within a CBA and in particular Section 12.7 outlines '*Measurement issues specific to SPDCEs*', however this section will provide some practical advice on the costing elements of this process.

Paying particular attention to the '*nature*' of health care attributes is a key consideration for measurement of resources within a CBA using SPDCE-derived benefits. As discussed in Chapter 12, the nature of attributes will influence the validity and generalizability of the resulting CBA depending upon the following: how they are defined; the context within which they are defined; the timescale associated with the health state or effect; the unit in which the attribute is defined; and whether the attribute is static or dynamic. Dynamic health care attributes may be associated with differing time periods; for instance, particular diseases will be associated with differing health states over time. This then leads to the usual challenges associated with adjusting for differential timing of costs and benefits, but crucially for CBAs using SPDCEs or WTP measures further consideration of the *context* within which preferences for the health states were elicited and the validity of results when used in differing time periods. All these issues have implications for the resource use being measured. Where the intervention (or health state) being evaluated lasts into the future then discounting of resource use costs and 'preferences' should also be considered (see Section 4.4.1). In addition however assumptions will have to be made regarding the time period over which SPDCE-derived preferences are valid. Hence, it will therefore be important to ensure that the resource use required/removed achieving the given welfare gain/loss are also measured and valued in line with the valid time period. Chapter 12 recommends that explicit 'time periods' be incorporated directly into the context setting of the SPDCE survey to improve the validity of preferences over the time period of interest and this process will also help to identify the appropriate resource use time period. The extent to which resources and hence costs are also divisible is a further consideration. It may be that an attribute in a SPDCE relates to a resource which is not divisible and hence the appropriate full opportunity cost of that resource needs to be included in the costing exercise. This is an important matter when it comes to the reporting and presenting of the CBA results. The aggregated CBA may provide a better opportunity to reflect the true opportunity costs of resources as a result of the divisibility problem as opposed to a patient level or study level CBA. As shown in downloadable Table 10.1 (www.herc. ox.ac.uk/books/cba/support) a number of attributes are reported in terms of probabilities, e.g. 'chance of complications following operation' or 'probability of retreatment with hysterectomy' and within the CBA the resource cost associated with this probability would also have to be measured accordingly. In majority of cases the expected cost, i.e. the cost multiplied by the probability of occurrence will be appropriate however the divisibility of some capital items and other resources may pose some further challenges in some evaluations. Some SPDCEs have a large number of attributes, e.g. chemotherapy-related attributes: social, emotional, cognitive, pain, fatigue, insomnia, anorexia, nausea, constipation – all attributes related to chemotherapy. While the cost of chemotherapy must be attributed so must the expected cost of the side effects and all within the time frame of the preference elicitation exercise.

4.6 Costing example: The costs of an intensive home visiting programme for vulnerable families

Home visiting programmes are now being used extensively in countries such as the USA (40) and Australia (41), and this development reflects a growing recognition of the importance of the first 3 years of life not only in preventing a range of adverse health outcomes but also in promoting optimal mental and physical health in infancy, childhood, and adulthood. A recent HDA review of reviews shows that these programmes are associated with a range of benefits including better rates of breast-feeding, reduced accidents, improved detection, and management of postnatal depression and improvements in parenting and the home environment (42). It is not, however, clear that their use is justified from an economic perspective. There have been few economic evaluations of health visiting services (43–50), most of which have been conducted in the US, have diverse economic objectives and many of which have been beset by methodological problems including the lack of a societal perspective. The results of these economic analyses have been variable with some studies showing that the costs of such services are offset by savings from reduced inpatient care etc (45–47;49), and some showing increased expenditure on home visiting with no savings (48).

4.6.1 Costing methods

A multicentre RCT was conducted in which women identified as being 'at risk of poor parenting' were randomly allocated to a home visiting arm ($n = 67$) or a standard treatment control arm ($n = 64$). Further details of the development of the home visiting service, RCT methods (51) and full cost effectiveness analysis (52) are reported elsewhere. Data on resource use were identified and measured within the RCT. The resource-use data were collected as an integral part of the trial data collection forms. A section entitled '*Your use of Services*' (available to download from: www.herc.ox. ac.uk/books/cba/support) was included in the trial forms and women were asked to recall their use of services such as visits to the GP for the antenatal period till 2 months postnatally, 2–6 months postnatally, and finally from 6 to 12 months postnatally. To aid recall the women were asked to keep a '*Diary of service use*', which they used as an aid to completing the resource-use form. Where such data were not completed women were asked to return their diary so that some estimate could be obtained of service use. Unit costs (2003/2004) adjusted by appropriate quantities were then attached to the items of resource-use to obtain a study cost. These study costs were summed for each individual in the study and the mean difference in costs between the two arms of the trial estimated. Private costs incurred to women such as childcare costs, over-the-counter medicines, and use of private practitioners was also measured. Unit costs were attached to all resources measured to allow reporting of variances in cost arising through economic significance as well as statistical significance. The majority of unit costs were obtained from Netten and Curtis (53), Netten and Curtis (54), and the 'New NHS' 2004 reference costs (55). Where unit costs required inflating to 2004 prices, the readily available Hospital and Community Health Services (HCHS) and PSS inflationary indices were used. Recommended discount rates of 3.5% were used for both costs and benefits where applicable (56). A societal perspective was adopted such that costs to the health service, social services, legal costs, local authority housing costs, and private costs to women were included. However, in line with the NICE reference case costs were disaggregated so that health service and PSS only costs could be identified.

4.6.2 Results

Thirty-three items of potential resource-use services for this group of high-risk women were originally identified and included in the resource-use proforma for women to complete. The results reveal that 29 of these resource services had been used as well as a number of 'other' services. The resources identified along with their unit costs are listed in Table 4.2. This table shows the range of costs used by these women and the importance of the broad multi-sector nature of the costing exercise.

The extent to which the resource-use quantity and cost for the entire period differs between the two arms is shown in Table 4.3. The total cost variable is produced from

Table 4.2 Summary of main resources and unit costs

Resource item	Unit cost[1]	Study cost (2004)[2]
Family doctor (GP)	£26.00[3]	£26.66[14]
Home visitor (home)	£76.00[3]	£77.94[15]
Home visitor (clinic)	£53.00[3]	£27.18[16]
Home visitor (phone)	£22.00[3]	£3.76[17]
Social worker (home)	£76.00[3]	£79.50[18]
Social worker (clinic)	£30.00[3]	£31.38[19]
Social worker (phone)	£30.00[3]	£5.23[20]
Midwife (home)	£44.00[4]	£44.00[21]
Midwife (hospital)	£62.00[4]	£62.00[22]
Antenatal class	£37.00[3]	£3.70[23]
Alcohol/drug support	£87.00[4]	£91.00[24]
Paediatrician	£105.00[4]	£105.00[25]
Obstetrician	£84.00[4]	£84.00[26]
Audiology	£59.00[4]	£59.00[27]
Opthalmology	£49.00[4]	£49.00[28]
CPN	£62.00[3]	£63.58[29]
Child and family team	£27.69[3]	£27.69[30]
Hospital A & E Department	£65.67[4]	£67.34[31]
Psychologist	£66.00[3]	£67.68[32]
Family centre	£27.69[3]	£2.77[33]
Sure-start	£27.69[3]	£27.69[34]
Home-start	£76.00[3]	£77.94[35]
Housing department	£12.50[5]	£12.50[5]
Women's aid	£93.00[6]	£46.50[36]
Legal aid	£93.00[6]	£46.50[37]
CAB	£12.50	£12.50[38]
Psychologist	£66.00[3]	£67.68[39]
Psychiatrist	£210.00[3]	£215.36[40]
Foster care	£593.00[3]	£620.28[41]
Adoption services	See[7]	See[7]
Local advice centre	£12.50	£12.50[42]
Parent–toddler group	£2.00[8]	£2.00[8]
Court hearing	£945.00[9]	£945.00[43]
Social services case conference	£258.00[10]	£450.58[10]

Resource item	Unit cost[1]	Study cost (2004)[2]
Crèche	£4.50[11]	£4.50[11]
Playgroup	£2.00[11]	£2.00[11]
Private child care	£35.00[11]	£35.00[11]
Police attendance	£12.00[12]	£12.00[13]

[1] Published unit cost: [2] Unit cost multiplied by quantity of resource-used in study and inflated to 2004 prices using HCHS or PSS Inflationary indices where relevant: [3] Netten and Curtis (53;54) : [4] NHS Reference Cost (2004) (Online spreadsheets: http://www.doh.gov.uk) (55) : [5] 2004 costs personal communication, Business Manager, Housing Customer Services, Oxford City Council: [6] Legal aid costs http://www.gov.uk: [7] 'Costs of Adoption', Selwyn et al. (2004) in Netten and Curtis (54). Costs include: post placement unit costs per year of £6,070 (2003); Post-adoption unit cost per year £2,334 (2003); Carer and legal costs of the adoption process of £252 (2003): [8] Average for Oxfordshire (2004): [9] http://www.courtservice.gov.uk: [10] Assumption: 2 hr social worker time[3] plus 2 hr social worker assistant[3] plus 2 hr home visitor[3] plus 2 hr legal aid time[6]: [11] Average for Oxfordshire (2004): [12] http://www.homeoffice.gov.uk: [13] £12 per hour according to ready reckoner: Assume 1 hr contact time: [14] Per clinic consultation lasting 12.6 min: [15] Per 1 hr client contact for home visit: Assume 1 hr for study cost: [16] Assume 30 min contact time for study cost: [17] Unit cost of £22 per hour non-contact: Assume 10 min phone call: [18] Per 1 hr client contact for home visit: Assume 1 hr for study cost: [19] £30 per hour of client related work in clinic: [20] £30 per hour of client related work in clinic: Assume 10 minute phone call: [21] Midwifery postnatal visit cost (55): [22] Midwifery outpatient appointment cost: [23] NHS Reference costs Antenatal Support (55): Assume 10 women attend each class – individual cost of £3.70: [24] NHS Reference costs (2004) Mental health Services: booked appointments data for alcohol and drug counselling (55): [25] Paediatric outpatient appointment (55): [26] Obstetric outpatient appointment (55): [27] Audiology outpatient appointment (55): [28] Ophthalmology outpatient appointment (55): [29] Community Psychiatric Nurse (CPN) (53): [30] Netten and Curtis (53); Per hour of client contact: Assume 1 hr for study cost: [31] NHS Reference cost (55): Assumption: Average cost of referred/discharged/transferred: [32] Per 1 hr client contact with a clinical psychologist: [33] Session at a local authority nursery as proxy (£27.00; Netten and Curtis (53)): Assume 10 women attend each session: [34] Session at a local authority nursery as proxy (£27.00; Netten and Curtis (53)): [35] Home Start is a home visiting service, run by a charity: Assumption – resources are the same as home visiting. [36] Assume same cost as legal aid (see[37]): [37] Based on the cost of a legal aid solicitor, Legal aid costs £93 per hour, assume a 30 min appointment: [38] Assume average local authority service unit cost: [39] £66 per hour of client contact with a clinical psychologist: [40] £21– per hour patient contact with a consultant psychiatrist: [41] Netten and Curtis Local Authority foster care costs per week (53) (individual cases varied according to number of weeks in foster care, emergency removal or standard, social worker time, case conference costs, and court hearing costs: [42] Assume average local authority service unit cost: [43] Assume court hearing for emergency child protection order, Assume Band 2 Grade B summary assessment fees (Oxfordshire Solicitors Court Fees)*2 = £145*2, plus Counsel's fees of 0.5 day hearing on Queen's bench (£655), total = £945.

a societal level whereby all costs to all parties are included, as would be the case if a CBA was being carried out. Home visiting training costs were also included pro-rata in the costs of each woman allocated to the intervention arm. In addition to this, where infants were placed in foster care or for adoption additional resource-use information for such events were individually identified from the relevant home visitor records including type of removal (i.e. emergency or routine), foster care duration, adoption expenses, court cases, child protection resources, legal costs, and social care involvement.

A mean cost estimate per woman per arm of the trial was computed. The cost data distributions for both arms were not normally distributed hence the 95% confidence interval for the difference was therefore obtained using non-parametric bootstrapping methods. The mean costs in the control and intervention arms were: £7,120 vs £3,874,

Table 4.3 Mean cost and quantity differences arising between arms of the trial

Resource	Control	Home visiting	Mean cost difference (SE)	P
Mean no. of clinic visits to a health visitor	14.24	8.82		
Mean cost (£)	£383.48	£237.07	−£146.41 (£56.60)	0.01
Mean no. of phone calls to a health visitor	6.94	10.34		
Mean cost (£)	£25.86	£38.41	£12.55 (£5.27)	0.019
Mean no. of home visitor home visits	10.30	40.63		
Mean cost (£)	£797.54	£3,128.05	£2,330.51 (£136.33)	0.000
Mean no. of social worker office visits	0.5	1.55		
Mean cost (£)	£15.86	£47.72	£31.85 (£26.75)	0.23
Mean no. of midwife hospital visits	2.8	3.9		
Mean cost (£)	£177.58	£245.21	£67.62 (£48.93)	0.16
Mean no. of alcohol/drug counsellor visits	1.2	0.78		
Mean cost (£)	£107.51	£69.88	−£37.63 (£94.64)	0.69
Mean no. of A&E visits (mother)	0.65	0.41		
Mean cost (£)	£43.38	£27.31	−£16.06 (£14.67)	0.27
Mean no. of A&E visits (infant)	0.83	0.43		
Mean cost (£)	£54.87	£28.35	−£26.52 (£16.31)	0.10
Mean no. of Psychologist appointments	0.08	0.98		
Mean cost (£)	£5.73	£65.40	£59.66 (£26.85)	0.028

Mean no. of Psychiatrist appointments	0.50	0.95		0.259
Mean cost (£)	£106.69	£202.70	£96.01 (£84.75)	
Mean no. of visits to an Obstetrician	2.20	1.36		0.49
Mean cost (£)	£184.30	£114.19	−£70.12 (£102.79)	
Mean no. of family centre visits	6.13	7.67		0.63
Mean cost (£)	£166.97	£209.79	£42.81 (£89.08)	
Mean no. of Home Start visits	0.53	1.7		0.25
Mean cost (£)	£41.25	£129.07	£87.82 (£76.40)	
Mean no. of visits to the housing department	6.17	4.75		0.37
Mean cost (£)	£76.34	£58.70	-£17.64 (£19.70)	
Children entering foster care/adoption	0	4		0.15
Mean cost (£)	£0	£776.53	£776.53 (£536.04)	
Home visiting training cost apportionment per woman (£)[1]	(n/a)	(n/a)		0.000
Mean cost (£)	£0.00	£29.63	£29.63 (£1.05)	
Total cost (all resource-use data)[2]	**£3,874**	**£7,120**	**£3,246**	0.000
			95% CI[3]: **£1,645 - £4,803**	

[1] This cost was an apportioned cost to account for the beneficial effect of the home visiting training on all the other women home visited by the home visitors who were not in the trial.

[2] The total cost variable includes all costs and not only those which were statistically significantly different. This allows cost differences to be economically significant although not statistically so.

[3] The 95% confidence interval for the cost difference was obtained using non-parametric bootstrapping to account for the skewed nature of the cost data in each arm of the trial.

a difference of £3,246 (95% confidence interval for the cost difference: £1,645 – £4,803). The total costs of the intervention arm as shown in Table 4.3 are statistically significantly greater due to increased home visits, phone calls to a home visitor, home visitor training costs and appointments with a psychologist. Costs incurred, though not reaching statistical significant include: foster care and adoption costs; social worker office visits; hospital visits to a midwife; appointments with a psychiatrist; visits to family centres; and Home Start visits. However, Table 4.3 also reveals significant cost savings arising due to the home-visiting intervention in the form of reduced costs of *clinic* health-visiting costs. Further cost savings arising in the intervention arm, although not statistically significant arose in the following categories: alcohol and drug counselling costs; obstetric costs; A & E costs for both mother and baby; obstetrician appointment costs; and local authority housing department costs. Although many of the additional costs did not reach formal levels of statistical significance when all resources were combined within a 'total cost' variable, the mean incremental cost in the home visiting arm of £3,246 was statistically significant ($p = 0.000$) with 72% of this incremental cost being due to the extra costs of the home visiting intervention, and 24% due to the costs of the infants being removed from parental care and entering foster care and/or the adoption process (resources involved with infants being removed from parental care involved social workers, police, solicitor, and court costs, foster care and adoption placement costs).

In summary, the main challenges arising with the economic evaluation of home-visiting interventions, as documented by researchers such as Olds (40) and Byrd (57) are firstly that whilst the costs of such services can be easily identified and measured the resulting benefits and cost savings are more complex to identify and measure since they may occur in sectors of government beyond health care including social services, education, crime, and housing. It is clearly the case that there is a need for such interventions to be evaluated using broader frameworks such as CBA. Indeed, 24% of the incremental costs of the home-visiting intervention in this study were due to non-health service costs. Secondly, the benefits and cost savings may accrue over a longer time period than is often accommodated for in trials, and this combined with the multi-sectors affected by this intervention makes for a complex economic evaluation process. Decision modelling methods for CBA studies are recommended to extrapolate the costs and welfare effects beyond the end of the trial where the data provide appropriate hypotheses. For a summary of such decision modelling methods, see the first book in this series of handbooks, Briggs *et al.* (58).

4.7 **Summary**

The aim of this chapter was to outline key applied costing methods for economic evaluation and more specifically to outline those specific costing issues which have particular relevance to CBA studies. It is generally accepted that costing methodology is the same no matter what the economic evaluation technique being used however with new developments in the benefit assessment methodology in CBA such as Stated Preference Discrete Choice Experiments (SPDCE) there are a number of considerations when costing specifically for a CBA study. These considerations relate to the appropriate identification and measurement of costs specific to the timescale and context within which benefits are elicited. It is also important to align the cost units with the benefit data and matters such as divisibility of costs and their appropriate opportunity cost should also be considered accordingly. In addition to this the use of decision models to extrapolate costs and welfare effects beyond the end of a trial period, taking into account issues of preference timescale, etc. would be a useful development to the CBA approach.

References

1. Donaldson, C., Hundley, V., and McIntosh, E. 1996. Using economics alongside clinical trials: why we cannot choose the evaluation technique in advance. *Health Economics* **5**: 267–269.

2. Glick, H., Doshi, J.A., Sonnad, S.S., and Polsky, D. 2007. *Economic evaluation in clinical trials*. Oxford: Oxford University Press.

3. Gold, M.R., Siegel, J.E., Russell, L.B., and Weinstein, M.C. 1996. *Cost-effectiveness in health and medicine*. New York: Oxford University Press.

4. Johnson, K., Buxton, M.J., Jones, D.R., and Fitzpatrick, R. 1999. Assessing the costs of healthcare technologies in clinical trials. *Health Technology Assessment* **3**(6): 1–76.

5. Drummond, M.F., Sculpher, M.J., Torrance, G.W., O'Brien, B., Stoddart, G.L. 2005. *Methods for the economic evaluation of health care programmes*. 3rd ed. Oxford: Oxford University Press.

6. National Institute for Health and Clinical Excellence (NICE) 2009. *Guide to the methods of technology appraisal*. London: NICE.

7. Sugden, R. and Williams, A. 1978. *The principles of practical cost-benefit analysis*. New York: Oxford University Press.

8. Basu, A., Paltiel, D., and Pollack, H.A. 2008. Social costs of robbery and the cost-effectiveness of substance abuse treatment. *Health Economics* **17**: 927–946.

9. Wordsworth, S., Ludbrook, A., Caskey, F., and Macleod, A. 2005. Collecting unit cost data in multicentre studies: creating comparable methods. *European Journal of Health Economics* **50**: 38–44.

10. Evans, C. and Crawford, B. 1999. Patient self-reports in pharmacoeconomic studies. their use and impact on study validity. *Pharmacoeconomics* **15**(3): 241–256.

11. Petrou, S., Murray, L., Cooper, P., and Davidson, L. 2002. The accuracy of self reported healthcare resource utilisation in health economic studies. *International Journal of Technology Assessment in Health Care* **18**(3): 705–740.

12. van den Berg, B. and Spauwen, P. 2006. Measurement of informal care: an empirical study into the valid measurement of time spent on informal caregiving. *Health Economics* **15**: 447–460.

13. Chapko, M.K., Liu, C.F., Perkins, M., Li, Y.F., Fortney, J.C., and Maciejewski, M.L. 2009. Equivalence of two healthcare costing methods: bottom-up and top-down. *Health Economics* **18**(10): 1188–1201.

14. Baker, J.J. 1995. Activity-based costing for integrated delivery systems. *Journal of Health Care Finance* **22**(2): 57–61.

15. Carey, K. and Burgess, J.F. 2000. Hospital costing: experience from the VHA. *Financial Accountability and Management* **16**(4): 289–308.

16. Kaplan, R.S. 1988. One cost system isn't enough. *Harvard Business Review* **66**(1): 143–160.

17. Knapp, M. and Beecham, J. 1993. Reduced list costings: Examination of an informed short cut in mental health research. *Health Economics* **2**: 313–322.

18. Graves, N., Walker, D., Raine, R., Hutchings, A., and Roberts, J.A. 2002. Cost data for individual patients included in clinical studies: no amount of statistical analysis can compensate for inadequate costing methods. *Health Economics* **11**: 735–739.

19. www.dh.gov.uk. New NHS 2004 reference costs. http://www.dh.gov.uk . 2004.

20. Department of Health. 2008. NHS Costing Manual 2007/2008.

21. Curtis, L. 2008. *Unit costs of health and social care*. Canterbury: University of Kent at Canterbury.

22. James, M. and Stokes, E. 2006. *Harnessing information for health economics analysis*. Oxford: Radcliffe Publishing.

23. Neuhauser, D. and Lewicki, A.M. 1975. What do we gain from the sixth stool guaiac? *New England Journal of Medicine* **293**: 226–228.

24. Clement, F.M., Ghali, W.A., Donaldson, C., and Manns, B.J. 2009. The impact of using different costing emthods on the results of an economic evaluatin of cardiac care: microcosting vs gross-costing approaches. *Health Economics* **18**(4): 377–388.

25. Drummond, M.F., Sculpher, M.J., Torrance, G.W., O'Brien, B., and Stoddart, G.L. 2005. *Methods for the economic evaluation of health care programmes*. 3rd ed. Oxford: Oxford University Press.

26. HM Treasury. 2004. *The green book: appraisal and evaluation in central government*. 2nd ed. London: HMSO.

27. Smith, D. and Gravelle, H. 2000. *The practice of discounting economic evaluation of health care interventions*. York: CHE, University of York. Report No.: 19.

28. Van der Pol, M. and Cairns, J. 2000. Negative and zero time preferences for health. *Health Economics* **9**(2): 171–175.

29. Cairns, J. 1992. Discounting and health benefits: another perspective. *Health Economics* **1**(1): 76–79.

30. Briggs, A.H. 2001. Handling uncertainty in economic evaluation and presenting the results. In: Drummond, M.F., and McGuire, A., editors. *Economic evaluation in health care: merging theory with practice*.Oxford: Oxford University Press, pp. 172–214.

31. Tan, S.S., Redekop, W.K., and Rutten, F. 2008. Costs and prices of single dental fillings in Europe: A micro costing study. *Health Economics* **17**: S84–S93.

32. Herrero, C. and Moreno-Ternero, J.D. 2009. Estimating production costs in the economic evaluation of health care programs. *Health Economics* **18**: 21–35.

33. Brouwer, W., Rutten, F., and Koopmanschap, M.A. 2001. Costing in economic evaluations. In: Drummond, M.F. and McGuire, A., editors. *Economic evalaution in health care: merging theory with practice*. Oxford: Oxford University Press, pp. 68–93.

34. Rice, D.P. and Cooper, B.S. 1967. The economic value of human life. *American Journal of Public Health* **57**: 1954–1966.

35. Koopmanschap, M.A., Rutten, F., van Ineveld, B.M., and van Roijen, L. 1997. The friction cost method for measuring indirect costs of disease. *Journal of Health Economics* **6**: 253–259.

36. Johannesson, M. and Karlsson, G. 1997. The friction cost method: a comment. *Journal of Health Economics* **6**: 249–255.

37. Liljas, B. 1998. How to calculate indirect costs in economic evaluations. *Pharmacoeconomics* **13**(1 part 1): 1–7.

38. Pritchard, C. and Sculpher, M. 2000. *Productivity costs: principles and practice in economic evaluation*. London: Office of Health Economics.

39. Roemer, J.E. 1998. *Equality of opportunity*. Cambridge, MA: Harvard University Press.

40. Olds, D.L., Eckenrode, J., Henderson, C.R., Kitzman, H., Powers, J., Cole, R., *et al.* 1997. Long term effects of home visitation on maternal life course and child abuse and neglect: Fifteen-year follow up of a randomized trial. *Journal of the American Medical Association* **278**(8): 637–643.

41. Brown, K. 2004. *Evaluation of family home visiting program*. 2nd ed. Australia: Government of South Australia.

42. Bull, J., McCormick, G., Swann, C., and Mulvihill, C. 2004. *Ante and post-natal home-visiting programmes: a review of reviews*. London: HDA.

43. Brooten, D., Kumar, S., Brown, L.P., Butts, P., Finkler, S.A., Bakewell-Sachs, S.A., *et al.* 1986. Randomized clinical trial of early hospital discharge and home follow up of very low birth weight infants. *New England Journal of Medicine* **315**: 934–939.

44. Hardy, J.B. and Streett, R.R. 1989. Family support and parenting education in the home: an effective extension of clinic-based preventive health care services for poor children. *Journal of Pediatrics* **115**: 927–931.

45. Olds, D.L. and Henderson, CRPCKH. 1993. Effect of pre-natal and infancy nurse home visitation on government spending. *Medical Care* **31**(2): 155–174.

46. Archbold, P.G., Steward, B.J., Miller, L.L., Harvath, T.A., Greenlick, M.R., Van Buren, L., *et al.* 1995. The PREP system of nursing interventions: a pilot test with families caring for older members. *Research in Nursing and Health* **18**: 3–16.

47. Miller, L.L., Hornbrook, M.C., Archbold, P.G., and Stewart, B.J. 1996. Development of use and cost measures in a nursing intervention for family caregivers and frail elderly patients. *Research in Nursing and Health* **19**: 273–285.

48. Brown, J. 1992. Screening infants for hearing loss. *Journal of Epidemiology and Community Health* **46**: 350–356.

49. Yanover, M.J., Jones, D., and Miller, M.D. 1976. Perinatal care of low risk mothers and infants: early discharge with home care. *New England Journal of Medicine* **294**: 702–705.

50. Morrell, C.J., Siby, H., Stewart, P., Walters, S., and Morgan, A. 2000. Costs and effectiveness of community postnatal support workers: randomised controlled trial. *British Medical Journal* **321**: 593–598.

51. Barlow, J., Stewart-Brown, S., Callaghan, H., Tucker, J., Brocklehurst, N., Davis, H., *et al.* 2003. Working in partnership: The development of a home visiting service for vulnerable families. *Child Abuse Review* **12**: 172–189.

52. McIntosh, E., Barlow, J., Davies, H., and Stewart-Brown, S. 2009. Economic evaluation of an intensive home visiting programme for vulnerable families: a cost-effectiveness analysis of a public health intervention. *Journal of Public Health* **31**: 423–433.

53. Netten, A. and Curtis, L. 2003. *Unit costs of health and social care*. Canterbury: Personal Social Services Research Unit, University of Kent at Canterbury.

54. Netten, A. and Curtis, L. 2004. *Unit costs of health and social care*. Canterbury: Personal Social Services Research Unit, University of Kent at Canterbury.

55. New NHS 2004 reference costs. http://www.dh.gov.uk; 2004.

56. HM Treasury. 2003. *The green book*. London: The Stationery Office, HMSO.

57. Byrd, M.E. 1997. A typology of the potential outcomes of maternal child home visits: A literature analysis. *Public Health Nursing* **14**(1): 3–11.

58. Briggs, A.H., Sculpher, M.J., and Claxton, K. 2007. *Decision modelling for health economic evaluation*. Oxford: Oxford University Press.

Chapter 5

Valuation and cost–benefit analysis in health and environmental economics

F. Reed Johnson and W.L. (Vic) Adamowicz

5.1 Introduction

Environmental economists pioneered non-market valuation methods in the 1970s and 1980s. Health economists began adapting these methods to health valuation about a decade later. Unlike environmental economics, instances where such estimates actually have been used in a CBA to inform health care policy or other decisions are relatively rare. Torrance (1) observes in a recent article the curious fact that health economics, particularly health-economic evaluation, is 'the only application of economics that does not use the discipline of economics'. Torrance notes that if it did, health economists would be experts in CBA, and routinely employ monetary values to evaluate improved health. In fact, many health economists have little or no training in economics, at least not in welfare economics, which provides the conceptual basis for CBA.

Gold's widely cited book on cost-effectiveness analysis (CEA) in health notes two reasons why CEA, the preferred approach in health economics, is superior to CBA: 1. CBA presumes to put a dollar figure on the value of human life and uses controversial methods to do so and 2. monetizing the price of life introduces ethical concerns that are avoided by CEA (2). An environmentalist similarly asked how we can place a value on environmental quality. 'Its value is inestimable. We must value it beyond whatever price we put on it, by respecting it, by taking good care of it'. (3)

The Gold CEA guidelines for health technology assessment have won official acceptance in many countries, while the intellectual and institutional orthodoxy in environmental economics has favoured CBA despite similar ideological objections to monetizing environmental and health values. The differences in accepted practice between health economics and environmental economics have their origins in quite different intellectual, regulatory, and institutional circumstances. These circumstances have made it possible for many non-economists to practise health economics, but virtually impossible for non-economists to practise environmental economics.

One of the key differences between non-market valuation in environmental cases and health cases is that the former tend to examine public goods while the latter tend to examine private goods that often are publicly provided, such as preferences for medical treatments, testing, and screening programmes, health-care delivery systems, and health insurance. Development of methods for valuing public goods was strongly influenced by several historical developments in environmental economics for which there are no corresponding events in health economics. In 1974, Karl-Göran Mäler published a systematic welfare-theoretic basis for early empirical valuation studies, beginning with Robert Davis' original contingent-valuation study of the Maine Woods 10 years earlier in 1963. In 1981, Ronald Reagan issued Executive Order 12291, which has been re-issued by all subsequent U.S. presidents, requiring federal agencies to conduct CBA for all significant government regulations (currently Executive order 12866, as amended) (71). The order requires monetization of non-market environmental values in assessing the impact of major environmental, transportation, food safety, and workplace regulations. This mandate made significant resources available to the U.S. Environmental Protection Agency for funding environmental-valuation methods research in the 1980s. Mitchell and Carson published their definitive book on empirical methods in 1989 (72).

Natural resource damage assessment (NRDA) provided a separate impetus for methods development in non-market valuation. In 1989, the Exxon Valdez oil tanker spilled 11 million gallons of crude oil in Prince William Sound, Alaska. The subsequent Oil Pollution Act of 1990 and the high stakes involved in subsequent litigation on the Alaska oil spill and other oil and chemical-contamination cases made considerable resources available to researchers and significant methodological advances were achieved in these studies. The resources devoted to high-profile contingent-valuation cases on environmental issues resulted in distinguished economists, statisticians, and survey researchers applying their skills to valuation methods, including survey design (4;5), valuation theory, econometric analysis (6, 69), experimental economics and strategic behaviour (7;8). NRDA cases have set the bar quite high for acceptable practices involving survey design, information provision, treatment of strategic behaviour, and econometric analysis in contingent valuation applied to environmental issues. Federal rules for conducting such studies were issued in 1994.

In the health context, there has been no corresponding impetus to obtain high-quality monetary health values, either as the result of government regulatory mandates or litigation. The lack of such research incentives and resources probably has slowed the convergence of methodological standards in the two fields. In contrast to environmental economics, health assessments often are conducted by clinicians with little economic training, decision makers attach low weight to 'uninformed' patient preferences, and resource-allocation decisions are dominated by equity concerns(9). As a consequence, environmental and other non-health applications of CBA methods often are rather more sophisticated than health applications.

5.2 Similarities between health and environmental contexts

While there are important differences in the institutional and regulatory contexts in which health economics and environmental economics are practised, these two areas of applied economics share important similarities in the kinds of problems they analyse and methods available for such analysis. We will discuss similarities between health and environmental contexts and the implications for CBA with regard to the 'publicness' of health and environmental services, resource scarcity, altruism, uncertainty, and benefit latency.

5.2.1 Public goods and public provision of private goods in health and the environment

Environmental goods and services generally have public-goods characteristics. Benefits of wilderness or protected areas can be viewed as non-rival and non-excludable in a fashion that is very close to the textbook definition of public goods (see Chapter 3, Section 3.3.6). Improvements in air or water quality have some public-goods characteristics in that publicly provided air and water quality can be non-rival and non-excludable to a certain degree. Outdoor recreation services, while privatized to a certain extent in some parts of the world, most often retain some public-good components, subject to congestion, crowding, or other aspects that move recreation services along the continuum away from pure public goods. The public-good nature of environmental goods and services leads to the call for government intervention in their provision and maintenance, and leads to processes like CBA for the evaluation of projects and NRDA to address impacts that reduce the quality of these goods and services.

Similarly, provision of some health care services can be viewed as having public-good characteristics. The ability to benefit from the existence of a health care system or public health programmes may be to a degree non-rival and non-excludable. For example, vaccination programmes that provide herd immunity provide benefits that are not excludable and not rival. Individual treatments within a health care system, however, can be excludable and rival, much like the recreation case in environmental economics.

An important concern in CBA is determining who provides the services (public or private sector). While there are few true public goods, there are many goods and services for which technology, custom, or preferences lead to collective provision through governments rather than the market. The failure of market processes to allocate scarce resources requires economic analysis to guide resource-allocation decisions (see Chapter 3, Box 3.2 for causes of market distortions). In these cases, economic valuation examines preferences for different combinations of public production, including choices between and within alternative categories of public expenditure such as health, environment, and education. It is these goods that Carson and Hanemann (10) refer to when they state:

> Nowhere has this need been more pressing than with public goods, where the major impediment to performing a benefit–cost analysis[1] in many fields of applied economics is the lack of monetary values for the outputs of government policies.

(p. 829)

---

[1] The term 'benefit–cost' analysis is more common in environmental economics, while 'cost–benefit' analysis is conventionally used in health economics.

In both health care and environmental or natural-resource cases there are opportunities for both private provision of services, such as private health insurance or well water, and public provision of similar services, such as publicly financed health systems or municipal water systems. Public provision may be chosen in such instances because of equity or altruistic judgements. Quantifying the value of the services themselves apart from the equity or altruistic values of public provision poses conceptual and methodological challenges for CBA. Total value can include both the willingness to pay (WTP) for a non-market public or publicly provided private good itself and the willingness to contribute to the government provision of a good or service for reasons unrelated to its direct, intrinsic value. Economists' interest in separating these different sources of value may explain much of the resistance to CBA in health economics, where equity concerns often dominate efficiency concerns.

Choice of valuation methods can depend on the degree of 'publicness' of the health or environmental service and what type of values are of interest. A case in point is valuing health effects from water-quality improvements. One could identify values associated with water-borne risk reductions in a purely private context by assessing expenditures on water filters, bottled water, and other private purchases. One also could assess the value individuals have for improving public provision of water treatment by their willingness to vote for higher taxes to finance water programmes. Individuals may have a positive value for improved public water-quality programmes because their private costs of protection may decrease if public protection increases. They also may have a value for improved public programmes because they believe everyone has a right to better-quality water. The private-expenditure or averting-behaviour approach excludes these altruistic values, while the voting or referendum approach may combine both personal and altruistic values.

One aspect of environmental valuation that differs from typical health analysis is that environmental valuation has tended to focus on WTP for avoiding a negative externality. In contrast, much of health valuation has focused on the value of the public or insured provision of services or programmes rather than correcting a market failure. Analysis of health and environmental problems overlap in the case of health externalities of environmental quality, such as the effects of air-pollution exposures on respiratory illness (11) and the effects of water-pollution exposures on gastro-intestinal illness (12).

5.2.2 Competition for scarce resources

The ultimate role of CBA is to aid in allocating scarce resources. In health and environment cases, where governments play a role in provision, CBA provides information on the 'how much is enough' question. That is, there are scarce government resources for the provision of health or environmental services and decisions have to be made regarding the extent to which these services will be provided. Of course there are equity and efficiency dimensions of these decisions, and CBA and valuation can help provide information to inform judgements involving both dimensions.

In environmental valuation, funding for environmental services, recreation attributes, and other aspects of environmental quality often are in competition with other demands on public funds. Increased environmental quality requirements through regulation result in a different type of tradeoff – impacts on economic activity. Similarly, provision of enhanced health services competes with other demands for public resources.

The implications for CBA and valuation vary depending on the context. In the case of regulatory assessment, the onus is on the benefit–cost analyst to identify the benefits of the improvements and to trace out the benefits function so that marginal benefits can be compared to marginal costs. Such an approach is illustrated by the assessment of the benefits of the Clean Air Act Amendments in the U.S. In this case, the regulatory amendments were evaluated in terms of whether the benefits realized through the regulations exceeded the costs (retrospectively and prospectively). The benefits assessment was conducted using measures of the value of statistical life, and various other non-market value estimates (values of recreation impacts, visibility impacts, etc.). Such regulatory assessment is relatively common in the U.S. and typically employs estimates of value, rather than cost-effectiveness measures. Given the general methodological consensus in environmental economics, it is puzzling that resource assessments in health rarely use valuation metrics and rely instead on cost-effectiveness measures. The lack of requirements for more rigorous efficiency analysis of health investments implies that health investments do not compete with scarce public and private resources in the same way as investments in environmental quality.

5.2.3 **The role of altruism**

As mentioned above, CBA in either health or environmental cases often involves goods and services whose value is influenced by altruism. This is a very important concern in CBA. If altruistic preferences are paternalistic, then they should be included in the CBA whereas if the preferences are non-paternalistic, including them will result in double counting (13;14).

Altruism has received relatively little attention in either environment or health areas. This is most likely due to the challenges of assessing motives that underlie values. It seems clear that altruism forms a component of existence values for environmental resources such as endangered species. Individuals often respond that one of their reasons for investing in programmes is so that future generations can benefit from these resources. Similarly, there is some evidence that individuals are willing to pay for public-health programmes because of their preferences over others' well-being. The provision of services (drinking water, public health, etc.) often is motivated by altruistic preferences. What is less clear is whether these are paternalistic or non-paternalistic and how large these altruistic values are relative to private values. This is certainly an area for future research as the implications for CBA could be significant.

A related issue is interdependence in preferences and the effect on value estimates. In most areas of empirical economics, interdependence has been ignored because of the complexity in identifying interdependence in econometric models (70). There have been some attempts to incorporate interdependence in environmental valuation (15) and in health contexts (16). The results in this literature often show that treating households as single utility-maximizing units oversimplifies the decision-making behaviour and could result in incorrect policy prescriptions. This may be particularly important in health care decisions involving treatments for children.

5.2.4 **Uncertainty**

In both health and environmental cost–benefit analyses, there is a significant amount of uncertainty in both the cost and benefit estimates. Often this is due to uncertainty in the underlying biological processes, but a great deal of uncertainty also arises in the assessment of preferences and tradeoffs. This has been represented in empirical work by presenting statistical confidence intervals around welfare measures, but the problem is deeper than this. Stated-preference valuation exercises often are presented as if the outcome of the choices is known with certainty, or at least by a well-defined probability distribution, while it seldom is this certain in reality. Respondents' attempts to factor in their perception of the uncertainty may influence value estimates in unobserved ways. In valuations involving health risks, researchers devote considerable effort to help respondents understand the nature of the risk and the possible outcomes of health interventions. Several issues continue to challenge researchers, including respondents' abilities to manipulate probabilities and developing effective presentation mechanisms to 'teach' probability concepts (17). Researchers must cope with the challenge of overcoming widespread innumeracy without over-conditioning respondents so they no longer are representative of the population of interest. Incorporating uncertainty into valuation and CBA in a more rigorous fashion is an area for future research in both health and environmental economics, see Chapter 12.

5.2.5 **Benefit latency**

A final area of similarity between health and environmental cases is that there often is a time lag between the programme and the realization of the benefits or costs. Environmental improvement programmes may take years to generate the benefits of programmes to improve water and air quality. Similarly, preventative efforts in health care or public-health interventions take time to achieve the desired results. Given that there often is a significant time difference between programme implementation and the benefits that the programme promises, it is important to investigate the effect of benefit latency on measured environmental or health values. There have been some recent efforts to incorporate latency directly into benefit assessments. Analogously to Gafni et al.'s (18) healthy-year equivalent generalization of QALYs, Cameron and DeShazo (19) develop the concept of the Value of Statistical Illness Profiles (VSIP) that incorporates latency and duration of illness into the valuation context. Their results show that cases with different degrees of latency will produce significantly different values and that these responses to latency are dependent on demographic factors.

5.3 **Application of environmental economics practices to health economics**

Contingent valuation applications in environmental and resource economics have been traced back to the early 1960s, with some attributing Ciriacy-Wantrup's text in 1947 (19a) as the origin of the approach. Significant numbers of papers appeared in the economics literature in the 1980s with rapid growth in the 1990s (see (20)). In contrast, health economics applications appear to have begun in the 1980s, growing in the 1990s but with considerably fewer studies than in the environmental and resource economics area (21).

It is difficult to construct a rigorous comparison of applications of contingent valuation over time in the two fields. The following are generalizations that arise from following the literature in the fields over the past decades. Practice in environmental economics was heavily influenced by the Exxon Valdez case and the NOAA panel report. While for some researchers NRDA simply induced methodological standards such as closed-ended techniques, scope tests, and advanced statistical modelling, for those involved in actual natural resource damage litigation support NRDA, involved significant increases in investments time and effort in survey design, data collection, and econometric analysis. The NRDA context resulted in a high standard of practice including effort in focus groups, pre-testing, and other investments in data quality. It also meant that economists teamed up with survey research experts to benefit from cross-disciplinary expertise. The theoretical basis underlying valuation was enhanced by Hanemann's work on random utility representations (e.g. (22)), and other contributions that built on his framework (for example, (23)). Econometric analysis also increased in rigor especially in the area of analysis of discrete-choice responses. Techniques for testing for scope, mitigating strategic behaviour, and other contingent-valuation design features were mostly developed in environmental applications.

Applications in health economics, while sometimes citing the NOAA panel recommendations and advanced statistical methods, have taken longer to adopt methodological advances arising from environmental applications. For example, Diener *et al.* (21) report that between 1990 and 1996 approximately 30% of the health valuation studies they examined used open-ended and payment-card elicitation formats and 35% used bidding games, while the discrete-choice approach, preferred in environmental applications since the late 1980s, appeared in 36% of the studies. Open-ended and payment-card elicitation formats continue to appear in published health-economics studies (for example, (24)).

Another illustration of the time lag in transferring valuation techniques between environmental and health applications is the analysis of discrete-choice versus payment-card methods. A study conducted by Ryan *et al.* (25) is an application to health cases that is parallel to studies published in the mid-1990s in environmental economics (26;27); Watson and Ryan's (28) analysis of double-bounded contingent valuation parallels DeShazo's (29) work and other similar efforts. Health researchers argue that health outcomes are much different than those studied in environmental economics and thus replications of studies published a decade or more earlier in the environmental area are necessary. However, these replications rarely produce results different from the original environmental studies.

A careful evaluation of the health-economics research agenda might ask whether well-established validity and reliability results in environmental economics are a result of the specific type of good being valued or the basic cognitive processes respondents employ in answering valuation questions in general. The consensus in environmental economics may favour the latter interpretation, since it is difficult to publish a replication of a standard methodological result simply because it is applied to a different kind of environmental or natural-resource commodity. Shifting the research focus from replicating results in environmental economics to understanding how subjects in non-market valuation studies answer discrete-choice questions and developing better statistical techniques for analysing such data would make the health-economics research agenda more consistent with that of environmental economics.

5.4 Opportunities for additional 'hybridization'

5.4.1 Risk valuation

Environmental-health studies have blurred the distinction between the two kinds of applications. For example, there is a great deal of literature on estimating the value of a statistical life (VSL) for use in environmental-policy and food-safety regulatory analysis. Contingent valuation in this area has rigorously applied survey and analysis methods employed in environmental valuation (e.g. 30) to cases of health-risk reductions. However, health economists have only rarely expressed an interest in such estimates (24;31). Extending the scope and application of VSL estimates is a potential opportunity for methodological cross-fertilization.

Figure 5.1 depicts an indifference curve where the horizontal axis is the probability of surviving the current period, and the vertical axis is the wealth available for spending on other things. Under conventional assumptions, it has the shape shown in the figure. VSL simply is the rate of substitution between wealth and some small change in mortality risk. Thus, Δw is the WTP for the associated Δp which keeps the individual on the same indifference curve.

$$VSL = \frac{WTP(\Delta p)}{\Delta p}.$$

So, for example, if the mean WTP is $7,000 for a 0.001 decrease in mortality risk, then VSL equals $7 million, which is the value the U.S. Environmental Protection Agency currently uses for regulatory CBAs.

While it is convenient to assume a constant VSL, the marginal rate of substitution between wealth and risk varies, depending on where it is measured on the indifference

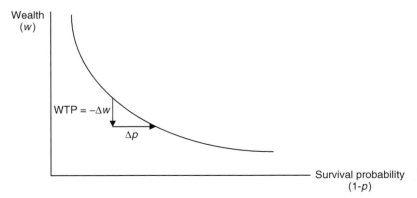

Fig. 5.1 Indifference curve between wealth and survival.

curve in Figure 5.1. At higher wealth levels and lower risk levels, theory predicts that WTP is large for a given change in risk, while at lower wealth levels and higher risk levels, WTP is small for the same change in risk. The shape of indifference curves also will vary among individuals depending on their risk tolerance relative to consumption. The question of how VSL varies systematically with age or not is an important policy question, but the empirical evidence is mixed.

Although widely misunderstood to mean the value of a human life, VSL is a useful concept when applied appropriately. It actually is an aggregate measure of WTP to reduce mortality risks in a given population. If mean WTP is V to reduce risk by $1/N$ in a population of size N, then VSL is the total $WTP = N \cdot \$V$. Some health economists have borrowed VSL estimates from the environmental-economics literature to suggest possible WTP per QALY thresholds, while others have criticized this practice (24;32;33). To convert VSL to an annual value comparable to a QALY, they divide VSL estimates by the average life expectancy to obtain the value of a statistical life-year (VSLY). For example, if VSL is about $5 million and life expectancy is 40 years, then VSLY = $1.25 million, more than twice the threshold commonly used in CEA.

Dividing VSL by life expectancy (or discounted life expectancy) is difficult to justify on either theoretical or empirical grounds, if the appropriate valuation concept is what people would pay to reduce their own risk of dying. There is no empirical evidence to suggest that the VSLY is constant, or that the VSL declines in proportion to remaining life expectancy, which the constant VSLY implies. Finally, QALYs as conventionally measured may not be conceptually compatible with the utility-theoretic and welfare-theoretic rational behind WTP measures (33).

VSL estimates can be obtained from two kinds of data: labour-market wage differentials and stated preferences. Labour-market or hedonic-wage studies estimate compensating wage differentials in risky occupations or industries as a function of risk levels. In principle, workers will require higher wages to compensate them for work-related risks. Stated-preference studies employ contingent-valuation or discrete-choice experiments to directly elicit hypothetical risk-money tradeoffs to estimate marginal rates of substitution to estimate VSL.

Hedonic wage studies resolve various conceptual and empirical problems in different ways (see 34). VSL estimates thus vary, depending on how each problem is solved.

- Hedonic wage studies require that we assume that labour markets function efficiently and that workers have accurate information on risk exposures.

- The required data to estimate a hedonic wage equation are mortality risk rates, worker pay, and worker characteristics. Inconsistencies among different data sources on workplace fatalities, compensation, and covariates often have to be harmonized before merging the data.

- Compensation presumably accounts for both fatal and nonfatal risks. These risks generally are highly correlated and various researchers deal with this problem in different ways.

- As is the case with all regression models, results often are sensitive to researcher judgements on model specification, such as whether the model includes a quadratic term in risk or interactions between risk and other variables.

There are several concerns about using VSL estimates based on hedonic-wage studies to evaluate health benefits of environmental policies. First, the population for which WTP is estimated generally is younger and healthier and their risk exposures are higher than the policy-relevant population. For example, the primary populations of interest for air-pollution exposures are older people in frail health or people with respiratory conditions. Even for these vulnerable groups, mortality risks from air-pollution, controlling for other risk factors, are lower than risk exposures in many occupations. In addition, there is considerable evidence that people care as much or more about characteristics of risks other than probability (35). It is unlikely that people would evaluate death from a workplace accident the same as a heart attack from breathing fine-particulate air pollution or cancer from drinking pesticide-contaminated groundwater, even if the probabilities were identical. Thus, applying wage-hedonic VSL estimates requires extrapolating outside the range of the data in several respects.

Stated-preference (SP) studies are not subject to the same restrictive assumptions as revealed-preference hedonic-wage studies. However, direct value-elicitation methods such as contingent valuation and discrete-choice experiments simply have a different set of limitations. The most important of these is that respondents evaluate hypothetical scenarios. Because the hypothetical context does not involve real tradeoffs between money and risk, many economists are skeptical of the validity of the resulting WTP and VSL estimates. Stated-preference studies have been subjected to 25 years of validity testing in environmental economics (e.g. (69)). This literature has identified various sources of vulnerability in designing SP survey instruments, administering surveys, and analysing the resulting data. While many of these problems have been resolved to some degree, many economists have persistent concerns about the usefulness of SP studies.

5.4.2 Design and evaluation of public-health programmes

While environmental and health valuation studies generally deal with different kinds of commodities or services, public-health programmes also offer opportunities for hybridization. To a certain degree such analysis is ongoing. Recent papers on the 'health of nations' use measures of values of statistical life or statistical life years to assess the investment in medical research and practice and find the return on these investments to be substantial (36; 73). Analysis of the impact of regulatory changes in health areas could be conducted in the same fashion as analysis of regulatory changes for environmental quality. The economic analysis of the benefits and costs of the US Clean Air Act Amendments, for example, provides a case in point. This CBA examined the prospective and retrospective benefits and costs of the changed regulation – to assess whether they were in the public interest.

While economic evaluations of public-health programmes are common (for example, (37)), these studies generally employ cost-effectiveness approaches rather than CBA. Furthermore, challenges to valid valuation estimates that have been investigated in the environmental-economics literature also are relevant to public health programmes. For example, our previous discussion of altruistic motives is as important for valuations of public-health programmes as it is to pollution-control programmes. Adequately treating risk type or context should be important considerations in public-health programme analysis. If mortality-risk values vary within an affected population because of the effect of demographic differences or kind of mortality risk, for example, then the values associated with public-health interventions will have to be adjusted according to the context and should not rely on naïve, direct benefit transfers alone. 'Illness profiles' that include discounting considerations, illness type, and latency (38) also affect the value of the intervention. Value differences based on the affected group will also affect the outcome. Impacts on children, for example, appear to be valued quite differently than impacts on adults (39;40). There is also considerable debate about values as a function of the age of the individual affected (30;41). While these are politically charged issues, improved understanding of them would help in evaluating public-health programme investments.

Examples of contingent valuation studies of public-health programmes that are strongly influenced by environmental-valuation methods include Phillips *et al.* (42), Marshall *et al.* (43), and Johnson *et al.* (44). Phillips *et al.* (42) used a choice-format stated-preference survey or discrete-choice experiment to estimate WTP for HIV testing programmes for a sample of at-risk subjects in public clinics in San Francisco. Marshall *et al.* (43) and Johnson *et al.* (44) used similar methods to estimate WTP for alternative colorectal cancer screening programmes and to determine whether the willingness to pay of subjects at high risk for diabetes was great enough to offset the costs of a public-health intervention designed to reduce the risk.

Hybridization of the literatures in this case could include more systematic assessment of the elements of public-health programmes in a public-goods context that environmental researchers are more familiar with. In addition, blending of the literatures on valuing risk reductions, use of risk communication tools, and econometric assessment of risk contexts and demographic factors affecting values of risk reductions will help improve the quality of research in this area.

5.4.3 Calibration and triangulation

In environmental economics, there has been a significant amount of calibration and triangulation of benefit estimates. Comparisons of stated-preference (SP) and revealed-preference (RP) analysis, or combined RP – SP analyses have been conducted to assess the extent to which assessment methods provide the same value and/or preference functions. Homegrown value experiments using experimental auctions or similar mechanisms (45;46) have been used extensively to examine strategic behaviour or hypothetical bias. There has been some exploration of these methods in health valuation (for example, Mark and Swait's (47) RP/SP study; Blumenschein *et al.*'s (48) experiments to address hypothetical bias), but there are relatively few studies of this nature. The limited use of RP/SP triangulation and/or data fusion in health valuation is somewhat surprising because several of the applications in health are private programmes for which there are market products or products with similar attributes.

Many CBAs for assessing the impacts of environmental regulations employ value information obtained in other studies to provide estimates of the economic benefits of the programmes. Environmental economists have undertaken extensive formal analysis of the validity of such 'benefits-transfer' techniques (49;50), but we are unaware of any such studies in health economics. This literature has evolved from relatively simple comparisons of value to structural models of benefit transfer (16). Benefit transfers are particularly difficult in environmental applications because of the diversity of environmental conditions associated with use values such as recreation and because of the uniqueness of passive-use values for natural environments or species.

In health, a commonly applied analogue to benefits transfer is QALYs. Experience from environmental economics suggests that simple transfers of such value equivalents often have dubious validity. Therefore, the notion of transferring 'generic' health values deserves careful scrutiny. Hybridization in the area of benefits transfer would require moving away from such generic notions of transfer values and defining the limits for using existing prior estimates as an acceptable source of value information.

5.4.4 Econometric analysis

A component of the history of environmental valuation is that training in the area typically included analysis of both SP and RP data using random-utility models and hedonic-price methods. This more general approach to valuation has meant that environmental economics has benefited from hybridization across valuation methods, including transfer of econometric methods across economic sub-disciplines. Combining RP and SP data, for example, requires relatively advanced econometric methods that involve an understanding of both travel-cost models and contingent valuation (51) or choice experiments (52). The high-profile nature of NRDA cases also has brought non-environmental econometric specialists to the problem of environmental valuation and elevated the application of econometric methods (for example, Train (6) and the incorporation of heterogeneity into random-utility analysis). There also has been the transfer of methods from marketing research to environmental economics and to analysing RP and SP data (53).

There appear to be similar opportunities for hybridization of econometric approaches between environmental and health fields. The use of discrete-continuous models or Kuhn–Tucker models (54) as applied in environmental valuation likely have considerable applicability to cases in health, especially for analysing treatment demand. Bayesian econometric methods as applied in marketing research (55) and environmental economics (e.g. 56) provide tools for analysing discrete-choice data that include interdependence and scale or variance effects – two complications that are equally challenging in health and environmental applications. One specific area of potential hybridization is the investigation of non-compensatory responses – a challenge facing analysis of preference data in many fields, including transportation (57) and marketing research (58). In all of these cases, methods applied to specific fields could provide significant benefits if transferred to applications in other areas.

5.4.5 Experimental design in stated-preference studies

One of the most active areas of hybridization among health economics, environmental economics, and market research is techniques for the experimental designs required for SPDCE studies (see Chapters 10 and 11). In a SPDCE study, respondents evaluate a series of tasks in which they are asked to choose among hypothetical alternatives.

The term 'experimental design' refers to the combinations of treatment attributes that appear in each set of treatment profiles that define the preference-elicitation tasks. Experimental design is crucial for obtaining valid estimates of choice parameters of interest to the researcher (59–61). The combination of attribute levels in each treatment profile, as well as the pairings of different profiles in each tradeoff task, is key to obtaining valid estimates of the relative importance of all attribute levels.

A flawed experimental design can affect the accuracy of preference estimates and lead to incorrect interpretations of the data (62). Statistically efficient designs satisfy conditions of level balance and orthogonality that minimize D-error or the 'average variance' of parameter estimates and thus ensure that the trade-off data yield the greatest possible unbiased information for samples of a given size (63). Street and Burgess (64) recently have proposed an alternative approach to D-efficient designs that promises even better statistical performance in some applications.

SPDCE studies in environmental, transportation, and health applications have benefited from advances in experimental-design technology in market research. Researchers such as Hensher, Swait, and Louviere who have conducted high-quality SPDCEs in all three areas have helped to disseminate design and analysis methods across application specialties (65). Such hybridization has been facilitated by software that has made advanced experimental-design techniques readily available to both seasoned and novice researchers. Programs that facilitate constructing best-practice experimental designs include Sawtooth Software, Warren Kuhfeld's SAS design macros, and Deborah Street's experimental-design website (64;66;67).

Estimation precision, however, depends on both the statistical properties of the experimental design and measurement error resulting from inattentive respondents. Evaluating tradeoffs in each task often requires a relatively high level of cognitive effort, depending on the number of attributes and the number of alternatives to be evaluated. These cognitive demands may be burdensome for some respondents and result in error-prone evaluations of the choice task. Minimizing cognitive burden by simplifying the tradeoffs inevitably comes at the expense of statistical efficiency (60). Devising SPDCEs that minimize joint statistical and measurement error is another potential area of common research interest in both health and environmental economics.

5.5 **Future directions**

This chapter describes a number of parallels between environmental valuation and health valuation and the uses of valuation in CBA in environment and health fields. The parallels are not surprising since both areas deal with decisions involving public goods, quasi-public goods, or publically provided goods that can benefit from economic evaluation. Arrow and colleagues (68) recognized these similarities and argued for improved use of CBA and valuation in policy and management. What is perhaps surprising is the somewhat divergent paths the two areas have taken – environmental economics following a more traditional welfare-economics orientation and health taking a cost-effectiveness path. While there clearly are institutional reasons for the divergence, we believe both applications of economics and statistical analysis would benefit from a stronger economic conceptual framework and higher analytical standards.

In terms of research, there has been considerable effort in health to assess the extent to which findings in environmental economics apply to health care cases. Many of the same principles apply. The literatures would benefit from collectively addressing problems in understanding revealed and stated choice behaviour, and identifying tools that can help in assessing tradeoffs. There are several areas where crossovers or hybridization can occur, including risk valuation, evaluation of public programmes, and methodological, econometric, and experimental-design tool development.

Many advances in environmental economics occurred as a result of institutional arrangements that arose largely outside of the discipline such as Reagan's executive order and the Exxon Valdez incident. Recent debate in the United States over a larger public role in health care may or may not provide similar opportunities for exploring alternative valuation approaches. In any case, methodological advances in health evaluation will require that health economists argue from within their discipline for adopting rigorous economic methods and techniques. As Arrow et al. (68) state 'Because society has limited resources to spend on regulation, benefit-cost analysis can help illuminate the trade-offs involved in making different kinds of social investments. In this regard, it seems almost irresponsible to not conduct such analyses, because they can inform decisions about how scarce resources can be put to the greatest social good' (p. 221).

References

1. Torrance, G.W. 2006. Utility measurement in healthcare: the things I never got to. *Pharmacoeconomics* **24**(11): 1069–1078.
2. Gold, M.R., Siegel, J.E., Russell, L.B., and Weinstein, M.C. 1996. *Cost-effectiveness in health and medicine*. New York: Oxford University Press.
3. Berry, W. 1986. Home economics – analysis of U.S. agricultural policy. *Whole Earth Review* Summer: 75–76.
4. Krosnick, J.A., Holbrook, A.L., Berent, M.K., Carson, R.T., Hanemann, W.M., Kopp, R.J. *et al.* 2002. The impact of "no opinion" response options on data quality: Non-attitude reduction or an invitation to satisfy? *Public Opinion Quarterly* **66**: 371–403.
5. Chapman, D.J. and Hanemann, W.M. 2001. Environmental damages in court: The American Trader case. In: Heyes, A., editor. *The law and economics of the environment*, pp. 319–367. Cheltenham: Edward Elgar Publishing.
6. Train, K.E. 1998. Recreation demand models with taste variation over people. *Land Economics* **74**: 230–239.
7. Cummings, R.G., Harrison, G.W., and Rutström, E.E. 1995. Homegrown values and hypothetical surveys: Is the dichotomous choice approach incentive compatible? *American Economic Review* **85**(1): 260–266.
8. List, J.A. 2001. Do explicit warnings eliminate the hypothetical bias in elicitation procedures? Evidence from field auctions for sportscards. *American Economic Review* **91**(5): 1498–1507.
9. Johnson, F.R. 2008. Why not ask? Measuring patient preferences for healthcare decision making. *The Patient* **1**(4): 245–248.

10. Carson, R.T. and Hanemann, W.M. 2005. Contingent valuation. In: Mäler, K.-G. and Vincent, J.R., editors. Volume 2 of *Handbook of environmental economics*, pp. 822–936. Amsterdam: Elsevier/North–Holland.

11. Johnson F.R., Banzhaf, M.R., and Desvousges, W.H. 2000. Willingness to pay for improved respiratory and cardiovascular health: A multiple-format stated-preference approach. *Health Economics* **9**: 295–317.

12. Carson, R.T. and Mitchell, R. C. 2006. Public preference toward environmental risks: The case of trihalomethanes. In: Alberini, A., Bjornstad, D., and Kahn, J.R., editors. *Handbook of contingent valuation*. Northampton, MA: Edward Elgar.

13. Flores, N.E. 2002. Non-paternalistic altruism and welfare economics. *Journal of Public Economics* **83**: 293–305.

14. McConnell, K.E. 1997. Does altruism undermine existence value? *Journal of Environmental Economics and Management* **32**: 22–37.

15. Dosman, D. and Adamowicz, W. 2006. Combining stated and revealed preference data to construct an empirical examination of intrahousehold bargaining. *Review of Economics of the Household* **4**: 15–34.

16. Smith, V.K., Van Houtven, G.L., and Pattanayak, S.K. 2002. Benefit transfer via preference calibration: "Prudential algebra" for policy. *Land Economics* **78**: 132–152.

17. Corso, P.S., Hammitt, J.K., and Graham, J.D. 2001. Valuing mortality-risk reduction: Using visual aids to improve the validity of contingent valuation. *Journal of Risk and Uncertainty* **23**(2): 165–184.

18. Gafni, A., Birch, S., and Mehrez, A. 1993. Economics, health and health economics: HYEs (healthy-years equivalent) versus QALYs (quality-adjusted live-year). *Journal of Health Economics* **12**: 325–339.

19. Cameron, T.A. and Deshazo, J.R. 2005. Valuing health-risk reductions: Sick-years, lost life-years, and latency. CCPR-053-05, On-Line Working Paper Series, California Center for Population Research.

19a. Ciriacy-Wantrup, S.V. 1947. Capital returns from soil conservation practices. *Journal of Farms Economics* **29**: 1180–1190.

20. Adamowicz, W. 2004. What's it worth? An examination of historical trends and future directions in environmental valuation. *Australian Journal of Agricultural and Resource Economics* **48**(3): 419–443.

21. Diener, A., O'Brien, B., and Gafni, A. 1998. Health care contingent valuation studies: A review and classification of the literature. *Health Economics* **7**: 313–326.

22. Hanemann, M. 1981. Applied welfare analysis with quantal choice models, Working Paper, Department of Agricultural and Resource Economics, paper 173, CUDARE Working Papers, University of California Berkeley, Berkeley, CA, 38 pp.

23. Cameron, T. A. 1988. A new paradigm for valuing non-market goods using referendum data - maximum-likelihood estimation by censored logistic-regression. *Journal of Environmental Economics and Management* **15**(3): 355–379.

24. Gyrd-Hansen, D., Halvorsen, P.A., and Kristiansen, I.S. 2008. Willingness-to-pay for a statistical life in the times of a pandemic. *Health Economics* **17**: 55–66.

25. Ryan, M., Scott, D.A., and Donaldson, C. 2004. Valuing health care using willingness to pay: A comparison of the payment card and dichotomous choice methods. *Journal of Health Economics* **23**: 237–258.

26. Holmes, T.P. and Kramer, R.A. 1995. An independent sample of yea-saying and starting point bias in dichotomous-choice contingent valuation. *Journal of Environmental Economics and Management* **29**: 121–132.

27. Ready, R.C., Buzby, J.C., and Hu, D. 1996. Differences between continuous and discrete contingent value estimates. *Land Economics* **72**: 397–411.

28. Watson, V. and Ryan, M. 2007. Exploring preference anomalies in double bounded contingent valuation. *Journal of Health Economics* **26**: 463–482.

29. DeShazo, J.R. 2002. Designing transactions without framing effects in iterative question formats. *Journal of Environmental Economics and Management* **44**(1): 123–143.

30. Krupnick, A., Alberini, A., Cropper, M., Simon, N., O'Brien, B., Goeree, R., *et al.* 2002. Age, health, and the willingness to pay for mortality risk reductions: A contingent valuation survey of Ontario residents. *Journal of Risk and Uncertainty* **24**: 161–186.

31. Hirth, R.A., Chernew, M.E., Miller, E., Fendrick, A.M., and Weissert, W.G. 2000. Willingness to pay for a quality-adjusted life year: In search of a standard. *Medical Decision Making* **20**: 332–342.

32. Kenkel, D. 2006. WTP- and QALY-based approaches to valuing health for policy: Common ground and disputed territory. *Environmental & Resource Economics* **34**: 419–437.

33. Johnson, F.R. 2005. Einstein on willingness to pay per QALY: Is there a better way? *Medical Decision Making* **25**: 607–608.

34. Freeman, A.M. 2003. *The measurement of environmental and resource values.* Baltimore, MD: Resources for the Future Press.

35. Fischhoff, B., Slovic, P., Lichtenstein, S., Read, S., and Combs, B. 1978. How safe is safe enough? A psychometric study of attitudes towards technological risks and benefits. *Policy Sciences* **9**: 127–152.

36. Nordhaus, W.D. 2002. The health of nations: The contribution of improved health to living standards. NBER Working Paper No. W8818.

37. Rush, B. and Scheill, A. 2002. Annotated bibliography of economic evaluations of public health interventions (1990–2001). Department of Community Health Sciences and Centre for Health and Policy Studies, University of Calgary, Alberta.

38. Bosworth, R., Cameron, T.A., and DeShazo, J.R. 2006. Preferences for preventative public health policies with jointly estimated rates of time preference. School of Public Health and International Affairs, North Carolina State University, Raleigh, NC.

39. Dickie, M. 1999. *Willingness to pay for children's health: A household production approach.* Proceedings of the Second EPA Workshop in Environmental policy and economics, valuing health for environmental policy with special emphasis on children's health issues. Silver Spring, MD, March 24–25.

40. Hoffmann, S., Krupnick, A., and Adamowicz, W. 2006. Uncertainties in valuing reductions in children's environmental health risks. In: *economic valuation of environmental health risks to children,* pp. 207–238. France: OECD Publishing.

41. Viscusi, W.K. and Gayer, T. 2005. Quantifying and valuing environmental health risks. In: Mäler, K.-G. and Vincent, J.R., editors. Volume 2 of *Handbook of environmental economics,* pp. 1030–1103. Amsterdam: Elsevier/North Holland.

42. Phillips, K.A., Maddala, T., and Johnson, F.R. 2002. Measuring preferences for health care interventions using conjoint analysis: An application to HIV testing. *Health Services Research* **37**: 1681–1705.

43. Marshall, D.A., Johnson, F.R., Phillips, K.A., Marshall, J.K., Thabane, L., and Kulin, N.A. 2007. Measuring patient preferences for colorectal cancer screening using a choice-format survey. *Value in Health* **10**: 415–430.

44. Johnson, F.R., Manjunath, R., Mansfield, C.A., Clayton, L.J., Hoerger, T.J., and Zhang, P. 2006. High-risk individuals' willingness to pay for diabetes risk-reduction programs. *Diabetes Care* **29**: 1351–1356.

45. Shogren, J. 2006. Valuation in the lab. *Environmental and Resource Economics* **34**: 163–172.

46. Harrison, G. 2006. Experimental evidence on alternative environmental valuation methods. *Environmental and Resource Economics* **34**: 125–162.

47. Mark, T.L. and Swait, J. 2004. Using stated preference and revealed preference modeling to evaluate prescribing decisions. *Health Economics* **13**: 563–573.

48. Blumenschein, K., Johannesson, M., Yokoyama, K.K., and Freeman, P.R. 2001. Hypothetical versus real willingness to pay in the health care sector: results from a field experiment. *Journal Health Economics* P.R.: 441–457.

49. Desvousges, W.H., Johnson, F.R., and Banzhaf, H.S. 1998. *Environmental policy analysis with limited information: Principles and applications of the transfer method.* Northampton, MA: Edward Elgar.

50. Navrud, S. and Ready, R. 2007. *Environmental value transfer: Issues and methods.* Dordrecht, The Netherlands: Springer.

51. Cameron, T.A. 1992. Combining contingent valuation and travel cost data for the valuation of nonmarket goods. *Land Economics* **68**: 302–317.

52. Adamowicz, W.L., Louviere, J. and Williams, M. 1994. Combining stated and revealed preference methods for valuing environmental amenities. *Journal of Environmental Economics and Management* **26**: 271–292.

53. Swait, J. and Adamowicz, W. 2001. The influence of task complexity on consumer choice: A latent class model of decision strategy switching. *Journal of Consumer Research* **28**: 135–148.

54. von Haefen, R.H. and Phaneuf, D.J. 2003. Estimating preferences for outdoor recreation: A comparison of continuous and count data demand system frameworks. *Journal of Environmental Economics & Management* **45**: 612–630.

55. Allenby, G.M., Bakken, D.G., and Rossi, P.E. 2004. The HB revolution: How Bayesian methods have changed the face of marketing research. *Marketing Research* **16**: 20–25.

56. Moeltner, K., Boyle, K.J., and Paterson, R.W. 2007. Meta-analysis and benefit-transfer for resource valuation: Addressing classical challenges with Bayesian modeling. *Journal of Environmental Economics and Management* **53**: 250–269.

57. Swait, J. 2001. A non-compensatory choice model incorporating attribute cutoffs. *Transportation Research Part B* **35**: 903–928.

58. Gilbride, T.J. and Allenby, G.M. 2004. A choice model with conjunctive, disjunctive, and compensatory screening rules. *Marketing Science* **23**: 391–406.

59. Carlsson, F. and Martinsson, P. 2003. Design techniques for stated preference methods in health economics. *Health Economics* **12**: 281–294.

60. Maddala T., Phillips, K.A., and Johnson, F.R. 2003. An experiment on simplifying conjoint analysis designs for measuring preferences. *Health Economics* **12**(12): 1035–1047.

61. Viney, R.C., Savage, E.J., and Louviere, J.J. 2005. Empirical investigation of experimental design properties of discrete choice experiments in health care. *Health Economics* **14**(4): 349–362.

62. Huber, J. and Zwerina, K. 1996. The importance of utility balance in efficient choice design. *Journal of Marketing Research* **33**: 307–317.

63. Kuhfeld, W.F., Tobias, R.D., and Garratt, M. 1994. Efficient experimental de-sign with marketing applications. *Journal of Marketing Research* **31**(4): 545–557.

64. Street, D. and Burgess, L.B. 2007. *The construction of optimal stated choice experiments: Theory and methods.* Hoboken, NJ: Wiley.

65. Louviere, J., Hensher, D., and Swait, J. 2000. *Stated choice methods: analysis and applications in marketing, transportation and environmental valuation.* Cambridge: Cambridge University Press.

66. Kuhfeld, W.F. 2009, Marketing research methods in SAS: Experimental design, choice, conjoint, and graphical techniques. MR-2009 SAS 9.2 Edition. Access July 21, 2009. http://support.sas.com/techsup/tnote/tnote stat.html#market

67. Chrzan, K. and Orme, B. 2000. An overview and analysis of design strategies for choice-based conjoint analysis. Sawtooth Software Inc. Research Paper Series. Accessed July 21, 2009. http://www.sawtoothsoftware.com/download/techpap/desgncbc.pdf

68. Arrow, K.J., Cropper, M.L., Eads, G.C., Hahn, R.W., Lave, L.B., Noll, R.G., *et al.* 1996. Is there a role for benefit-cost analysis in environmental, health and safety regulation? *Science* **272**: 221–222.

69. McFadden, D. 1996. *Computing willingness-to-pay in random utility models.* Working Papers 011, University of California at Berkeley, Econometrics Laboratory Software Archive.

70. Brock, W. and Durlauf, S. 2001. Discrete choice with social interactions. *Review of Economic Studies* **68**: 235–260.

71. Executive order 12866, 58 Fed. Reg. 51735 (Sept. 30, 1993), *as amended by* Exec. Order No. 13258, 67 Fed. Reg. 9385 (Feb. 26, 2002), *as further amended by* Exec. Order No. 13422 72 Fed. Reg. 2763 (Jan. 18, 2007).

72. Mitchell, R.C. and Carson, R.T. 1989. *Using surveys to value public goods.* Washington, DC: Resources for the Future Press.

73. Murphy, K.M. and Topel, R.H. 2006. The value of health and longevity. *Journal of Political Economy* **114**: 871–904.

Chapter 6

Benefit assessment for cost–benefit analysis studies in health care using contingent valuation methods

Emma J. Frew

6.1 Introduction

In this chapter, we describe how the contingent valuation (CV) method can be used to measure benefits for CBA studies. We will focus on the design of CV studies considering each of the methodological components of CV in turn. In particular, we discuss how information should be presented to respondents with reference to the scenario description, payment vehicle, and appropriate perspective. We review in detail the biases potential within CV studies and how these can be overcome with good study design. Consideration is given to how respondents form preferences and the implications for the elicitation of CV values. Finally, we discuss the aggregation of CV values and their use to inform evidence for policy decision-makers.

6.2 Overview

6.2.1 Contingent valuation

The CV method is a stated preference approach designed to directly estimate welfare gains/losses as appropriate. Individuals are asked to consider a hypothetical scenario where they are asked to imagine that a market exists for the benefits or losses of a public programme. The exercise proceeds on the hypothetical contingency that such a market exists. Various design instruments can then be applied to ask individuals to state their willingness to pay (WTP) to ensure that a welfare gain occurs or their willingness to accept (WTA) to tolerate the welfare loss from the programme. The WTP or the WTA amount is then taken as a measure of the individual's perceived value of the programme (i.e. the demand) which is then aggregated across all individuals. If individuals state a high (low) WTP amount, then it is inferred that the demand for that programme is high (low). CV has the potential to offer advantages over other methods of eliciting community values (including methods such as QALYs), and if well designed, has potential to measure non-health enhancing aspects of the process of care and other consumption benefits like provision of information (1–3).

6.2.2 Brief history of CV

The application of the CV method to assign values to benefits for goods without clearly defined demand curves has been traced back to 1958 (4) and was first applied in a health care context in a study to avoid heart attacks (5). From 1985 onwards, there has been a steady growth in the number of published papers using the CV method within health care (6). The number of published CV studies in the last 5 years has almost doubled that published in the preceding 15 years (7). This increase in the application of the CV technique has brought about an intensification of debate regarding the methodological qualities of the method. There exists no formal guidelines on the appropriate design of a CV study within health care only that which has been published in the environmental literature (8) and it is not clear how transferable these guidelines are to the health care context (9), see Chapter 5.

6.3 Scenario description

The first stage of designing a CV study is the scenario description. The scenario description contains information on all relevant aspects of the product/service being valued and is what the respondents will read/listen to prior to the CV task. As respondents are typically asked to consider goods or services that are not routinely available in the market, there is often little or no familiarity with the product being evaluated and thus (prior to the study), no opportunity to think about the product and form preferences and values. The scenario description therefore has to be realistic to the respondent and in a form that is both informative and understandable (10). This is often referred to in the literature as content validity and relates to the content of the survey instrument and related materials. If the scenario is not presented correctly, then any subsequent analysis of the CV data will be meaningless as it is likely that the respondent will have misunderstood what it is that they have been asked to value.

6.3.1 Scenario presentation (risk communication)

Normally, within a health care context, the goods/services being valued using the CV methodology are complex and require some thought as to how they should be presented to avoid confusion. Mitchell and Carson (11, p. 192) suggest that one should ask the following questions when evaluating the content validity of a CV study (11):

◆ *Does the description of the good and how it is to be paid for appear to be unambiguous?*

◆ *Is it likely to be meaningful to respondents?*

◆ *Are the property rights and the market for the good defined in such a way that the respondents will accept the WTP/WTA format as plausible?*

◆ *Does the scenario appear to force reluctant respondents to come up with WTP amounts?*

Ensuring that the scenario description is correct is a two-stage process. First, we need to check that the description contains all relevant informations such as details on the attributes of the product, who is going to provide the product, how it will be provided and paid for. Second, we need to ensure that this is communicated well so that the respondent has understood and digested everything to enable them to form a WTP/WTA value (10). Usually, scenarios contain information concerning the probability of an event or an uncertain outcome that the respondent is required to understand. The manner in which a respondent perceives risk is guided by heuristics and is prone to bias (12). Respondents can therefore be inconsistent in the way that they interpret risk. For example, the use of probabilities can lead to a different response to when the information is presented as an absolute or relative risk. Gigerenzer argues for the use of absolute frequencies as this is what respondents are more accustomed to when making decisions in everyday life (13). Below are examples of how to present risk information using first, probabilities, and second absolute frequencies.

Scenario 1 (probabilities): Assume you are buying a new car and your choice is between two equally priced and similarly desirable models, but one car has proven to reduce the chance of dying from 3 in 100 to 1 in 100 crashes. How much would you be willing to pay for the additional protection? $_____ (Source: Muller and Reutzel, 1984) (14)

Scenario 2 (absolute frequencies): If 6,000 lives per year could be saved by requiring new cars to have better crash protection, how much would you be willing to add to your monthly car payment for such protection? $_____(Source: Muller and Reutzel, 1984) (14)

Lloyd argues that there is a need to investigate empirically the extent to which individuals employ decision-making heuristics when responding to CV tasks (12). Research into this area is ongoing and until any conclusive recommendations result from this work, the CV analyst needs to be aware of the effects of presenting risk information differently.

6.3.2 Payment vehicle

The payment vehicle refers to the type of payment being asked of the respondent, e.g. additional income tax, charitable donation, monthly payments, etc. The choice of the payment vehicle has to be one that respondents can easily understand and fit into the scenario being described (or product being evaluated) and this has to be established through pilot work. The payment vehicle should not cause any undesirable reactions, i.e. respondents may object to being asked to pay more through income taxation in a tax-financed health care service. Evidence shows respondents to be sensitive to the choice of payment vehicle (15;16). The timing of the payment structure is just as important as the vehicle as respondents need to know if the payment being made is a one-off payment, if so, when is it to be paid or, alternatively, will it be made in stages. To avoid misunderstandings, the scenario should make this clear to the respondent.

The choice of payment vehicle will depend upon the objective of the survey and the survey environment. In the environmental literature, NOAA recommends the use of the taxation measure as this is what respondents are most familiar with in tax-financed health care systems. Interestingly, a recent review showed virtually no use of tax payments in the UK and the same to be the case for insurance payments in the US (10). The payment vehicle has to fit in well with the survey environment to encourage respondents to engage with the CV task. Once the payment vehicle has been chosen, it is vital to ensure that it is clearly explained to respondents (and fully understood) so the final WTP/WTA value is truly reflective of the respondents' welfare gain/loss.

6.3.3 Equivalent and compensating variation/ WTP versus WTA

The effects of the product/service being valued can be measured using either the compensating or the equivalent variation. Both methods measure the monetary amount required to keep utility levels constant. The compensating variation measures the amount starting from the original utility level, the equivalent variation measures it from the utility level after the change has taken place. The direction of payment, i.e. WTP or WTA, depends on whether a welfare gain or loss can, or is at risk of occurring. From a practical perspective it is useful to think about the direction of measurement in these terms when considering the CV survey as one that is either taking an ex ante (before) or an ex post (after) perspective. When an ex ante perspective is taken, WTP/ WTA is elicited prior to the event happening, i.e. prior to treatment being provided or services reorganized. The change in utility (welfare loss/gain) has not yet occurred therefore a compensating variation is being measured. With an ex post perspective, the change in welfare has happened and the WTP/WTA is being elicited from the utility level after the change has happened thus is an equivalent variation. Table 6.1 outlines different scenarios to demonstrate these different perspectives.

Where there is an uncertainty around the outcome, it is generally accepted that the most appropriate perspective is the ex ante perspective (11). Klose argues that there is a twofold uncertainty within health care which makes the distinction between an ex ante and an ex post perspective more complex than this (21). As well as there being uncertainty around the morbidity risk of becoming ill, there is also uncertainty around the efficacy of health care treatment meaning there are three health states to potentially consider:

Health state 1: Uncertainty of becoming ill and requiring treatment (ex ante state)

Health state 2: Diagnosis confirmed, treatment not started: uncertainty in the efficacy of treatment (intermediate state)

Health state 3: Treatment received: no uncertainty (ex post state)

Table 6.1 Direction of measurement

Scenario	Ex ante/ex post perspective	Compensating/ equivalent variation	WTP/ WTA	Source
Measuring heart patients WTP for changes in angina symptoms	Ex post	Equivalent	WTP	(17)
WTA for a community-based prevention programme	Ex post	Equivalent	WTA	(18)
Loss in utility among potential losers from a fluoridation programme	Ex ante	Compensating	WTA	(19)
Value placed on protection of minor illness for mother and baby in Taiwan	Ex ante	Compensating	WTP	(20)

Table 6.2 Ex-ante and ex-post perspectives

Scenario	Uncertainty	Perspective
Morbidity risk of becoming ill and requiring treatment in the future	Yes	Ex ante
Diagnosis confirmed, treatment not yet started	Yes	Ex ante
Treatment already started or completed	No	Ex post
Consideration of proposed service reorganization	Yes	Ex ante
Consideration of certain changes in health state	No	Ex post

The appropriate perspective is clear with health states 1 (ex ante) and 3 (ex post). In the intermediate state, uncertainty still exists in the efficacy of the treatment so in this state, the ex ante perspective is the most appropriate. Table 6.2 outlines the possible scenarios and the appropriate perspective to be taken.

6.4 **Whose values**

Theoretically, a CBA should take a societal perspective where all subjects that stand to lose or benefit from the health care intervention are included in the sample. If this sample is too large, then a representative sample is appropriate. If we ask subjects that benefit indirectly as well as directly, in theory, all externalities produced by the health care intervention will be incorporated into the analysis. However, it may be easier to access patients in a WTP survey as they are a convenient population to capture (22;23). Alternatively, a combined sample can be used as in the study by Ortega *et al.* that used both patients and the general population when investigating the WTP for erythropoietin in the prevention of chemotherapy-induced anaemia (24). The patients were asked how much they would be WTP for the drug as a direct payment, whereas the WTP question was framed as an increase in health insurance premiums for the general population. The question of whose values should be sought is not just relevant to CBA. Economic guidelines for the practice of cost-effectiveness analysis for decision-making by NICE within the UK, stipulate that general population values for valuing health states should be used (24a). This is based on the premise that when working within a tax-financed health system such as the UK NHS, it is the general population who are paying for the provision of health care and therefore should be a part of resource allocation decisions. Patients on the other hand are the best judge of their own well-being and as a consequence will be best placed to measure the quality of life of the health state that has been directly experienced. The question of the appropriate viewpoint is a normative one (24b), recent debate has suggested that the best way forward is to use general population values where the sample has been well-informed about what it is like to be living in the health state being valued (24c). Scenario descriptions should provide lots of information with respect to health state descriptions, and the size and nature of adaptation experienced by patients over time.

6.5 **Instrumentation technique**

The choice of the appropriate instrumentation technique has been debated a great deal in the CV literature (25). Direct face-to-face interviews are generally regarded as the 'gold standard' and are particularly beneficial if the health care intervention being valued is difficult to communicate. With this method, any of the elicitation formats (WTP question design) can be applied and there is scope to include a large amount of qualitative research if deemed necessary. There is a risk however that the respondent may become influenced by other aspects of the interview situation rather than on the relevant economic parameters (interviewer bias). Telephone interviews provide an economical alternative to face-to-face interviews both in time and in money and still offer the opportunity to choose any elicitation format and to probe further if misunderstandings occur. Mail surveys provide the most economical option overall and scope to achieve a large sample size (relative to face-to-face/telephone interviews) but are limited in that only certain elicitation formats can be used and there is minimal opportunity to describe the scenario in great detail. The choice of the instrumentation technique is a trade off between the ability to describe things in detail and gain reassurance that the respondent has understood the task versus the ease and ability to achieve large sample sizes. As a general rule, face-to-face interviews are regarded as the best form of instrumentation but this will always be subject to resource constraints.

6.6 **Elicitation format**

The elicitation format refers to the style of questioning to elicit the WTP/WTA value. There are a number of different formats to choose from, each with its own strengths and weaknesses, and there is little consensus in the health care literature concerning which is superior. Below is a brief summary of the most common formats used within CV with an illustrative example of each. The environmental economics literature provides guidelines for the environmental context (NOAA Panel Guidelines) (25a).

6.6.1 **Open-ended question**

The open-ended question is the 'simplest' of the elicitation designs. This question asks for the WTP for a health care intervention without any prompts or cues from the questionnaire or interviewer. Usually, the respondents are provided with a space (a line to write on) for their final maximum WTP value. An example of an open-ended question is provided in Box 6.1.

Box 6.1 **Example of an open-ended question**

What is the maximum that you would be willing to pay to have the (health care intervention being valued) available to you?

Please write in the space provided.   £_____

6.6.2 Iterative bidding technique

This elicitation format is termed the 'bidding game' and first originated in environmental economics having been introduced by Davis (26). The question is designed so that it resembles an auction as the respondent enters a bargaining process with the interviewer. The process can be likened to a 'haggle' technique that happens in real-life markets making it more familiar to the respondents. The respondent is presented with a first-bid and depending on whether they accept or reject that bid; it is either raised or lowered till eventually the respondent's maximum WTP is reached. The amount by which the bids are raised or lowered is governed by a pre-determined algorithm to ensure that each respondent participates in the same bidding process. Once the 'top' bid is reached in the algorithm the question reverts to an open-ended question. An example of three such algorithms is contained in Box 6.2 where the starting bid is varied between £10, £200, and £1000.

Some researchers claim that this technique is advantageous as the bidding process is more likely to measure consumer surplus (it will capture the highest price that consumers are WTP) (27) and it is more likely that the respondent will give consideration to the value of the amenity (28). Others believe that it gives respondents more time to consider their preferences (29).

Box 6.2 Example of the iterative bidding technique

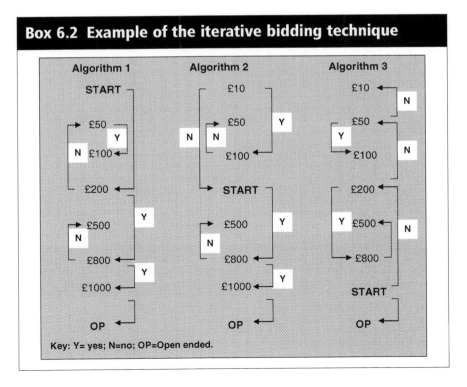

Key: Y= yes; N=no; OP=Open ended.

Box 6.3 Example of the payment scale/card elicitation format

Typical payment card design:

£10
£15
£20
£25
£30
£40
£50
£100
£200
£_____

6.6.3 Payment scale/card

The payment scale question design was developed by Mitchell and Carson in 1981 and 1984 as an alternative to the bidding game approach (30;31). The payment scale question presents respondents with a range of values to choose from. A typical design presents respondents with a series of bid amounts, in a vertical list from the lowest bid (top) to the highest bids (bottom) in increments. Box 6.3 provides an example of the payment scale/card elicitation format.

If the maximum WTP is greater than the highest bid in the list, then the question defaults to an open-ended question design. Typically, respondents are requested to put a tick mark next to the amounts that they are sure they would pay, put a cross mark next to the amounts they are sure they would not pay, and circle their maximum WTP.

6.6.4 Closed ended/dichotomous choice/discrete question

Closed-ended questions are designed to lead to a yes/no response. This method was developed by Bishop and Heberlein (32). Respondents are presented with a bid and are asked if they are WTP that amount. Box 6.4 provides an example of the closed-ended format.

The bid levels are varied across the sample so that it is possible to estimate the percentage of respondents who are WTP as a function of the bid. Several motivations for

Box 6.4 Example of the closed-ended WTP elicitation format

Do you think that having the health care intervention is worth 'bid value' (e.g. £100):

(please tick the appropriate box)

❏   Yes   ❏   No

using the dichotomous choice approach have been offered in the literature. It is thought that the question design resembles a 'real-life' situation whereby respondents are presented with a 'price' at which they decide whether or not they want to buy the product/service, as consumers are accustomed to facing offers of a good at given prices, it is argued to be a logical way to ask the question. Given its simplistic nature, the closed-ended design is recommended by Mitchell and Carson as being suitable for a mail questionnaire survey (11). It is also claimed that the question design is less stressful to the respondent (33;34).

6.6.5 **Closed ended with follow-up question**

The closed ended with follow-up approach was proposed by Carson, Hanemann, and Mitchell (35). This technique is an extension of the closed-ended method, to obtain more information from each respondent; a follow-up open-ended question is inserted. Box 6.5 provides an example of the closed ended with follow-up elicitation format.

The design therefore is a form of bidding that is truncated at two bids. The use of additional follow-up bids, or even triple bounded discrete questions have also been explored (36). Using a follow-up question lessens the need for such a large sample size as you get more information per respondent.

6.6.6 **Marginal approach**

The marginal approach (37) asks individuals to firstly consider what treatment or service they prefer and then to reveal their maximum WTP value to have their preferred option over their less preferred option. Therefore, instead of the absolute WTP being elicited, it is the relative WTP that is being revealed. Box 6.6 provides an example of this approach.

Box 6.5 Example of the closed ended with follow-up elicitation format

A. Are you willing to pay £100 for intervention? If yes go to B and if no go to C.

B. Are you willing to pay £200 for intervention? Answer yes or no.

C. Are you willing to pay £50 for intervention? Answer yes or no.

Box 6.6 Example of the marginal approach elicitation format

What is the maximum amount of money you would be prepared to pay to receive your most preferred option instead of your least preferred option?

(Please write your answer in the space provided) £_____

Some question formats are better suited to certain instrumentation methods. For example, the iterative bidding question design involves a lot of interaction between the respondent and the researcher making a personal or a telephone interview the most appropriate setting. Each elicitation design comes with its own strengths and weaknesses and the debate concerning the most appropriate format is far from resolved. Mitchell and Carson claim that the open-ended format leads to an unacceptably large number of non-responses or protest zero responses to the WTP question (11). Johannesson *et al.* in 1991, in a study that investigated the WTP for antihypertensive therapy also criticized the open-ended approach as resulting in low-response rates (38). However, Nabro and Sjostrom used the open-ended design to examine the WTP for obesity treatment and found that the question design led to a response rate of 99% which they claim is equal to, or higher, than response rates of other question formats (39). Ramsay *et al.* demonstrated the difficulty in using a bidding game design when the study design used a mail survey. The study investigated the WTP for antihypertensive care. Mail questionnaires were issued with a WTP question that contained ten separate WTP 'bids' ranging from $25 to $250, in $25 increments. They found that even at the highest bid, 24% of the sample responded with a 'yes' result and given that the design was a mail questionnaire, there was no scope to investigate this further (40). When a comparison was made between the closed ended and closed ended with follow-up questions (for the WTP for the alleviation of arthritis symptoms), the authors found that the two question designs produced significantly different WTP amounts (DKK637 versus DKK 1,268). They suggest that the inclusion of a follow-up question increases the precision of the results (41).

From a practical perspective, when selecting the elicitation design, consideration needs to be made to the potential for pilot research prior to the CV survey as well as the resources available for the instrumentation method. Certain elicitation designs such as the iterative bidding method and the closed-ended method require knowledge of the potential 'WTP distribution' to inform the researcher of what bid values to use within the questions. Table 6.3 summarizes each of the designs with this in mind.

Table 6.3 Choice of elicitation design

Elicitation design	Pilot research required on bid levels	Instrumentation method
Open ended	No	Mail or interview
Payment scale	Yes	Mail or interview
Closed ended	Yes	Mail or interview
Closed ended with follow-up	Yes	Interview
Iterative bidding	Yes	Interview
Marginal approach	No	Mail or Interview

6.7 **Value cues**

With the exception of the open-ended elicitation format, all elicitation designs provide respondents with value cues. Whilst these cues have the benefit of guiding the respondents and encouraging them to consider their maximum WTP, they can also have the disadvantage of overly influencing the respondent to reveal a WTP value that is more in accordance with the cues rather than their true maximum WTP value. This type of bias is commonly classified as either the 'anchoring effect' or 'range bias' and with good CV design the effects of each can be minimized. Each of these is discussed in turn below.

6.7.1 **Anchoring effect**

When the iterative-bidding design is adopted, the survey has the potential to be susceptible to starting point bias. The final maximum WTP value can be influenced by the starting bids used in the bidding algorithm. We can easily detect this by varying the starting bid across respondents to establish if those who start at high bids give significantly higher WTP values compared to a sub-group of respondents who start on low bids. The evidence for starting point bias is equivocal; some studies have found it exists; others have not (42).

We can minimize the risk of a starting point bias by following the advice of Reardon *et al.* (25) and Eastaugh (43). Reardon *et al.* (25) suggests that randomly generated initial bids administered across the study may be helpful, and Eastaugh suggests randomly assigning 10% of the study sample to one-tenth of the starting bids (25;43).

An extreme form of starting point bias, referred to as 'yea-saying', can be found when the closed-ended question design is adopted. This happens when respondents agree to pay regardless of the bid level offered. Many studies have found the final mean WTP to be much higher with the closed-ended design than with the open-ended format suggesting that 'yea-saying' is a problem (44–48).

6.7.2 **Range bias**

Another type of value cue bias is known as range bias and is usually encountered in payment scale question designs. Range bias is similar to starting point bias only instead of being influenced by the starting point bid; the respondent is influenced by the range of values chosen for the payment scale question design. Usually, respondents are presented with a range of values starting from the lowest (usually £0) to the highest (usually approximately £1000), if the study design adopts a different range, i.e. £0–100, then a change in the overall WTP results is likely (49). It is also plausible that respondents may be sensitive to the positioning of the values within the range. This effect has received limited empirical attention within the CV literature so the full impact of its effect is unclear. It is an important finding however and should be borne in mind when considering the range of values to include within the payment scale design. Similar to the solution for starting point bias above it may be necessary to design several payment scales with different ranges and randomly allocate these across the study sample.

6.8 **Strategic bias**

Strategic bias involves the respondents deliberately overstating or understating their true WTP value. If the respondent feels that the intervention will be implemented if they provide a high WTP value but that this will not affect how much they will actually have to pay for the intervention, then there is an incentive to overstate the true value. Authors such as Hoehn and Randall (1987) argue that the closed-ended question design provides an incentive for individuals to eschew strategic behaviour and respond truthfully (28). There is little empirical evidence to support the hypothesis of strategic bias in CV studies (50–52).

Protest responses can be classified as an extreme form of strategic bias and happen when respondents protest to the process of investigation by stating either a zero response or an unreasonably high or low response. Respondents may state no WTP value, even though they care about the intervention, if they feel that it is some-one else's responsibility to pay, i.e. the NHS. It is difficult to detect protesters in a CV survey without the elicitation of qualitative information alongside the CV values. Such qualitative information can provide valuable insight into the respondents thought processes and may help to separate the respondents who are protesting from those who are genuinely not willing to pay. Diamond and Hausman (53) claim that it should be a standard practice to eliminate protest zeros as this type of zero is not a credible response. They argue that if the respondent has answered all other questions in a manner that indicates that they do put a positive value on the intervention, but they have responded with a zero value, then they should be removed from further analysis. Dalmau-Matarrodona however argues that it may not be correct, statistically, to remove all respondents who have protested (54). There is a potential cost to the loss of information and these respondents may have different characteristics to the rest of the sample therefore you may inflict sample bias. With every CV survey, a qualita-tive question should be inserted into the CV survey design to allow the CV analyst to select with confidence the respondents who are true protestors (if any exist). The characteristics of these 'protestors' should then be checked against the rest of the sample to ensure that there is no sample bias from removing them from further analysis. If there are no differences then this sub-sample can be safely removed ensur-ing that this is clearly reported in a transparent fashion. If however their characteristics are different, then it is a good practice to firstly analyse the full sample (with the protes-tors included) then conduct the same analysis again with the protestors removed as a form of sensitivity analysis on the overall CV results. Both sets of results should then be reported.

6.9 **Question order**

Theoretically, the response to a CV question should not be influenced by the order of questions in the survey. The same response should be given if the CV question is asked by itself or with other questions. Respondents however can be influenced by question order when different bids are used in subsequent WTP questions. For example, if asking for a WTP value for two competing alternatives the WTP revealed for the first alternative can unduly influence the WTP for the second alternative. Some authors describe the ordering effect as one of 'fading glow', whereby the first programme in any sequence captures much of the utility associated with giving (55). This can be easily minimized by randomly varying the question order across respondents.

6.10 Embedding effect

The embedding effect was first analysed systematically by Kahnemann and Knetsch (56) and happens when respondents find it difficult to isolate a specific case from overall considerations when they are deciding on their maximum WTP value. For example, if the respondent is asked to consider two alternative treatments for the same disease and they give the same WTP value for both, they may be considering the treatment of the disease generally and not the different aspects of the two alternative treatments. A good way to overcome this problem is to ask a follow-up question, asking respondents if they would be WTP for alternative treatments. This alternative health care treatment could substitute the treatment valued in the initial WTP question. Respondents would then be encouraged to consider the total value of the WTP amount stated in the first question in relation to their total WTP for treatment of the disease.

6.11 'Warm-glow' feeling

Respondents may respond to the CV question in a manner that does not reflect their true preferences. Individuals can experience a 'warm-glow' from expressing support for a good cause (57) and get some kind of moral satisfaction when deciding upon their WTP response (58). This theory is based on the 'impure altruism' model that individuals contribute towards the health care intervention for two reasons:

1. They simply demand more of the good.

2. Gain benefit from their contribution per se, like a warm-glow.

Andreoni has proved the model of impure altruism to be a straightforward but powerful predictor of the act of giving and that it is consistent with empirical observations (57). It is reasonable to assume that preferences will include a combination of both the altruistic and the warm-glow effect as individuals actually care about the good but also contribute to receive a warm-glow as well. Alternatively, the respondent may feel some moral obligation towards the scenario being valued and may give a WTP value so that they feel they are 'doing their fair share' (59). The warm-glow feeling is closely related to the embedding effect. If respondents get pleasure from contributing to the health care programme to help the community, the WTP for this warm glow is not determined by the *particular* health care intervention being valued.

6.12 Preference formation

The CV method rests on the theory that consumers have well-formed preferences that are easily accessible when asked to value a health care intervention (see Chapter 1, Section 1.4.5, 'Theory of preferences'.). There is clear evidence available however that has proven this not to be the case (60). A classic example of this is preference reversal concerning decisions relating to P- and $- bets. The P bet offers a relatively large chance of a modest prize while the $ bet offers a smaller chance of a larger prize. When the individual evaluates each of these alternatives, the classic tendency is to indicate a preference for the P-bet but then place a higher value on the $-bet. Loomes and Sudgen (1982) (64) first proposed regret theory as an explanation of preference reversal whilst the psychologists believe that preferences are context sensitive. That is, preferences are formed during the performance of tasks and there are different preferences for different classes of task (61). This means that the process of choosing your preferred category and then attaching a monetary value to it involves two different thought processes. Individuals tend to place high valuations on gambles that generate large prizes, even if the probability of winning is low.

Theoretically all respondents have what is known as reference prices (r) for products and when asked if they would be WTP a bid amount (b) for that product they will say 'yes' if $b < r$ and 'no' if $b > r$. If respondents answer in this manner, then they are being consistent with their preferences. However, in a hypothetical framework (such as a WTP survey), it is difficult to determine if the respondent is answering in an equivalent way to that in a real-life framework. The literature on CV points to many reasons why subjects may be inconsistent with their real preferences (62), Box 6.7 provides a summary of these reasons.

CV surveys should be designed to try and achieve responses that are identical or as close to that revealed under a real-life scenario. When the respondents depart from what they would do under a real-life setting and do not answer the survey questions truthfully then the affect this group can have on the overall survey results can be huge and present a real problem. The elicitation of qualitative information alongside the WTP/WTA data can provide an insight into respondent behaviour which can help to establish the validity of response. After the WTP/WTA values have been elicited, the reasons for that WTP/WTA value can then be revealed. Ideally, this question

Box 6.7 Reasons for inconsistency in preferences

1. A misunderstanding of the question or the scenario being presented to the respondent.

2. A protest response.

3. Failure to consider the substitutes (private or public) available for the good being valued. This will lead to an invalid positive response.

4. The 'warm-glow' effect.

5. Strategic bias.

6. The interviewer effect.

7. The embedding effect.

should be in the form of an open-ended question to allow the respondent flexibility in revealing their true reasons for their chosen value (or response to a closed-bid question). Alternatively however the question can be framed as one where respondents are asked to choose from a list of reasons. Shiell believes that, 'If we are to understand better what people mean by the answers that they give to economic surveys then we need to learn from and trust the insights that come from qualitative research techniques' (63). The reasoning behind a CV response can help to determine, among others, the protestors to the survey design, people who have the 'warm-glow' feeling, subjects who have attempted to estimate the resource costs of the product, and all those that have produced an embedding effect. This qualitative data can then be used to either validate or invalidate the quantitative response.

The most common technique to analyse qualitative reasons within CV research is to use content analysis whereby the analyst reads through the reasons and codes them into themes or categories. These codes can then be used as a validation tool and as a predictor of WTP/WTA in subsequent regression analysis. This process will be described in more detail in Chapter 7.

The underlying assumption within CV survey methodology is that with every respondent a complete set of preferences exist and with a good survey design these preferences can be revealed by CV responses. However, there is doubt about whether individual preferences are well formed. According to Fischhoff, values only come to be recognized when an individual has the opportunity to act upon them and reflect on the consequences of their decisions (65). It is probable that individual values may be constructed during the elicitation process, that is, the act of eliciting the values that people attach to different states of the world may in itself prompt a process of 'value clarification'. This has an important implication when measuring the 'performance' of elicitation techniques. Fischhoff argues that the individual may 'try on' a value in order to see how it fits, they then reflect on their answer, and possibly revise their response. The process of elicitation therefore may aid the construction of preferences as well as elicit them and any resulting discrepancies may be a function of a deliberate process of reflection and revision as opposed to measurement error (63).

6.13 **Overall survey design**

This chapter has focused on the methodological properties of the CV method drawing attention to possible biases inherent within a CV study. Whilst these biases are important some of them are functions of surveys in general and not just related to CV surveys. As Hanemann points out when considering the effects of these biases within the world of CV, it is important to keep a sense of proportion as many surveys such as the Current Population Survey, Consumer Expenditure Survey are also sensitive to these effects and this has not led to economists stopping using them for data (34). Whilst Hanemann makes a relevant point with respect to general survey effects, some of the biases within CV surveys that have been discussed within this chapter can be eliminated or at best reduced with good survey design. Table 6.4 summarizes each of the methodological points discussed in this chapter.

Table 6.4 Components of a CV survey design

Methodological component	Description	What to consider
Scenario description	Contains information on all relevant aspects of the product/service being valued	1. Realistic, informative, and contains all relevant information about the attributes of the product/service. 2. Check respondent has fully understood the scenario.
Payment vehicle	Type of payment asked within the elicitation design, e.g. charitable donations, tax payments, etc.	Should not cause any undesirable reactions. Choose vehicle that fits into the context. The timing of the payment also has to be clearly stated.
Perspective	WTP or WTA/equivalent or compensating variation	Dependent upon context of study, whether there is a welfare loss or gain and whether it is prior to or after the alteration in welfare levels (product/service has been implemented).
Elicitation format	1. Open ended 2. Payment scale 3. Iterative bidding 4. Closed ended 5. Closed ended with follow-up 6. Marginal approach	The appropriate elicitation design will depend upon predicted sample size, scope for pilot work, place of survey, and chosen instrumentation method.
Instrumentation method	1. Face-to-face interviews 2. Telephone interviews 3. Mail surveys 4. Focus group discussion	This will depend on time and resources. Ideal is face to face interviews but offset against loss in sample size and potential interview effect. Not all elicitation formats can be adopted with mail surveys.
Scope effect	Sensitivity of WTP to size of good being valued	The levels of the good should be varied to assess if the WTP values move in the direction expected.
Ordering effect	Sensitivity of WTP to order of questions	The WTP values should in theory, not be sensitive to the ordering of questions. Randomly vary the order of questions within the sample.
Range bias	Influence on the WTP values by range of values inserted into the payment scale design.	Vary the scales within the sample to check for strength of this effect.
Embedding effect	Tendency for respondents to consider the global good being valued instead of the individual alternatives.	Encourage the respondent to digest and understand the differences between alternative goods being asked to value.

Methodological component	Description	What to consider
'Warm glow' effect	Tendency to state any WTP value due to moral satisfaction element of WTP.	Elicitation of qualitative reasons for WTP will help to identify these respondents. Encourage reflection of values to get the respondent to consider true WTP.
Strategic bias	Deliberate over/understatement of WTP due to perceived influence on policy	Encourage the respondent to 'think aloud' to deter this from happening. Explain clearly that the exercise is hypothetical.
Consistency	Consistency between direction of preference and WTP values	Raise query with respondent about any 'preference reversals' to ensure that the respondent understands WTP exercise.

6.14 Sampling and aggregation

Theoretically, the CV method is applied for the use of measuring outcomes in monetary units in a conventional CBA. Costs are then weighted against the perceived benefits to evaluate if the programme or intervention is worth implementing (subject to the budget constraint). The results of a CBA are then presented as a net social benefit (NSB) for the intervention or product being valued (or the benefits minus the costs). In situations where there is no fixed budget, if the benefits exceed the costs then the product or the intervention should be implemented. The circumstances change however under conditions of a fixed budget as instead of implementing everything with a NSB > 0, the goal is to maximize the monetary benefits and use the net social benefit to rank projects that have a net social benefit greater than zero.

In practice, very few CV studies combine WTP values with cost. Occasionally CV studies report the cost of the interventions they are valuing separately in the paper but it is rare for a full CBA to be presented in health care (7). Refer to Chapter 8 for a full CBA in spinal surgery and Chapter 9 for a CBA in screening. For CV to be accepted and used by policy makers there needs to be a movement towards improving the manner in which CV studies are reported. Sach *et al.* found that despite there being a growing improvement in the reporting methods of CUA, the standard of reporting for CBA has been deteriorating over time (7). The poor reporting of CV studies makes it difficult to draw conclusions about the relative worth of various interventions that have been valued. To better facilitate the reporting of CV surveys, Table 6.5 provides a guide of the type of information that should, at the very least, be included in a CV study report. By including this information, it will help to better communicate study methods more generally and indeed facilitate comparisons across interventions that have been evaluated as part of a CBA. Also refer to Chapter 12 for a practical guide to reporting and presenting stated preference results within a CBA.

Table 6.5 Checklist for reporting a CV survey

Elements of study	What should be reported
Study design	
1. Statement of objective	There should be a clear statement of the objective of the study with respect to whether a full CBA is being conducted or whether CV is being used solely as a measure of value.
2. Scenario description	Details of information provided to frame the scenario and communicate risk to the respondent.
3. Payment vehicle	Details of the type of payment asked of respondent and the timing of the payment structure.
4. Perspective	The perspective of the survey should be clearly stated with details on whether an equivalent or compensating variation is being measured.
5. Facilitation method	There should be a clear description of the type of facilitation method.
6. Sample recruitment	The rationale for the chosen sample, e.g. patients/general population should be clearly explained.
7. Country of origin	For facilitation of comparison of CV studies the country of origin along with currency should be clearly stated.
8. Price year	The year in which the study was conducted along with the price year should be clearly stated.
9. Elicitation method	The type of elicitation method should be specified and justified.
Data collected	
10. Socio-demographic and economic characteristics	All socio-demographic and economic characteristics collected should be clearly explained.
	Details on how information on 'ability to pay' was collected should be specified.
11. Qualitative information	Methods for collecting qualitative information should be transparent.
Analytical methods	
12. Qualitative information	Methods for analysing qualitative data should be transparent and it should be clear how the data has been used to understand/predict CV values.
13. Regression model	All regression methodology should be described and based on justifiable statistical methods.
	Details on how data has been coded for the regression should be clearly specified.
14. Average CV values	Methods applied to calculate average CV values from data, where appropriate, should be transparent and based on justifiable statistical methods.
Results	
15. Average CV values	Both mean and median WTP values should be reported along with data to allow the reader to understand the distribution of data.
16. Costs	Depending on the objective of the study, the costs of the intervention/programme should be reported to facilitate computation of the NSB.
17. Net social benefit (NSB)	Where appropriate, details of the NSB should be reported.

References

1. Gerard, K., and Mooney, G. 1993. QALY league tables: handle with care. *Health Economics* **2**(1): 59–64.

2. Mooney, G. 1994. *Key issues in health economics*. London: Harvester Wheatsheaf.

3. Ryan, M., and Shackley, P. 1995. Assessing the benefits of health care: how far should we go? *Quality in Health Care* **4**(3): 207–213.

4. Hanemann, W.M. 1992. In: Navrud, S., editor. *Preface. Pricing the European environment*. Oslo: Scandinavian University Press.

5. Acton, J.P. 1976. *Evaluating public programs to save lives: the case of heart attacks*. Santa Monica: RAND Corporation. Report No.: R950RC.

6. Olsen, J.A., and Smith, R.D. 2001. Theory versus practice: a review of 'willingness to pay' in health and health care. *Health Economics* **10**: 39–52.

7. Sach, T.H., Smith, R.D., and Whynes, D.K. 2007. A 'league table' of contingent valuation results for pharmaceutical interventions. A Hard pill to Swallow? *Pharmacoeconomics* **25**(2): 107–127.

8. Arrow, K., and Solow, R., *et al*. 1993. *Report of the NOAA panel of contingent valuation*. Federal Register Washington, DC **58**(4601): 4614.

9. Smith, R.D. 2000. The discrete-choice willingness-to-pay question format in health economics: Should we adopt environmental guidelines? *Medical Decision Making* **20**: 194–206.

10. Smith, R.D. 2003. Construction of the contingent valuation market in health care: a critical assessment. *Health Economics* **12**: 609–628.

11. Mitchell, R., and Carson, R. 1989. *Using surveys to value public goods: the contingent valuation method*. Washington, DC: Resources for the Future.

12. Lloyd, A.J. 2003. Threats to the estimation of benefit: are preference elicitation methods accurate? *Health Economics* **12**: 393–402.

13. Gigerenzer, G. 1996. The psychology of good judgment: frequency formats and simple algorithms. *Medical Decision Making* **16**: 273–280.

14. Muller, A., and Reutzel, T.J. 1984. Willingness to pay for reduction in fatality risk: An exploratory survey. *American Journal Public Health* **74**: 818–812.

15. Brookshire, D., and d'Arge, R., *et al*. 1981. Experiments in valuing public goods. In: Smith, V., editor. *Advances in Applied Microeconomics*. Connecticut: JAI Press.

16. Greenley, D.A., Walsh, A.G., and Young, R.A. 1981. Option value: empirical evidence from a case study of recreation and water quality. *Quarterly Journal of Economics* **95**: 657–673.

17. Chestnut, L., Keller, L., *et al*. 1996. Willingness to pay for changes in angina symptoms. *Medical Decision Making* **16**: 248–253.

18. Lindholm, L., Rosen, M., *et al*. 1994. Are people willing to pay for a community-based preventative program. *International Journal of Technology Assessment in Health Care* **10**: 317–324.

19. Dixon, S., and Shackley, P. 1998. *Using contingent valuation to elicit public preferences for water fluoridation*. Galway: Oral Presentation at the Health Economists Study Group Conference (HESG).

20. Liu, J.T., Hammitt, J.K., Wang, J.D., and Liu, J.L. 2000. Mother's willingness to pay for her own and her child's health: A contingent valuation study in Taiwan. *Health Economics* **9**: 319–326.

21. Klose, T. 1999. The contingent valuation method in health care. *Health Policy* **47**: 97–123.

22. Neumann, P., and Johannesson, M. 1994. The willingness to pay for in vitro fertilisation: a pilot study using contingent valuation. *Medical Care* **32**: 686.

23. O'Brien, B., and Viramontes, J.L. 1994. Willingness to pay: A valid and reliable measure of health state preference? *Medical Decision Making* **14**: 289–297.

24. Ortega, A., Dranitsaris, G., and Puodziumas, A.L.V. 1998. What are cancer patients willing to pay for prophylactic epoetin alfa? *Cancer* **83**: 2588–2596.

24a. NICE, 2004. *Guide to the methods of technology appraisal*. National Institute for Health and Clinical Excellence: London.

24b. Brazier, J., Akehurst, R., Brennan, A., *et al.* 2005. Should patients have a greater role in valuing health states. *Applied Health Economics and Health Policy* **4**(4): 201–208.

24c. Mann, R., Brazier, J., and Tsuchiya, A. 2009. A comparison of patient and general population weightings of EQ-5D dimensions. *Health Economics Letters* **18**: 363–372.

25. Reardon, G., and Pathak, D.S. 1989. Contingent valuation of pharmaceuticals and pharmacy services – Methodological considerations. *Journal of Social and Administrative Pharmacy* **6**(2): 83–91.

25a. Arrow, K., Solow, R., Portney, P., Leamer, E., Radner, R., and Schuman, H. 1993. *Report of the NOAA panel on contingent valuation*. Washington: National Oceanic and Atmospheric Administration.

26. Davis, R.K. 1964. *The value of big game hunting in a private forest*. Transactions of the 29th North American Wildlife and Natural Resources Conference, Washington, DC: Wildlife Management Institute.

27. Cummings, R.G., Brookshire, D.S., *et al.* 1986. *Valuing environmental goods: a state of the arts assessment of the contingent valuation method*. Totwa, NJ: Rowman & Allanheld.

28. Hoehn, J.P., and Randall, A. 1987. A satisfactory benefit cost indicator from contingent valuation. *Journal of Environmental Economics & Management* **14**: 226–247.

29. Bateman, I., Willis, K., and Garrod, G. 2004. *Consistency between CV estimates. A comparison of 2 studies of UK national parks*. Report No.: working paper 40.

30. Mitchell, R.C., and Carson, R.T. 1981. *An experiment in determining willingness to pay for national water quality improvements*. Washington, DC: U.S. Environmental Protection Agency.

31. Mitchell, R.C., and Carson, R.T. 1984. *A contingent valuation estimate of national freshwater benefits: Technical Report to the US Environmental Protection Agency*. Washington, DC: Resources for the Future.

32. Bishop, R.C., and Heberlein, T.A. 1979. Measuring values of extra market goods: are indirect measures biased? *Natural Resources Journal* **23**: 619–633.

33. Cameron, T.A. 1988. A new paradigm for valuing non-market goods using referendum data: maximum likelihood estimation by censored logistic regression. *Journal of Environmental Economics and Management* **15**: 355–379.

34. Hanemann, W.M. 1994. Valuing the environment through contingent valuation. *Journal of Economic Perspectives* **8**(4): 19–43.

35. Carson, R.T., Hanemann, W.M., *et al.* 1986. *Determining the demand for public goods by simulating referendums at different tax prices*. San Diego, CA: University of California.

36. Langford, I.H., Bateman, I.J., *et al.* 1996. A multilevel modelling approach to triple bounded dichotomous choice contingent valuation. *Environmental and Resource Economics* **7**: 197–211.

37. Donaldson, C., Hundley, V., and Mapp, T. 1998. Willingness to pay: A method for measuring preferences for maternity care? *Birth* **25**(1): 32–39.

38. Johannesson, M.B., Jonsson, B., *et al.* 1991. Willingness to pay for antihypertensive therapy: results of a Swedish pilot study. *Journal of Health Economics* **10**: 461–474.

39. Narbro, K., and Sjöström, L. 2000. Willingness to pay for obesity treatment. *International Journal of Technology Assessment in Health Care* **16**(1): 50–59.

40. Ramsey, S.D., Sullivan, S.D., Psaty, B.M., and Patrick, D.L. 1997. Willingness to pay for anti-hypertensive care: Evidence from a staff-model HMO. *Social Science and Medicine* **44**(12): 1911–1917.

41. Slothuus, U., Larsen, M.L., and Junker, P. 2000. Willingness to pay for arthritis symptom alleviation. *International Journal of Technology Assessment in Health Care* **16**(1): 60–72.

42. Stalhammer, N. 1996. An empirical note on willingness to pay and starting point bias. *Medical Decision Making* **16**: 242–247.

43. Eastaugh, S.R. 2000. Willingness to pay in treatment of bleeding disorders. *International Journal of Technology Assessment in Health Care* **16**(2): 706–710.

44. Boyle, K., Bishop, R., *et al.* 1985. Starting point bias in contingent valuation bidding games. *Land Economics* **61**: 188–194.

45. Brown, T.C., Champ, P.A., *et al.* 1996. Which response format reveals the truth about donations to a public good? *Land Economics* **62**: 478–488.

46. Kealy, M.J., and Turner, R.W. 1993. A test of the equality of closed-ended and open-ended contingent valuations. *American Journal of Agricultural Economics* **75**: 321–331.

47. Seller, C., Stoll, J.R., *et al.* Validation of empirical measures of welfare change: A comparison of nonmarket techniques. *Land Economics* **61**: 156–175.

48. Frew, E.J., Whynes, D.K., and Wolstenholme, J. 2003. Eliciting willingness to pay: comparing closed-ended with open-ended and payment scale formats. *Medical Decision Making* **23**: 150–159.

49. Whynes, D.K., Wolstenholme, J.L., and Frew, E. 2004. Evidence of range bias in contingent valuation payment scales. *Health Economics* **13**: 183–190.

50. Bohm, P. 1972. Estimating demand for public goods: an experiment. *European Economic Review* **3**: 111–130.

51. Milon, J. 1989. Contingent valuation experiments for strategic behaviour. *Journal of Environmental Economics and Management* **17**: 293–308.

52. Smith, V.L. 1979. An experimental comparison of three public good decision mechanisms. *Scandinavian Journal of Economics* **81**: 198–215.

53. Diamond, P.A., and Hausman, J.A. 1994. Contingent valuation: is some number better than no number? *Journal of Economic Perspectives* **8**(4): 45–64.

54. Dalmau-Matarrodona, E. 2001. Alternative approaches to obtain optimal bid values in contingent valuation studies and to model protest zeros. Estimating the determinants of individuals' willingness to pay for home care services in day case surgery. *Health Economics* **10**: 101–118.

55. Stewart, J.M., O'Shea, E., Donaldson, C., and Shackley, P. 2002. Do ordering effects matter in willingness-to-pay studies of health care? *Journal of Health Economics* **21**: 585–599.

56. Kahnemann, D., and Knetsch, J.L. 1992. Valuing public goods: the purchase of moral satisfaction. *Journal of Environmental Economics and Management* **22**: 57–70.

57. Andreoni, J. 1989. Giving with impure altruism: applications to charity and ricardian equivalence. *Journal of Political Economy* **97**: 1447–1458.

58. Andreoni, J. 1990. Impure altruism and donations to public goods: A theory of warm-glow giving. *Economic Journal* **100**: 464–477.

59. Diamond, P.A., and Hausman, J.A. 1992. *On contingent valuation measurements of non-use values*. Massachusetts, MIT Working Paper.

60. Slovic, P. 1995. The construction of preference. *American Psychology* **50**(5): 364–371.

61. Cubitt, R., Munro, A., and Starmer, C. 2004. *Preference reversal: An experimental investigation of economic and psychological hypotheses*. Working paper at UEA.

62. Bassett, G.W. 1997. *The St Petersburg paradox and bounded utility. Expected utility, fair gambles and rational choice*. Cheltenham: Elgar Reference Collection, pp. 181–187.

63. Shiell, A., Seymour, J., Hawe, P., and Cameron, S. 2000. Are preferences over health states complete? *Health Economics* **9**: 47–55.

64. Loomes, G., and Sugden, R. 1982. Regret Theory: An alternative theory of rational choice under uncertainty. *Economic Journal* **92**(368): 805–824.

65. Fischhoff, B., Bostrom, A., and Quadrel, M.J. 1993. Risk perception and communication. *Annual Review of Public Health* **14**: 183–203.

Chapter 7

Benefit assessment for cost–benefit analysis studies in health care: A guide to carrying out a stated preference willingness to pay survey in health care

Emma J. Frew

7.1 Introduction

Chapter 6 focused upon the design elements of constructing a contingent valuation (CV) survey with particular emphasis upon the biases inherent within the survey method. This chapter will discuss and illustrate the techniques that are useful for the analyses of CV data. Illustrative examples of the methods that can be used to analyse different types of CV data are provided with particular emphasis upon the presentation of socio-demographic and economic variables, preference groups, qualitative information, regression analyses, and average willingness to pay (WTP).

Throughout this chapter, we will be using a series of WTP sample datasets that are available to download from the website of the Health Economics Research Centre at the University of Oxford (www.herc.ox.ac.uk/books/cba/support).

These datasets have been adapted from survey data collected as part of a study designed to measure the value of colorectal cancer (CRC) screening in the UK (1). The datasets have been purposively adapted to demonstrate the unique features of WTP data and to provide examples to illustrate the methods required for WTP analyses.

7.2 Background to the study

To understand the rationale behind the analytical methods that are described in this chapter, we will begin by providing a brief background into the study whose sample data will be used for the analyses. This study elicited WTP values for two different screening tests for CRC: faecal occult blood testing (FOB) and flexible sigmoidoscopy (FS). Briefly, the FOB protocol provides screening once every 2 years from the age of 50–74 years old. The tests are carried out at home and require small stool samples to be taken, placed on special paper within the test kit and then returned to the patient's local General Practitioner. The FS protocol involves a one-off screen for all people aged

60–65 years and is a thin flexible sigmoidoscope that is inserted into the colon to look for bowel polyps. This is done at the local hospital clinic and no anaesthetic is required. Both these screening protocols have the same objective (detecting CRC) but have quite different processes of care, e.g. differences in patient time (amount of time required to complete test) and invasiveness (home versus hospital). The objective of the study therefore was to explore attitudes towards CRC screening in general and more specifically towards each of the two screening tests. The following sections describe a step-by-step process of designing, analysing, and presenting the results of this CV survey.

7.3 Description of study design

In the CRC study, we used a sample from the general population, data was collected using a mail-based questionnaire, CV values were elicited using the open-ended and payment scale method from an ex-ante, WTP perspective. Box 7.1 in Appendix 7.1 provides full details of the study design.

Within every CV study, it is standard practice to collect information on respondent socio-demographic and economic data so that we are in a position to draw inferences about what factors are influencing/determining the CV values. At the very least, these data will be on respondent age, gender, and ability to pay (ATP). A variety of different question formats have been used to collect information on ATP such as direct questions about personal income or on social class (to be used as proxy for ATP). In the CRC study, we framed the question to reveal information about household income, see Box 7.1.

We provided a 'tick box' option so that respondents do not feel that they are revealing too much information. Alternatively, if the CV study was designed to recruit students as the study population then a question on household income would be no longer relevant and a better way of framing the question would be as shown in Box 7.2.

There are always going to be sensitivity issues around questions related to ability to pay and this should be borne in mind when considering the best way of framing the question. Clearly, a trade off exists between direct open-ended questions about personal income versus vague questions that do not provide enough information. 'Tick box' responses are vague enough to place the respondent at ease whilst being suitably informative for data analysis.

Box 7.1 Annual income question

Could you please estimate the annual income of your household before deducting tax and national insurance? (If you receive any benefits or pensions include them as income).

(please tick the appropriate box)

❑   Less than £10,000
❑   £10,000 –20,000
❑   £20,001–30,000
❑   £30,001–above

Box 7.2 Alternative example of income question

Which of these statements best describes your situation with regards to money?
- ❏ I normally have enough money for anything I want
- ❏ I have enough money, so long as I plan my spending carefully
- ❏ I have enough money for basic things, but I can't afford anything unnecessary
- ❏ Sometimes it is hard for me to afford even the basic things I need

Other socio-demographic and economic information collected will relate to the objective of the survey and what factors are felt to have a potential influence upon WTP. Table 7.1 provides a list of all the socio-demographic and economic questions asked as part of the CRC study and with the exception of the questions relating to age, each were framed as 'tick box' questions for ease of response.

When reporting the CV survey, details of how these questions are asked (and also the rationale for asking them) should be clearly explained. If using 'tick box' questions, details of the scale used should be provided, e.g. in the CRC study individuals were asked to rate their own perceived health status using a four-point scale defined as: poor, fair, good, and excellent.

7.4 Response rate and sample characteristics

It is good practice with every study design to report details on the response rate and sample characteristics. However, what is unique to CV surveys and potentially very useful is to provide information on the specific response to the CV section of the survey. This is because it is possible for individuals to respond to all other sections of the questionnaire/interview but to leave the CV section blank, and it is interesting to explore who these individuals are and why they are responding in this manner. For example in the CRC study, 554 respondents (20%) failed to complete either of the CV questions and a further 293 (10.6%) completed only one. When comparing the

Table 7.1 Example of socio-demographic and economic questions

Respondent circumstances	Feelings/attitude towards health and screening
Gender	Experience with health problems
Age	Current health
Ethnic origin	Smoking status
Marital status	Number of GP visits in last year
Number of children	Number of dental visits in last 2 years
Employment status	Screening behaviour
Household income	Attitude towards exercising, eating healthily
Education age	Attitude towards bowel cancer

value placed on two alternative interventions (such as in the CRC study) it is important to check that there are no significant differences in terms of socio-demographic characteristics between the two preference groups. This can be done using standard statistical tests such as the Chi-squared, Fisher's exact test (categorical variables), and the ANOVA test (continuous variables).

7.5 Analysing the reasons for WTP

Before moving on to describe the quantitative analysis of WTP values, this section will explain how to analyse the qualitative reasons provided. After the CV section of the questionnaire, it is useful to include a question that asks respondents to provide reasons explaining why they are WTP for the good/service being evaluated. Ideally, this should be in the form of an open-ended question to allow the individual to respond freely. However, it can be designed as a 'tick box' question with possible reasons listed. Depending on the size of the survey this can produce a vast amount of data that has the potential to validate (or invalidate) the WTP response.

To describe the methods used to analyse qualitative reasons, we will use the CRC study as an example. This example by no means provides an exhaustive list of possible methodological techniques that can be used to analyse qualitative data, rather it gives one well-worked example of an application within the CV context. Before presenting the qualitative results, information on the numbers of respondents providing reasons needs to be provided. Within the CRC study, of the 1919 subjects who offered, a WTP for both FOB and FS testing, 1,270 (66.2%) entered a written explanation. Most of the reasons provided were brief and ranged from a few words to one or two sentences. To analyse these reasons, we used a technique known as 'content analysis' whereby each member of the research team read several hundred responses selected at random, identified themes or categories of explanation, and then endeavoured to position a new sub-sample within this framework. The themes were then repeatedly re-worked between the team members as and when individual inconsistencies in existing coding appeared to arise. In total, we identified nine broad categories of explanation and these are listed in Table 7.2 along with examples of the reasons provided for each category.

Once these reasons had been coded they were inserted back into the main SPSS database by creating a separate dichotomous variable for each reason (1 = reason given; 0 = otherwise). This then put us in a position where we could combine them with the full analysis. In the write-up of the study, we explained that the reasons reported in the table came from reasons offered from the entire sample thus included comments from respondents who had provided no or zero, as well as positive WTP values.

7.6 Quantitative WTP analysis: Open-ended and payment scale

7.6.1 Sorting the dataset

Regression analysis is often used to describe factors and socio-demographic variables that are influencing WTP. Survey data in its raw form usually requires some degree of sorting before being in a form ready for regression analysis. It is worth considering the

Table 7.2 Explanations of WTP valuations

Category	Type of explanation provided
E1	**Question deemed in-applicable, on the grounds of:** Subject's age Possession of private health insurance
E2	**Subject expressed difficulties in estimating WTP owing to:** Ignorance of cost Uncertainty of future financial circumstances *Difficult to answer* *You can't put a price on health* Other
E3	**WTP estimate based on a nominal amount** Token or arbitrary sum Guess
E4	**WTP reflects ability to pay (affordability)** Stated WTP constrained by pensioners' ability to pay Stated value is that which everyone ought to be able to pay Maximum affordable, given current income/unemployment An amount affordable within the subject's present means An affordable amount, without further specification
E5	**WTP reflects a fair, acceptable, or reasonable value** The NHS should pay but this would be an acceptable limit Subject is happy/willing to make this contribution to NHS costs An acceptable value, as everyone could afford this amount An acceptable amount, without further specification
E6	**WTP reflects costs of screening** Subject attempted to estimate likely resource costs required Current dental/optical charges used as comparator Other
E7	**WTP reflects perceived benefit of screening** Screening deemed worthwhile, given recognized benefits Reassurance and *peace of mind* *Screening offers early detection of disease* *Screening can save money for the NHS*
E8	**Reported familial experience of CRC**
E9	**Protest expressed at the idea of payment** *Having paid taxes, one shouldn't have to pay more* *Screening is vital and must be free* *The NHS should bear the costs* *The service should be free, to encourage use* *Free tests will benefit the NHS by cost saving*
Total	

type of variables collected as part of the survey and giving some thought as to whether they can be recoded for better use. 'Tick box' responses for example might be better recoded as dummy variables or as dichotomous variables. It may be useful to aggregate the responses to a group of questions to provide one common variable, for example in the CRC study a 'health motivation' score was created from responses to four questions related to: healthy eating, exercising, and importance placed on being screened regularly for breast and cervical cancer.

7.6.2 **The regression analysis**

This section will use the data stored within the 'WTP dataset_open-ended and payment scale' SPSS spreadsheet available to download from the Oxford University website (www.herc.ox.ac.uk/books/cba/support). Before embarking on the exercises below, it may be worth taking some time to familiarize yourself with the dataset and the coding of the variables. Each variable has been clearly labelled with the values specified.

The first stage of the analysis is to think about the classes of response to a WTP question. When using the open-ended and payment scale elicitation formats, there are three classes of response: 1. No WTP value offered (no response), 2. Zero WTP, and 3. Positive WTP. By employing multi-stage estimation (2), each class of response can become the dependent variable in a suite of regression models. Using the CRC dataset we will demonstrate how this is done. For each regression model a common set of independent variables as provided by the data capture instrument is used. The set comprised the following variables:

- Socio-economic data: gender, age, age on leaving full-time education, household income (four dummy variables, with that most frequently reported, £10,000–20,000, being excluded from the regression models).

- Attitudes towards prevention: number of visits to the dentist over the past 2 years, whether the subject smoked, health motivation score. As a working hypothesis, a more positive attitude towards preventative medicine generally (and therefore potentially towards screening for CRC in particular) would be signalled by increased frequency of dental visits, and/or being a non-smoker, and/or a higher health motivation score.

- Attitudes towards CRC: whether the subject was worried about the disease (dummy = 1 if no worries expressed) and whether they perceived their chances of contracting it to be above average (dummy = 1). Intuition would lead us to expect higher WTP values from those worried and/or perceiving themselves to be particularly at risk, ceteris paribus.

- Experience: whether or not the subject had previous experience of either type of colorectal screening (dummies for each).

- Preferences: as expressed over the choice of preferred screening test, FOB or FS (dummy = 1 if that particular test was preferred).

- CV format: open-ended or payment scale (dummy variable, payment scale = 1)

◆ Explanations: as from Table 7.2 (dummy variables for E1–E9, including an additional dummy for 'no reasons offered'). E4 was excluded from the models on the grounds that it was the reason most commonly cited and that affordability would be picked up by the income variables.

1. *Non response* and 2. *Zero CVs*

As outlined above, it is important to determine the characteristics of the respondents not responding to the WTP questions. These are individuals who have completed all parts of the questionnaire apart from the WTP section. To do this we need to run a logistic regression with the dependent variable reflecting the non-response to both the FOB and FS WTP question (labelled fob_resp and fs_resp in the dataset: 1= non-response; 0=otherwise). Box 7.3 provides the set of instructions to run the logistic regression within the SPSS dataset.

We also want to determine the characteristics of respondents who are providing zero WTP values for either the FOB or FS test. To do this run, the same model as explained in Box 7.3 only instead of inserting FOB_resp (FOB non-response model) and FS_resp (FS non-response model) insert zero FOB and zero FS as the dependent variables for the FOB and FS model, respectively. Throughout the models, the covariates remain the same. Table 7.3 illustrates the results for both sets of regressions.

Table 7.3 tells us that for FOB, no response was more probable if respondents had a preference for FS, if they deemed the WTP questions inapplicable or more difficult to answer and if they registered a protest vote. No response was less likely if they deemed their chosen WTP to be more acceptable, had more visits to the dentist and expressed a preference for FOB. Similar results are found for FS, with slight variations, respondents who regard their WTP to be a token amount and who are from a higher income bracket, who are non-smokers, and who believe that their chances of developing CRC are greater than average are more likely to respond to the WTP question. All these results appeal to intuition. We can interpret the results from Table 7.3 in a similar

---

Box 7.3 Performing a logistic regression on WTP response data

Click on analyse/regression/binary logistic.

Enter FOB_resp as the dependent variable.

Enter the following variables as covariates: gender, age, edu_age, dum_inc1, dum_inc3, dum_inc4, den_visi, dum_smok, h_motiv, dum_worr, dum_chanc, dum_fob, dum_fs, dum_prFOB, dum_prFS, op_pay, code_1, code_2, code_3, code_5, code_6, code_7, code_8, code_9

(All these variables cover the full list described above).

Enter method: Backward conditional. Click OK.

Follow the above instructions again inserting FS_resp as the dependent variable for the FS model.

Table 7.3 Logistic regression – predicting non-response and zero values

	Dependent: non-response (=1)						Dependent: zero WTP value (=1)					
	FOB			FS			FOB			FS		
	b	S.E.	exp(*b*)	*B*	S.E.	exp(*b*)	*b*	S.E.	exp(*b*)	*b*	S.E.	exp(*b*)
Format (payment scale = 1)	−1.427	0.225	0.240	−0.750	0.181	0.473						
	1.857	0.395	6.405	2.414	0.358	11.176						
E1 (applicable)	2.183	0.244	8.873									
E2 (difficulties)	−1.914	0.609	0.147	−1.129	0.633	0.323	−18.953	5343.87	0.000	−19.325	5302.31	0.000
E3 (token amount)	−0.576	0.334	0.562	−0.610	0.332	0.543	−18.541	3097.12	0.000	−2.643	1.021	0.071
E5 (acceptable value)							−1.515	0.609	0.220	−1.291	0.541	0.275
E6 (cost)	−0.594	0.325	0.552				−1.760	0.735	0.172	−2.067	0.737	0.127
E7 (benefit)	0.610	0.254	1.841	0.490	0.212	1.632	2.020	0.265	7.537	1.958	0.251	7.088
E9 (protest)	0.015	0.008	1.015	0.036	0.007	1.037	−0.017	0.265	0.983	−0.025	0.010	0.975
Age												
Income												
<£10 k				−0.553	0.254	0.575				0.598	0.292	1.818
>£30 k												
Age leaving education	−0.127	0.062	4.112	−0.099	0.054	0.906	−0.176	0.075	0.839	−0.184	0.074	0.832
Visits to the dentist	0.574	0.254	5.092	0.547	0.223	1.728						
Current smoker (1 = yes)	−0.457	0.232	0.633	−0.988	0.305	0.372						
Chances above average				0.880	0.305	2.410				0.550	0.243	1.733
Preference for FOB	0.739	0.283	2.095									
Preference for FS							−18.192	6481.38	0.000	−18.414	6805.91	0.000
Had FOB (1 = yes)	−2.362	0.537	0.094	−3.647	0.495	0.026	−1.507	0.590	0.222	−1.258	0.587	0.284
Constant	0.297			0.288			0.306			0.319		
Nagelkerke *R*²												

fashion for the zero WTP logistic regression drawing inferences about the characteristics of individuals who are more likely to respond with a zero valuation for FOB and FS screening. These results help us to understand what 'type' of respondent is more likely to provide a no or a zero response to the WTP question.

3. Positive WTP values

Once we have explored the non-responders and the zero WTP responders, the analysis progresses to explore the distribution of positive WTP valuations. To provide a clear presentation of the nature of the WTP distribution, standard descriptive statistics can be used such as the mean, median, mode, and coefficients of skew. For example, Box 7.4 describes the SPSS commands to derive the information contained within Table 7.4.

In this example, as is commonly the case with WTP information the distribution is skewed, therefore prior to regression analysis it is appropriate to transform the data to natural logarithms. Box 7.5 describes how to do this using the SPSS datasheet.

Box 7.4 WTP descriptive statistics

Click on analyse/descriptive statistics/frequencies. Select the WTP_FOB and WTP_FS variables into the variable box. Click on statistics and select mean, median, mode. Select percentile and specify 20 and 90. Select skewness.

Table 7.4 WTP distribution: descriptive statistics

Statistics	WTP for FOB (£)	WTP for FS (£)
Mean	104	88
Median	50	50
Mode	50	50
Coefficients of skewness	22	39
Percentiles		
• 20	10	10
• 90	200	200

Box 7.5 Transforming the WTP data to natural logarithms

Click on transform/compute. In the target variable box, type log_fob. Select the function 'Ln' and insert into the numeric expression box. Select WTP_FOB variable and insert into the numeric expression box: Ln(WTP_FOB). Click on OK. Perform the same steps for the WTP_FS variable calling the new variable, Log_FS.

Box 7.6 Running a linear regression on the WTP data

Click on analyse/regression/linear.

Enter log_fob as the dependent variable. Enter the following variables as independents: gender, age, edu_age, dum_inc1, dum_inc3, dum_inc4, den_visi, dum_smok, h_motiv, dum_worr, dum_chanc, dum_fob, dum_fs, dum_prFOB, dum_prFS, op_pay, code_1, code_2, code_3, code_5, code_6, code_7, code_8, code_9 (All these variables cover the full list described above).

Enter method: Backward. Click OK.

Follow the above instructions again inserting log_fs as the dependent variable for the FS model.

Table 7.5 Linear regression for positive WTP values (natural logarithms)

	FOB		FS	
	b	**S.E.**	**b**	**S.E.**
Constant	2.580	0.308	2.937	0.158
Elicitation format	0.259	0.073	0.600	0.066
Gender	0.188	0.078		
Education age			0.018	0.007
Income				
£20–30 k	0.250	0.091	0.316	0.082
>£30 k	0.388	0.097	0.464	0.086
Visits to dentist	0.052	0.023	0.045	0.021
Health motivation score	0.156	0.070		
	0.190	0.106		
Chances above average	0.493	0.120		
	0.228	0.099		
E2(difficulties)	0.440	0.095	0.331	0.086
E6 (cost)	0.588	0.188	0.530	0.170
E7 (benefits)	−0.288	0.090	−0.332	0.082
E8 (family experience)			−0.250	0.087
			−0.112	0.067
E9 (protest)	0.112		0.177	
Smoker				
Preference for FOB				
Adjusted R^2				

To describe the positive WTP values, standard linear regression analysis is applied using the log_WTP variables as the dependant variables and the same set of independent variables used for the logistic regression analysis listed earlier. To perform these linear regressions, follow the instructions in Box 7.6. The results are displayed in Table 7.5.

Despite the large sample size of our dataset alongside the log-transformation of the dependent variable, it is worth noting that the goodness-of-fit of the regression models is still remarkably low. It therefore appears that despite our inclusion of many potential explanatory variables, and the significant coefficients associated with those with intuitive appeal, there is a considerable amount of noise in the WTP data. To explore the WTP data further it is useful to plot the demand curves.

7.7 Demand curves using WTP data

The most straightforward method of producing a demand curve from WTP data is to use Microsoft Excel. For an example of how to do this, please download the Excel worksheet: WTP demand curve from the Oxford University website (www.herc.ox.ac.uk/books/cba/support). The data contained within this spreadsheet is from the CRC study and has been obtained from the SPSS dataset: open-ended and payment scale. To construct the demand curves, we require two sets of data from the SPSS dataset: 1. The WTP value and 2. The proportion WTP for FOB and FS. To obtain this information, we use the descriptive statistics command in SPSS and ask for the frequencies of the WTP_FOB and the WTP_FS variables. These tables can then be simply copied and pasted into the Excel spreadsheet. Once you have this information within the Excel spreadsheet, it is then simply a case of manipulating it to produce a column of values reflecting the total proportion of the sample that are WTP at each price level. So, the numbers will be arranged as shown in Box 7.7.

You will see from the Excel spreadsheet that for illustrative purposes for the graph, the range of WTP values have been restricted to £0–5000, this is of course optional and can be easily varied to include the full range of values. Using the graph function with Excel, the demand curve can be plotted and is illustrated in Figure 7.1.

Each demand curve has the appearance of a demand curve that is frequently encountered for normal goods providing reassurance that the WTP demand curve for CRC screening is not particularly unusual.

Box 7.7 WTP proportions

Value	Proportion WTP FOB	Proportion WTP FS
0	90.7%	88.9%
5	86.7%	85.4%
10	75.2%	77%
–	–	–
5,000	0.04%	0.05%

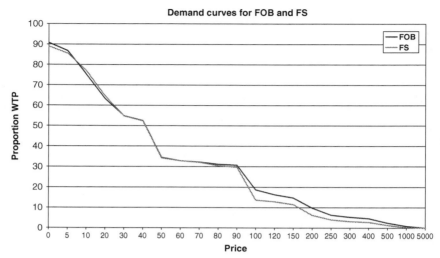

Fig. 7.1 WTP demand curve.

7.8 **Preferences and WTP**

Chapter 6 discussed the concept of preference reversal within the context of CV. It is logical to assume that to be consistent, all respondents must provide a greater WTP value for their most over their least preferred test. To explore this effect using data from the CRC study, we need to categorize the WTP values for each of the preference groups. Note that this analysis will only be done on those respondents who indicated a preference for a test and who provided a WTP value for both the FOB and the FS test ($n = 1,902$). This can be done within SPSS by using the Descriptive Statistics/Crosstabs function and by inserting WTP_direc and prefer variables.

Table 7.6 shows that for the 10% of respondents that preferred the FOB test, they were WTP more for the FS test and for the 3% that preferred the FS test, they were WTP more for the FOB test. Plausible reasons for an inconsistent response suggest that an attempt to estimate the resource cost of the test and difficulties in understanding the WTP task can increase the likelihood of inconsistency occurring (3). To explore this

Table 7.6 WTP for preference groups

Preference Group	Is WTP FOB > WTP FS?			
	No (%)	Equal (%)	Yes (%)	Total (%)
FOB	199 (10)	433 (23)	200 (10)	832 (44)
FS	82 (4)	125 (7)	49 (3)	256 (13)
No preference	185 (10)	442 (23)	187 (10)	814 (43)
Total	465 (24)	1,000 (53)	437 (23)	1,902 (100)

effect, we can isolate these responses from the rest of the sample and explore the qualitative reasons provided. However, it is equally plausible that these inconsistent responses arise through random error whereby the respondents answered in an inconsistent manner due to lack of concentration, attentiveness, or 'by mistake'. Harless and Camerer incorporate an error rate into their analyses of different theories to explain violations of expected utility theory in order to take account of systematic variation in responses that are inconsistent (4). If we assume that in both choice and valuation tasks there is a probability e that individuals will behave contrary to their true preferences. This means that in the choice task for example, and assuming that the true preference is for the FOB test, that the probability that the FOB test will be chosen is $1 - e$ and the probability that the FS test will be chosen is e. Taking both choice and valuation tasks together, there is therefore a $2e(1 - e)$ probability of responses being inconsistent between the tasks in either direction. We know from the above results that 10% of the sample chose FOB as their preferred test yet gave a higher WTP value for the FS test, and that 3% chose FS yet gave a higher WTP value for the FOB test. It therefore follows that if $2e(1 - e) = 13\%$ then the error probability within this study is equal to 7%. Thus using the Harless and Camerer account of behaviour, there is a 7% probability that individuals in this study will behave contrary to their true preferences.

7.9 WTP analysis: Further elicitation methods

So far, we have described a WTP analysis using the open-ended and payment scale format however these are just two means of eliciting WTP that can be measured using a variety of different formats. The following sections focus on the analysis of WTP when elicited using a closed-ended (CE) and an iterative bidding (IB) format (both described in Chapter 6). Throughout, the CRC example will continue to be used with the following SPSS datasets available to download from the website: (www.herc.ox. ac.uk/books/cba/support: WTP Dataset_closed-ended and WTP Dataset_iterative bidding). These datasets contain information derived from two further studies that sought to measure the WTP for CRC screening using the same set of questions as before (in the open-ended and payment scale study) with the only difference being the WTP elicitation design. The following sections will focus purely on the aspects of analysis that are particular to the CE and IB design and these methods should be combined with the general analysis already described above, i.e. analysis of respondent demographics, qualitative reasons, preference groups, etc. to form a full WTP analysis.

7.10 Closed-ended data

7.10.1 Choosing the bid values and distributing the questionnaire

When adopting the closed-ended format (CE), the rationale for the bid amounts chosen ideally should be based on a pilot study with one of the offer amounts being set at the median value elicited (5). In the case of the CRC example, the open-ended and payment scale data informed the basis of the bid values chosen for the closed-ended design. We chose the £50 median value as one of the offer values and four more, spaced more-or-less symmetrically across the distribution. These were £10, £25, £100, and £200, located at the 15th, 37th, 75th, and 90th percentile of the open-ended, payment scale data. Equal numbers of questionnaires at each of the five bid levels were distributed at random. Qualitative reasons for the WTP values were also sought and this was done separately for the FOB and the FS test.

7.10.2 'Yea-saying'

The CE format can be susceptible to the 'yea-saying' effect where respondents continually say 'yes' regardless of the bid value offered. This was found to be the case in the CRC example as analysis of the data revealed that even the largest offer value (£200) had attracted a very high proportion of acceptances. By using the descriptive statistics/cross tabs function within the SPSS dataset and entering the bid_value into the row and the wtp_fob and wtp_fs variables into the column section you will see that 88.4% and 72.5% of the sample are still saying 'yes' at £200 for the FOB and FS test, respectively. As a direct result of this response, more questionnaires were distributed in an identical manner, this time using bid values of £500 and £1,000. The data obtained from this additional element of the study was incorporated into the main closed-ended dataset.

7.10.3 Regression analysis: Closed-ended data

As the response to a CE question is dichotomous (i.e. yes/no response), a logistic regression can be applied in the manner equivalent to that run to predict non-response and zero WTPs within the OP and PS study. Thus, the variable 'wtp_fob' and 'wtp_fs' will be computed as the dependant variables with the same set of covariates used as that used within the OP and PS study. The regression results can then be interpreted in the same manner.

7.10.4 Estimating average WTP from closed-ended data

To estimate average WTP from closed-ended data we apply a simple non-parametric method (6), this method offers an advantage as it makes no distributional assumptions. We need to estimate the proportion accepting (p) for each bid (i), which is calculated from dividing the number of respondents accepting (k) (for each bid) divided by the bid sample (n): ($p_i = k_i/n_i$). As the bid level increases the probability for acceptance should progressively fall (monotonic sequence). If there is not a monotonic sequence, then the mean proportion across the bid levels needs to be estimated until a non-increasing proportion of acceptances is obtained. To see how this is done, open the Excel spreadsheet 'Closed-ended_average WTP' (www.herc.ox.ac.uk/books/cba/support). Here, the bid values are listed along with the number of acceptances (k_i), the bid sample (n_i) and the proportion of acceptances for each bid (p_i) (all have been obtained from the data within the SPSS closed ended database). Note that we have assumed that for both FOB and FS, 100% of the sample accept the bid £0. For FOB, we can see that $p_{200} > p_{100}$ therefore the sequence is not monotonic. To adjust for this, the following algorithm is applied (7):

$$(k_i + k_{i+1})/(n_i + n_{i+1}) \qquad (7.1)$$

and the procedure is repeated until the sequence is monotonic. Thus, within the Excel spreadsheet, we adjust the proportion accepting £100 and £200 using the algorithm above as shown below:

$$\text{Proportion accepting bid £100} = (37 + 38)/(47 + 43) = 0.8333 \quad (7.2)$$

(same adjustment is made for bid £200)

Once we have a monotonic sequence, we can then transfer these numbers into a new database in SPSS and run a linear interpolation (regression) to obtain the coefficients to calculate the median WTP. To see how this is done open the SPSS database 'Average WTP_closed ended' and run the following: 'Analyse/regression/curve estimation – request 'linear' and 'Display ANOVA table' – select the 'proportions accepting' as the independant variables and the 'bid levels' as the dependent variable'. The results of the ANOVA table are shown in Table 7.7.

The regression coefficients displayed within the ANOVA table can then be used to calculate the mean WTP as shown in Box 7.8

The results are illustrated in the regression worksheet in the Excel spreadsheet: 'Closed-ended average WTP', and for both FOB and FS are shown in Box 7.9.

For a linear interpolation the median WTP is also mean WTP.

Table 7.7 Results from the ANOVA

	Unstandardized coefficients		Standardized coefficients	t	Sig.
	B	Std. error	Beta	B	Std. error
Propn accepting	−1,947.112	180.430	−0.975	−10.792	0.000
(constant)	1,814.392	149.264		12.156	0.000

Box 7.8 Calculating mean WTP

For FOB:
$$y = \beta_0 + \beta_1 x$$
$$\text{Median WTP} = 1,814.392 + (-19,473.112(0.5))$$
$$= £840.84$$

Box 7.9 Closed-ended average WTP values

Regression	$y = \text{constant} + \text{beta}(x)$	
	FOB	FS
Constant	1,814.3	1,453.3
Beta	−1,947.1	−1,686.8
Proportion accepting	0.5	0.5
Median WTP	840.8	609.9

7.11 **The iterative bidding (IB) method**

As the IB method is prone to starting point bias, the CRC study adopted three different structured algorithms to elicit WTP. These were applied to ensure that each respondent received the same bidding process. Each of the algorithms are displayed in Appendix 7.2 and start from either £10, £200, or £1,000 (algorithms 1, 2, and 3, respectively). The data for this study is contained within the WTP_Iterative bidding dataset that contains equivalent variables to the previous datasets already discussed.

7.11.1 **Estimating average WTP from iterative bidding data**

By using the IB method, the respondent reveals a range of values where the maximum WTP will lie. For example, within algorithm 1, if the respondent said 'yes' to £10 and 'no' to £200 and then 'no' to £50 then the analyst knows that the maximum WTP lies somewhere between £0 and £49. We can either take the midpoint between £10 and £50 as the maximum WTP (£30), or we can take the lower bound (£10) and the upper bound (£49) and present the mean WTP as a range. Within the dataset, this has been done by including a variable that indicates the direction of bidding with each respondent. The upper, midpoint, and lower WTP values have then been estimated for each respondent. Standard descriptive statistics can then be used to derive the overall mean WTP for each algorithm for the FOB and the FS test (Table 7.8).

To identify the factors that are influencing WTP, the midpoint value for FOB and FS can be defined as the dependant variable and linear regression applied as in the OP and PS case. To determine the impact of the starting point, insert the starting bid variable into the regression as an independent variable.

7.12 **Cost–benefit analysis**

The results of the series of CRC CV surveys have shown the full extent of the influence of elicitation design upon final WTP results. The final task is to take the WTP values revealed from each of these studies and combine them with the cost of the screening protocols to achieve a full CBA. To do this, we need to estimate the cost of running each screening programme which has already been calculated to be £62 per subject for the

Table 7.8 Average WTP by bid algorithm

	FOB test			FS test		
	Lower	**Middle**	**Upper**	**Lower**	**Middle**	**Upper**
Algorithm 1	330.67	418.67	505.77	419.09	499.70	579.48
Algorithm 2	606.77	676.77	746.13	640.00	724.31	807.93
Algorithm 3	817.50	865.78	913.69	798.71	851.77	904.42

FOB protocol (8) and £56 per subject for the FS protocol (9). Comparing the WTP values with cost then reveals the following net social benefit values:

Elicitation method	FOB	FS	NSB
OP/PS	£42	£32	>0
CE	£841	£610	<0
IB*	£614	£655	<0

*Using the midpoint WTP value with algorithm 2.

We can see from the results that the policy decision would be different for each of these studies primarily due to the differences in the elicitation format adopted.

References

1. Whynes, D.K., Frew, E., and Wolstenholme, J.L. 2003. A comparison of two methods for eliciting contingent valuations of colorectal cancer screening. *Journal of Health Economics* **22**: 555–574.

2. Donaldson, C., Jones, A.M., and Mapp, T.J. 1998. Limited dependent variables in willingness to pay studies: applications in health care. *Applied Economics* **30**: 667–677.

3. Donaldson, C., Shackley, P., and Abdalla, M. 1997. Using willingness to pay to value close substitutes: Carrier screening for cystic fibrosis revisited. *Health Economics* **6**: 145–159.

4. Harless, D.W., and Camerer, C.F. 1994. The predictive utility of generalised expected utility tehroies. *Econometrica* **62**(6): 1251–1289.

5. Hanemann, W., and Kanninen, B. 1996. *The statistical analysis of discrete-response contingent valuation data*. University of California: Department of Agriculture and Resource Economics. Report No.: Working paper 798.

6. Kriström ,B. 1990. A non-parametric approach to the estimation of welfare measures in discrete response valuation studies. *Land Economics* **66**(2): 135–139.

7. Ayer, M., Brunk, H.D., Ewing, G.M., and Silverman, E. 1995. An empirical distribution function for sampling with incomplete information. *Annals of Mathematical Statistics* **25**(march): 641–647.

8. Frew, E., Wolstenholme, J., and Whynes, D. 2001. Willingness to pay for colorectal cancer screening. *European Journal of Cancer* **37**: 1746–1751.

9. Whynes, D.K., Frew, E.J., Edwards, R., and Atkin, W.S. 2003. The costs of flexible sigmoidoscopy screening for colorectal cancer in the United Kingdom. *International Journal of Technology Assessment in Health Care* **19**(2): 384–395.

10. Hardcastle, J.D., Chamberlain, J.O., Robinson, M.H.E., Moss, S.M., Amar, S.S., Balfour, T.W., *et al.* 1996. Randomised controlled trial of faecal-occult-blood screening for colorectal cancer. *The Lancet* **348**: 1472–1477.

11. Atkin, W.S., Hart, A., Edwards, R., McIntyre, P., Aubrey, R., Wardle, J., *et al.* 1998. Uptake, yield of neoplasia, and adverse effects of flexible sigmoidoscopy screening. *Gut* **42**: 560–565.

Appendix 7.1

Box 7.1 CRC study design

Our WTP data capture instrument was designed for self-completion without supervision. After initial construction, the instrument was piloted, revised, presented for ethical approval, and again modified accordingly. In addition to containing standard administrative details, such as contact information and a guide to completion, the opening pages of the instrument were devoted to descriptions of colorectal cancer, the principle of screening and the two screening options. With respect to the latter, we chose descriptions essentially similar to those which have been employed in inviting subjects to participate in the Nottingham-based English FOB trial (10) and the UK multi-centre FS trial (11). Following the descriptions, each subject was asked whether they would wish to undertake a screening test, were one to become generally available, and, if so, which test they would prefer.

Thereafter, each subject was invited to supply a valuation for each of the two screening options, FOB and FS. We asked for WTP amounts using an ex ante perspective. The payment was framed as a one-off payment. Two variants of the instrument were produced, differing only with respect to the format under which the CV was elicited. We chose to use the open-ended and payment scale format. The preamble to each of the CV questions was as follows.

One way of measuring the value of screening for colorectal cancer is to ask you what you would be prepared to give up to receive this service, i.e. how much money you would be willing to pay for it. Of course, if colorectal cancer screening did come into existence in the UK, the screening test would be provided free by the NHS. We believe that people should not have to pay for health care. This is a simply method of measuring how strongly you feel about having a new screening programme and how much you would value such a service. There are no right or wrong answers. The amount you say could be large or small. It is up to you. We are interested in your view.

In the open-ended format, the CV questions then ran:

What is the maximum amount of money you would be willing to pay for having the complete series of FOB tests every 2 years from the age of 50 until the age of 74 (please write in the space below).

£_____.

What is the maximum amount of money you would be willing to pay for the one-off Flexi-Scope test at the age of 60 (please write in the space below).

£_____.

In the payment scale format, the space provided in the open-ended variant was replaced with a vertically arranged list of 29 values. These values were, from top to bottom, £0, £5, and £10, thereafter to £100 in units of £10, to £200 in units of £20, to £500 in units of £50, and to £1,000 in units of £100. Subjects expressing a valuation in excess of £1,000 were requested to write in the appropriate amount (i.e. beyond the limit of the scale, the payment format defaulted to the open-ended format). Following common practice with payment scales, subjects were requested to encircle the maximum amount, whilst placing ticks against amounts they were sure they would not pay and crosses against amounts they were sure they would not.

The instrument was distributed on our behalf via a group of primary care physicians, themselves members of a regional collaborative research network. Each GP received a randomly shuffled pile of questionnaires, containing equal numbers of each CV format. The GPs were requested to offer a questionnaire (selected at random) to any patient during a normal consultation, subject to three forms of exclusion. These were, first, persons under approximately 25 years of age, on the grounds of perceived irrelevance of screening in that age group. Second, GPs were, at their discretion, to exclude any subject with a recent diagnosis of colorectal cancer in the family, on the grounds of minimizing distress. Finally, potential subjects with substantial reading, learning, or language difficulties were to be excluded, on the grounds of incapacity to complete the questionnaire.

Appendix 7.2

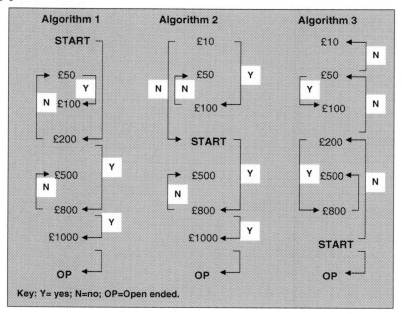

Key: Y= yes; N=no; OP=Open ended.

Chapter 8

Applied cost–benefit analysis in health care: An empirical application in spinal surgery

Emma McIntosh, Alastair Gray,
Mathias Haefeli, Achim Elfering,
Atul Sukthankar, and Norbert Boos

8.1 Introduction

Following on from the WTP survey design outlined in Chapter 6 and the applied WTP / CBA in Chapter 7, the objective of this chapter is to provide an applied example of a CBA in health care using a retrospective study design. By combining WTP estimates with cost estimates in a group of spinal surgery patients this example shows the viability of using CBA methodology in health care. The study design is a CBA feasibility study using a WTP survey with ex-post willingness-to-pay/-to-accept (WTP/WTA) questions. Much of this chapter is adapted from Haefeli *et al.* (38).

8.2 Background to the empirical study

Although increasing data are gathered on the societal costs of low back pain, little information is available on how patients 'value' the benefits of surgery or whether interventions in this area are indeed cost-beneficial. Costs for spinal surgery have risen substantially over the last two decades due to a variety of factors. Demographic changes, advances in technology, unclear indications, and financial incentives for the involved parties may have had synergistic effects (1). Despite the frequent use of spinal interventions, scientific evidence for their therapeutic efficacy compared to natural history and non-operative treatment is sparse. This is particularly true for instrumented fusion for degenerative disc disease, one of the most costly spinal interventions (2). In addition, there is little evidence on the valuations patients place on such surgery. Further, as per the topic of this book, limited health care resources make it a requirement that evidence is obtained not only on therapeutic efficacy of treatment modalities but also on costs.

Consequently, an increasing number of health-economic studies are being published in the field of spinal surgery. Recently, the cost-effectiveness and cost-utility of several spinal interventions has been explored (3–6). However, as in many areas of health care there are no other identifiable studies using formal CBA methodology in the field of spinal surgery.

8.3 Elicitation perspective

One important distinguishing feature of WTP methods, is the elicitation perspective, whether ex ante or ex-post. Table 6.2 in Chapter 6 provides a summary of the differing perspectives depending upon the level of health state certainty/uncertainty. Values are ex ante in the sense that the consumer's expected utility may differ from the realized utility of a particular good compared to ex-post values where the state of the world is known. O'Brien and Gafni (7) distinguish between an ex-post user-based perspective and an ex ante insurance based perspective where the ex-post user is assumed to be 'at the point of consuming some unit of the program being evaluated'. Shackley and Donaldson (37) note that, to be more specific, patients are defined as individuals who are 'currently diseased', i.e. individuals who may be in the process of consuming health care or are waiting to consume health care. O'Brien and Gafni (7) define an ex ante user as someone at risk of contracting a disease and therefore at risk of consuming the treatment programme of interest. In his review of contingent valuation studies in health care, Klose (9) states that whilst the use of ex ante WTP values are consistent with CBA, only about 20% of economic evaluations performed contingent valuation from such a state. Shackley and Donaldson (37) categorize the appropriate perspective depending upon whether data are collected from patients or the public and for a privately financed good or a publicly financed good. A useful discussion of the theoretical difference between ex-ante and ex-post WTP is provided by Johannesson (10).

While interest in WTP has substantially increased in many different areas in health care (7;11–13), in the field of musculo-skeletal disorders only a few studies have been performed, in studies of cervical spondylotic myelopathy (14), rheumatoid arthritis (15;16), and osteoarthritis (17;18). Most of them explored methodological aspects, and only one study has empirically assessed the benefits of a surgical intervention, i.e. joint arthroplasty for knee and hip osteoarthritis in a group of individuals operated on because of osteoarthritis(19). Further to this, no identifiable studies have tested the feasibility of using either ex ante or ex-post WTP values within a CBA in the field of musculo-skeletal disorders. Based on this, the aim of this study was to test the feasibility of the ex-post WTP approach for the most frequent spinal interventions (discectomy for disc herniation (20), spinal decompression for spinal stenosis (21), spinal fusion for degenerative disc disease (22)), i.e. whether or not patients are willing and able to answer such questions, and to make a first estimate from a patient's perspective of the economic net-benefit of these interventions within a formal CBA framework.

8.4 Sample and setting

A total of 115 consecutive patients with a mean age of 59.4 years (21–94 years) were included in the study. Inclusion criteria were: 1. posterior or anterior lumbar interbody fusion (PLIF/ALIF) for degenerative disc disease/spondylolisthesis ($n = 37$), lumbar discectomy for disc herniation ($n = 39$), or lumbar decompression for spinal stenosis ($n = 39$) between 2000 and 2003 in the Orthopaedic University Hospital, Balchrist, Switzerland; 2. Failed conservative treatment; 3. Followed-up for a minimum of 1 year after surgery as most of the changes after a spinal intervention occur within 1–2 years postoperatively (this is the generally accepted follow-up time for clinical orthopaedic studies); and 4. Sufficient knowledge of the German language. Included patients who had to be re-operated ($n = 9$) due to complications or recurrent symptoms remained included for all analyses. To reduce heterogeneity in the sample, patients with previous spine surgery, tumor, infection, or other consuming illness were not included; such patients are sometimes treated with similar operations to those investigated in this study, but have different diagnoses and prognoses that would hamper comparison.

All patients were sent a self-rating questionnaire in which patient characteristics and WTP information on the procedure they had experienced were collected. Those not answering within 4 weeks were contacted by telephone and encouraged to participate. To explore the plausibility of the results, 80 respondents were contacted for a post-hoc telephone interview in which they were informed of the average WTP across all respondents for the respective surgical procedure, and asked if they considered this figure to be realistic with respect to their perception of costs. Fifty-two patients additionally participated in a test–retest experiment to assess the reliability of the WTP questionnaire, in which they received identical WTP questions 4 weeks after the baseline survey.

In addition to items on socio-demographics, present complaints, and employment status, shown in Table 8.1, a set of WTP questions was included; see Vignette 8.1

Table 8.1 Variables collected from chart review and questionnaire

Variable	Scale
Socio-demographic data	
Age	Years
Gender	Male/female
Marital status	Never married, married, divorced, widowed
Individuals in household	Living alone, living with partner, living with partner and children, living with children, living with other persons
Children	Number
Educational level	University degree, high school, elementary school, none
Health insurance class	General, semi-private, private
Complaints (at follow-up)	
Present pain intensity (back/leg pain)	VAS[1]
Present pain index (pain at present, worst/best last 7 days)	VAS (composite score)
Frequency of medication	None, seldom, frequently, regularly
Type of medication	None, paracetamol, NSAID[2], narcotics
Work status	Full time, part time, lighter work, student/homemaker
Outcome variables	
Subjective assessment of surgery	Excellent, good, fair, poor, worse than before
Subjective rating of general care	Very satisfied, satisfied, undecided, dissatisfied, very dissatisfied
Relative postoperative improvement (at follow-up)	VAS

[1] VAS – Visual analogue scale

[2] NSAID – Non-steroidal anti inflammatory drug

Vignette 8.1 – WTP Questions used in the study

WTP Question	Response format
Suppose your insurance would not have covered the cost of the surgery. What would be the maximum amount you would have paid for the intervention out of your own pocket?	Absolute value Open-ended
Would you be willing to take on a loan, if you could not pay for the surgery?	Likert scale (yes, probably yes, probably no, no)
Suppose your household income was €5,769 and your wealth was €128,205. What would be the maximum you would have paid for the intervention out of your own pocket?	Absolute value Open-ended
Would you have renounced surgery for money? If yes, for how much?	Dichotomous (yes, no)
Imagine the surgery would cost €x Would you have chosen the operation? (x = 6,410 for discectomy, 12,821 for spinal decompression, 19,231 for spinal fusion)?	Likert scale (yes, probably yes, probably no, no)
How much do you estimate the total hospital costs for your intervention?	Absolute value Open-ended
What is your monthly gross household income?	Numerical rating scale (NRS)
Do you own real estate?	Dichotomous (yes, no)
Financial solvency: How easy is it for you to gather €32,051 in cash within short-term?	Likert scale (very difficult, difficult, rather difficult, rather easy, easy, very easy)

(also see Appendix 8.1 for full set of questions, item characteristics and reproducibility tests). The valuation was based on WTP at the time of the interview, i.e. at least 1 year postoperatively (ex-post).

The design of the WTP survey was evaluated using the following three steps before giving a final version to the study population:

1. In face-to-face interviews (n = 20) the general acceptance of the WTP questions were tested. Closed-ended (CE), open-ended (OE), and payment scale formats were explored (23). The face-to-face interviews were carried out during consultations in the outpatient clinics. Patients that were interviewed were planned for the similar interventions under investigation but were not part of our study population. The experience of the qualitative face-to-face interviews was used to design a pilot questionnaire.

2. In a structured interview with 20 additional patients from outpatient clinics this pilot questionnaire was then explored. The payment scale format was abandoned after this step due to evidence of strong starting point bias (see Chapter 6, Sections 6.7.1 and 6.7.2). Comments from the patients concerning question content and format resulted in further refinements.

3. The pilot questionnaire was then validated using the 'Delphi method' (24) by asking five peers in the field of economics, psychology, and medicine to comment on its design. This resulted in supplements and a re-phrasing of questions.

The final questionnaire included two OE WTP questions, one dichotomous WTA question (yes/no) and a closed ended four-point Likert scale 'take-it-or-leave-it' item (TIOLI). As we used an ex-post approach to assess WTP where patients had already undergone surgery, there was no information provided on success rates, risks, or alternatives incorporated. However, patients had been informed about the risks, possible improvement, and alternative treatment possibilities before surgery according to a general preoperative procedure of obtaining informed consent for the intervention. Patients who answered the WTA question with 'yes' were asked for how much money they would do so (open question). In the TIOLI question, respondents were asked if they would have surgery for a given hypothetical intervention cost. Patients were not informed that this hypothetical amount approximately equaled the actual intervention costs.

8.6 Costing the intervention

The price base year was set at 2003 because since then all costs arising during a hospital stay at the institution can be related to the corresponding patient (institutional full absorption cost accounting). As the costs for these interventions remained stable over the last years this permitted the estimation of all direct patient-related costs incurred during the hospital stay for our population. We chose 60 patients who underwent the interventions under investigation (20 each) in 2003 and used their cost data for our analysis. Prices are given in Euros (€).

Data analyses and statistics were carried out in five steps as follows:

1. Evaluation of the CV-questions: Acceptability was assessed as the proportion of each questionnaire item answered in relation to the number of returned questionnaires. Distribution was assessed by calculating skewness and kurtosis. Reliability was estimated by kappa statistics (25), and the intra-class correlation coefficient (26). Floor and ceiling effects were considered by calculating the relative number of individuals obtaining the lowest or highest scores possible for each scale/item.

2. Descriptive statistical analyses were carried out to explore frequencies mean-/median values, standard error of mean, and standard deviation.

3. Univariate correlative analyses of the clinical outcome parameters, income levels, health insurance status, and the WTP values were carried out to test the theoretical validity of the WTP data.

4. Multivariate linear regression analyses using the ordinary least square (OLS) approach was used to explore significant predictor variables for WTP/WTA. Due to the numerous covariates that might influence outcome, we chose to include only those parameters for which the univariate correlative analyses showed a significant relationship. Age, gender, household income, real estate, financial solvency, estimation of intervention costs, and health insurance class entered the

model as confounding covariates in the first step. In the second step, potential predictor variables were entered if significant in the correlative analysis.

5. Net benefits were estimated by subtracting the costs from the WTP values (net benefit = WTP – Cost); these data were then bootstrapped to generate 95% confidence regions around the estimates (the upper 97.5th and the lower 0.2.5th percentiles were the confidence values).

SPSS™ 11.5 and EXCEL™ were used for statistical analyses. The level of significance was set at 0.05, two-tailed.

8.7 **Results**

The response rate was 91.3% ($n = 105$). All but five patients were located. Three patients had died. Two patients found the questionnaire too personal or complicated and refused participation. The missing patients did not differ significantly from the participants in terms of age and distribution of gender. The average time elapsed since surgery was 32 months (range: 12–53). Nine patients had to be re-operated due to wound infection ($n = 1$), implant loosening ($n = 1$), failed fusion (pseudarthrosis, $n = 1$), recurrent disc herniation ($n = 4$), and newly occurred stenosis ($n = 2$) 1 week to 21 months after primary surgery. They valued the success of surgery significantly ($p < 0.021$) lower than the others. In all other economic and clinical outcome parameters no significant differences were found between the two groups.

A total of 22.9% of the study population had a monthly gross household income below €2,560, and 26.7% in the €2,560–€3,850 range, which is still below the average household income of €5,770 (median: €4,490) in Switzerland.

No significant differences were found between responders and non-responders in terms of age, gender, health insurance class, underlying diagnosis, rate of re-operation, and educational status. The TIOLI question led to higher response rates than the OE maximum WTP item (94.3% vs. 73.3%). Reasons for not answering specific questions were the hypothetical context in up to 10.5% of cases, the intimate character of the questions in up to 13.3% and not knowing the answer in up to 10.5% of the cases. In the OE WTP questions up to 11.4% of the patients mentioned that they would pay everything, or as much as necessary, for the surgery and therefore did not report a specific amount of money. Floor and Ceiling effects ranged from 1.0% to 71.4%. The questions on recommendation of surgery to family and friends showed the strongest ceiling effects with 71.4% and 58.1%. The weakest ceiling effect with 1% was found in the question on financial solvency. Kappa statistics exhibited fair to substantial reliability (0.35 and 0.74) and the ICC ranged from 0.49 to 0.81. 83.8% ($n = 67$) of respondents in the post-hoc telephone interview found the average WTP results presented plausible. 15% ($n = 12$) did not quite agree, and one patient (<1%) completely disagreed with the findings.

8.7.1 **Willingness to pay and willingness to accept**

Maximum WTP averaged €11,008 (95% CI: 7,211–16,186) for spinal fusion, €7,170 (95% CI: 4,423–10,256) for lumbar discectomy and €7,692 (95% CI: 5,513–10,128) for spinal decompression, see Table 8.2. In addition to this, with the hypothetically given average monthly gross household income (€5,770) and wealth (€128,205) of the population, maximum WTP increased to €21,427, €17,117, and €10,287, respectively. Two male (33 years, fusion and 83 years, decompression) and one female (84 years, decompression) participants were willing to hypothetically renounce surgery for money. They mentioned a WTA of €384,615, €32,051, and €3,205, respectively. Their WTP accounted for €6,500, €3,250, and €1,950, respectively. The two men

Table 8.2 Descriptive statistics on maximum willingness to pay, and effective hospital costs (€)

Surgery	Maximum WTP	Maximum WTP with given income	Effective hospital costs
Spinal fusion			
Valid numbers	29	27	20
Mean	11,007*	21,427†	13,779
S.E (Mean)	1,919	3,0924	758
Min–Max	0–51,282	1,603–64,103	10,221–24,767
St. Dev	10,335	16,070	1,467
Median	9,615	19,231	13,560
Discectomy			
Valid numbers	27	27	20
Mean	7,170*	17,117†	5,226
S.E (Mean)	1,285	4,776	247
Min–Max	0–25,641	0–128,205	3,901–7,948
St. Dev	6,674	25,819	1,107
Median	6,410	6,410	5,255
Spinal decompression			
Valid numbers	21	21	20
Mean	7,692*	10,287	6,969
S.E (Mean)	1,235	1,555	569
Min–Max	1,923–25,641	1,923–25,641	3,676–11,979
St. Dev	5,562	7,125	2,542
Median		6,410	6,226
Overall			
Valid numbers	77	75	60
Mean	8,758*	16,756	8,658
S.E (Mean)	927	2,131	578
Min–Max	0–51,282	0–128,205	3,676–24,767
St. Dev	8,134	18,460	4,476
Median	6,410	12,821	7,329
Group difference (Kruskal–Wallis test)	*p* = 0.204	*p* < 0.032	*p* < 0.001

No significant differences were found between maximum WTP and effective hospital costs

*Significant difference compared to estimated hospital costs

†Significant difference compared to maximum WTP

***Significant difference compared to effective hospital costs

Table 8.3 Descriptive results from the WTP survey

Item	Spinal fusion		Spinal decompression		Discectomy		Total	
	N	%	N	%	N	%	N	%
Would you be willing to take on a loan, if you could not pay for the surgery?								
Yes	20	54.1 %	12	35.3%	21	61.8%	53	50.5%
Probably yes	7	18.9%	7	20.6%	4	11.8%	18	17.1%
Probably no	4	10.8%	5	14.7%	2	5.9%	11	10.5%
No	5	13.5%	7	20.6%	4	11.8%	16	15.2%
Missing	1	2.7%	3	8.8%	3	8.8%	7	6.7%
I would have renounced the surgery for money?								
Yes	1	2.7%	2	5.9%	0	0%	3	2.9%
No	34	91.9%	28	82.4%	31	91.2%	93	88.6%
Missing	2	5.4%	4	11.8%	3	8.8%	9	8.6%
Would you recommend your type of surgery to family and friends?								
Yes	25	67.6%	25	73.5%	25	73.5%	75	71.4%
Probably yes	8	21.6%	4	11.8%	6	17.6%	18	17.1%
Probably no	3	8.2%	1	2.9%	1	5.9%	6	5.7%
No	0	0%	1	2.9%	1	2.9%	2	1.9%
Missing	1	2.7%	3	8.8%	0	0%	4	3.8%

Would you recommend your type of surgery to family and friends, even if they have to pay for it out of their own pocket?

Yes	22	59.5%	20	58.8%	19	55.9%	61	58.1%
Probably yes	10	27.0%	8	23.5%	10	29.4%	28	26.7%
Probably no	3	8.1%	2	5.9%	1	2.9%	6	5.7%
No	1	2.7%	1	2.9%	2	5.9%	4	3.8%
Missing	1	2.7%	3	8.8%	2	5.9%	6	5.7%

TIOLI: Imagine the surgery would cost €x. Would you have chosen the operation? (x = 6,410 for discectomy, 12,821 for spinal decompression, 19,231 for spinal fusion)

Yes	19	51.4%	13	38.2%	22	64.7%	54	51.4%
Probably yes	9	24.3%	11	32.4%	6	17.6%	26	24.8%
Probably no	6	16.2%	4	11.8%	3	8.8%	13	12.4%
No	2	5.4%	3	8.8%	1	2.9%	6	5.7%
Missing	1	2.7%	3	8.8%	2	5.9%	6	5.7%

Financial solvency: How easy is it for you to gather €32,051 in cash within the short term?

Very difficult	10	27.0%	9	26.5%	12	35.3%	31	29.5%
Difficult	11	29.7%	8	23.5%	8	23.5%	27	25.7%
Rather difficult	8	21.6%	6	17.6%	5	14.7%	19	18.1%
Rather easy	2	5.4%	3	8.8%	3	8.8%	8	7.6%
Easy	4	10.8%	3	8.8%	2	5.9%	9	8.6%
Very easy	0	0%	0	0%	1	2.9%	1	1.0%
Missing	2	5.4%	5	14.7%	3	8.8%	10	9.5%

Note – differences between groups were not significant

reported the success of surgery being satisfying while the woman reported an excellent success of surgery. All mentioned to have achieved a substantial pain-relief of 70–90%. Seventy-one patients (67.6%) stated they would be willing to take on a loan if they were unable to pay for the intervention. Ninety-three patients (88.5%) would recommend surgery to close friends and family and 84.8% would even do so if their relatives or friends had to pay for it out of their own pocket. 76.2% of the individuals mentioned that they would choose the operation for a given hypothetical intervention cost (TIOLI). No significant differences in the TIOLI – answers were found between the different treatment groups. WTP correlated positively with the willingness to have the operation for a given price (TIOLI; $r = 0.441, p < 0.001$).

8.7.2 Correlation analysis

Economic outcome variables (maximum WTP, WTP with given income/wealth, TIOLI, willingness to take on a loan, recommendation to friends/family) were correlated with the financial situation of the individuals ($r = 0.279$ to $0.379; p < 0.001$–0.050). Furthermore, the estimation of hospital costs ($r = 0.405$–$0.576; p < 0.001$) and insurance class ($r = 0.270$–$0.342; p < 0.019$–0.002) were significantly correlated with the OE WTP items. Among the health related parameters, relative pain improvement ($r = 0.203$–$0.355; p < 0.028$–0.001), present pain ($r = -0.208$ to $-0.257; p < 0.09$–0.011), frequency of pain medication intake ($r = -0.199$ to $-0.224; p < 0.048$–0.027) and disability ($r = -0.226$ to $-0.357; p < 0.049$–0.001) were significantly correlated in the expected direction. Age was significantly inversely correlated with the willingness to take on a loan ($r = -0.25; p < 0.013$).

8.7.3 Prediction of WTP

Relative pain improvement ($p < 0.014$), duration of hospital stay ($p < 0.047$), and the estimated intervention cost ($p < 0.001$) were significant independent predictors of WTP. Moreover, present pain ($p < 0.054$) and the frequency of painkillers ($p < 0.087$) also showed a strong tendency to significantly predict WTP (final regression model: $R = 0.811, R^2 = 0.657$, adj. $R^2 = 0.529, F = 5.146, P < 0.001$). Relative pain improvement ($p < 0.007$), present pain level ($p < 0.031$), and the SF-8 mental sub-score ($p < 0.026$) were significant predictors for the willingness to undergo the intervention with given costs (TIOLI) (final regression model: $R = 0.669, R^2 = 0.448$, adj. $R^2 = 0.295$, $F = 2.937, P < 0.001$). A recommendation of surgery to friends and family was predicted by relative pain improvement ($p < 0.042$), present pain levels ($p < 0.019$), and the duration of hospital stay ($p < 0.043$) (final regression model: $R = 0.639, R^2 = 0.408$, adj. $R^2 = 0.245, F = 2.499, P < 0.006$). Only the SF-8 mental sub-score significantly predicted the willingness to take on a loan for surgery ($p < 0.043$), while the EuroQol showed a tendency toward significant prediction ($p = 0.064$) (final regression model: $R = 0.568, R^2 = 0.323$, adj. $R^2 = 0.136, F = 1.726, P = 0.067$).

8.7.4 Costs of surgery

The actual mean costs of lumbar fusion (€13,778) were almost twice the costs for lumbar decompression (€6,969). Discectomy was least cost intensive, at €5,226.

Significant differences were found in costs between fusion and decompression/discectomy ($p < 0.001$) and between decompression and discectomy ($p < 0.012$). The main components of cost were wages for personnel and medical services, while implants accounted for 24.0% of the total costs in the fusion group.

8.8 Cost–benefit analyses

In the fusion group, maximum WTP was lower (-20%) than the actual procedure costs, while WTP exceeded costs in the discectomy and the decompression group by 37% and 10%, respectively. These differences were not statistically significant. Calculation of net benefits (net benefit = WTP − cost)showed that spinal decompression and discectomy are both within the realms of being cost-beneficial with positive net benefits whilst spinal fusion gave rise to a net welfare loss, see Table 8.4.

Figures 8.1–8.3 show the plots of these bootstrapped net benefits so that the welfare gain/loss can be seen clearly in each case.

Given a hypothetically average wealth and monthly household income of Switzerland's population, maximum WTP was substantially higher than the actual intervention costs (fusion: +55%; decompression: +47%; discectomy: +227%): these differences were significant for spinal fusion ($p < 0.023$) and decompression ($p < 0.020$).

Table 8.4 Net benefits and 95% CI of the different interventions

Intervention	Net benefit	95% CI
Spinal decompression	€723.58	€−426.65–€1'799.91
Discectomy	€1'943.52	€1'390.76–€2'372.88
Spinal fusion	€−2'771.27	€−4'351.98–€−1'495.74

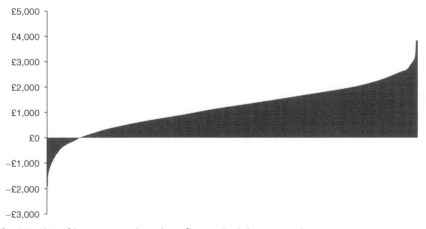

Fig. 8.1 Plot of bootstrapped net benefits – spinal decompression.

Fig. 8.2 Plot of bootstrapped net benefits – discectomy.

Fig. 8.3 Plot of bootstrapped net benefits – spinal fusion.

Beside the potential advantages of CBA over other economic evaluation methods, some methodological concerns about the questions used to assess WTP and the health care setting in which the investigation is taking place must be kept in mind before using the data as a basis for allocating resources. The way WTP values may be used depends on the perspective of the approach, i.e. whether the data was assessed from patients or from the public, ex-post or ex-ante, respectively according to O'Brien and Gafni (7). Furthermore, it will depend on whether the programme under investigation is privately financed or publicly financed (37). In the cases where values for a privately financed programme are elicited from patients or the public, the use of WTP is uncontroversial. But if the values are obtained for a publicly financed good it is often doubted that the conventional approach can be meaningfully applied. Shackley and

Donaldson (37) therefore suggested modified approaches to these two scenarios (8). As described earlier, the Swiss health care system is partly privately but mainly publicly financed. For a comparison of different treatments in such a setting, the modified approach suggests the assessment of a so-called 'marginal' WTP (see Chapter 6, Section 6.6.6): 1. patients are asked to state their preferred treatment alternative and 2. they are then asked to state their WTP for receiving their preferred treatment rather than the less preferable alternative. In a retrospective approach as in this study this would mean that patients had to value the incremental benefit of the preferred alternatives (surgery or preoperative conservative treatment) after a time span of at least 1 year. We believe that this may bias the valuation as the perception of pain and disability may change dramatically during time. It is for the same reason that retrospective pain assessment of more than 3 months is not recommended (27–29). Moreover, Haas *et al.* (30) found that pain and disability recall became more and more influenced by present pain and disability during a period of 1 year while the influence of actual relief and pain- and disability reporting at the initial consultation decreased. For this study, with the main objective being to test, the feasibility of the CV questions we believe that our procedure was appropriate. However, it would be interesting to include and explore the 'marginal' WTP approach in future studies.

Acceptability, validity, and reproducibility of a questionnaire are always important issues of concern. This study tried to address these topics from different directions. The acceptability in terms of response and completion rates of the CV-questions ranged from fair to very good depending on the question format. The OE WTP questions and those relating to the respondent's financial situation achieved lower response rates, in line with other reports in the literature on musculoskeletal disorders (15–19). Compared to a study on WTP for antihypertensive therapy by Johannesson *et al.* (31) who reported a non-response rate of 59% in OE WTP questions we achieved response-rates of around 71%. We could not confirm that older patients more often failed to answer the OE questions as reported by others (39;40). In our study, reduced acceptability of WTP questions is partly explained by the personal nature of these questions, objections to the hypothetical nature of the questions, and by the fact that 9.6% would have paid 'everything or as much as necessary' for surgery and therefore did not note a specific amount of money. As the majority of these patients suffered from an acute pain syndrome, i.e. disc herniation, we conclude that in this situation a TIOLI format may be more appropriate than an OE question which is also in agreement with other reports (32). Being given an amount for the costs seems to facilitate answering in the hypothetical context. Interpreting these results should respect the limited sample size which ideally should be higher for the TIOLI format (even though the positive correlation with WTP indicates internal consistency). To overcome the disadvantage of limited variance of answers in the CE TIOLI format and the questions on recommendation of surgery, we used four-point Likert scales which led to strong floor and ceiling effects. The question on recommendation really screens for those who are dissatisfied with treatment outcome, and would not make the same choice again irrespective of the chance within other treatment options. Fortunately, such dissatisfaction is rare. Therefore, ceiling effects are to be expected. Floor and ceiling effects refer to the proportion of patients obtaining the lowest or highest possible score for the given scale, and for whom any transition to an even more extreme status would therefore not be measurable with that scale. In longitudinal research floor and ceiling effects therefore restrict the measurement of change and recommendations are given to avoid floor or ceiling effects greater than 70% (61). However, in cross-sectional clinical research, items with floor and ceiling effects should be included, because they are not adverse but reflect that some items are endorsed by most patients and some by very few patients – which is valuable 'state of the art' information (61). Taking into consideration that the use of the current item on recommendation is primarily descriptive for cross-sectional purpose, floor and ceiling effects seem acceptable. However, to increase sensitivity in future studies, the response format could be expanded to seven points which would probably not damage scale reliability, while increasing scale sensitivity (62).

Content validity was addressed by applying the Delphi method in composing our questionnaire (24). It is felt that the resulting additions and modifications of content and format led to a substantially improved and broad-based questionnaire. However, lacking a gold standard, a conclusive assessment of content validity is very difficult to achieve. In the post-hoc telephone interview, 83.8% of respondents found the results plausible and in line with their expectations, estimating good respondent validity. This result may however be biased by some yea-saying effect (see Chapter 6, Section 6.7.1) and in future this might be addressed by offering different amounts of money and comparing the answers. The test–retest experiment revealed fair to substantial reproducibility. The majority of preference changes occurred within one category. None of the respondents completely changed side from yes to no or vice-versa. It should be noted that a minimum of four weeks follow-up is a difficult test of reproducibility, as some background variables may have changed during this period leading to deviating responses (50).

The monetary valuation of the perceived benefits by maximum WTP was greater than the actual intervention costs for discectomy and decompression but lower for spinal fusion. WTP increased substantially for all three interventions when patients were asked to imagine that they had the average monthly household income and wealth of Switzerland. This reflects the fact that the average financial situation of the patients in the study was well below average, with almost 50% of our patients reporting an average monthly household income of less than €3,846. The median values of €4,487 for the monthly income and €3,205 for the taxable wealth in our country make clear that only a small minority of wealthy people caused the high mean values. It seems that patients would pay more for surgery if they had the respective financial resources. This is particularly true for the aforementioned 50% of patients: this group reported a significantly higher relative increase of WTP when income and wealth were given (+152% vs. +52%; $p < 0.019$) indicating that they valued their perceived benefit higher than they could realistically afford. This and the fact that WTP with given income and wealth was somewhat higher than the estimated intervention cost in all three interventions indicates that patients perceived a substantial benefit of surgery. However, two patients with less monthly income than the suggested €5,770 – reported a lower WTP in the scenario with given income and wealth than they did in the simple WTP question. This is a critical point as it may indicate that the question was misunderstood or provoked protest answers. Three participants were willing to renounce surgery for money. Two male patients reported the success of surgery only as being satisfying and would have accepted an amount of money that was 10 and 60 times their WTP, respectively. One female patient reported an excellent success of surgery but reported a WTA of only 1.7 times of her WTP. All three achieved a substantial pain-relief of 70–90%, but the two male participants still reported actual pain levels of 6 and 9 on the VAS. This discrepancy remains unclear. The problems of pain recall may play a role here but one would expect a lower valuation of pain relief with higher actual pain levels (30). These individuals may simply have expected more from surgery in terms of pain and disability relief than they achieved. Another reason for the small number of 'acceptors' might be founded in the nature of the WTA-approach which is probably even more hypothetic than the WTP-approach in the current Swiss health system. On the other hand, those individuals reporting that they were not willing to renounce surgery for money might either not want to admit that they would choose money for health or they felt that they needed surgery in any case. Considering the patients' subjective rating of surgery, and the fact that all failed to improve substantially by conservative treatment, we feel that the latter is valid for most of our patients indicating that they perceived a valuable health-benefit from surgery.

Several studies have highlighted the dependence of the consumer's WTP on income (19;31). We not only assessed household income but also the possession of real estate and financial solvency as indicators of the individual financial situation. These two additional parameters revealed even stronger correlations with WTP than household income, indicating that the assessment of household income alone in WTP studies may lead to an underestimation of the influence of the individual's financial situation on WTP.

8.9 **Conclusions**

This study directly compared the valuation placed on benefits of spinal interventions with the treatment costs within a formal CBA framework and estimated net benefits. In the discectomy and spinal decompression groups the net benefit was positive (+37%/+10%). In the discectomy group, this might be due to the good treatment results after acute onset of the disease in a substantially younger and active population. In conclusion, the results from the CBA show that discectomy and spinal decompression appear to be cost-beneficial when considering the treatment costs during hospital stay. For an ALIF/PLIF procedure, our data do not seem to allow for a clear conclusion on the net benefit ratio of these interventions. Only six patients were willing to pay more than the actual cost of spinal fusion, and they differed significantly from other respondents in the possession of real estate and financial solvency but in none of the clinical outcome parameters. Seventy-eight percent of those who quoted a sum below the actual costs nevertheless exhibited a good or excellent result of surgery, and 87% were satisfied or very satisfied with the treatment. There was no significant difference between the answers to the TIOLI question and with a given income and wealth patients after fusion exhibited a WTP that was substantially higher than the effective hospital costs. While the isolated comparison of WTP and the effective costs indicates a net welfare loss, clinical parameters and the TIOLI results indicate a better ratio of costs and the perceived benefit.

This discrepancy may indicate a drawback to the OE WTP questions as outcome parameters when the effective costs are unknown to the patients.

8.9.1 **Limitations**

When interpreting the results of this feasibility study, some limitations should be considered. The retrospective study design did not allow for a comparison of the clinical status of the patients pre- and postoperatively and it was not possible to assess all treatment costs during the follow-up time (e.g. physiotherapy, pain medication, etc.). Therefore, the net-benefit results obtained must be seen in the light of the main objective of this study, i.e. to test the feasibility of this approach in spinal surgery. A more comprehensive cost assessment during the follow-up period including indirect costs is planned in future studies to allow for a full economic evaluation. The improvement in the patients' health status assessed by a prospective investigation of the clinical parameters would theoretically be a more reasonable predictor for WTP than only the actual clinical status. For this reason, further studies should include a prospective clinical assessment to investigate this point.

As discussed, a further limitation is the use of ex-post WTP values instead of ex-ante and whilst some justification has been provided in terms of the setting for these study future studies should consider the theoretical advantages of the ex-ante approach. Following the normative view of the Panel of Cost-Effectiveness in Health and Medicine, economic evaluations should be carried out from an ex-ante perspective. But as pointed out by Klose (9), only 20% of contingent valuation studies in the literature have used this ex-ante perspective, they include studies in cystic fibrosis and radiology (33;34). Some evidence in the literature comparing ex-ante and ex-post WTP show that ex-post values tend to be higher than ex-ante values (35;36). It was believed that in this study given the combination of patient values with the mainly publicly funded health care system that the ex-post approach was appropriate however future studies could compare ex-ante values with ex-post values in a surgical setting. In order to alleviate hypothetical bias, but to account for theoretical validity, further studies could use both approaches.

The results from this applied CBA show that discectomy and spinal decompression appear to be cost-beneficial when considering the treatment costs during hospital stay and the ability of patients to express their preferences using the WTP method worked effectively in this health care context. It is also clear however that there are still a number of methodological challenges within this area and the practice would benefit from explicit guidance on the minimum requirements for reporting and presenting the results of CV studies such as that provided in Chapter 6, Table 6.5. Further guidance on reporting and presenting the results of CBA studies using stated preference discrete choice experiments for the estimation of benefits can be found in Chapter 12, Appendix 12.2.

Acknowledgements

The example provided in this chapter is adapted from Haefeli *et al.* (38), the study was funded by a grant from the AO Spine, Grant number E-ORD 04/104. Further thanks go to Professors Semmer, Zweifel, Fehr, Hodler, and Scherer for their contribution to the questionnaire development. Special thanks also belong to Professor Fehr for his methodological inputs in this study. Permission from the International Society for Pharmacoeconomics and Outcomes Research (ISPOR) for reproduction of the contents of the article is acknowledged.

References

1. Deyo, R.A., Nachemson, A., and Mirza, S.K. 2004. Spinal-fusion surgery – the case for restraint. *New England Journal of Medicine* **350**: 722–726.

2. Gibson, J.N., Grant, I.C., and Waddell, G. 1999. The Cochrane review of surgery for lumbar disc prolapse and degenerative lumbar spondylosis. *Spine* **24**: 1820–1832.

3. Shvartzman, L., Weingarten, E., Sherry, H., Levin, S., and Persaud, A. 1992. Cost-effectiveness analysis of extended conservative therapy versus surgical intervention in the management of herniated lumbar intervertebral disc. *Spine* **17**: 176–182.

4. Fritzell, P., Hagg, O., Jonsson, D., and Nordwall, A. 2004. Cost-effectiveness of lumbar fusion and nonsurgical treatment for chronic low back pain in the Swedish Lumbar Spine Study: a multicenter, randomized, controlled trial from the Swedish Lumbar Spine Study Group. *Spine* **29**: 421–434; discussion Z423.

5. Malter, A.D., Larson, E.B., Urban, N., and Deyo, R.A. 1996. Cost-effectiveness of lumbar discectomy for the treatment of herniated intervertebral disc. *Spine* **21**: 1048–1054; discussion 1055.

6. Rivero-Arias, O., Campbell, H., Gray, A., *et al.* 2005. Surgical stabilisation of the spine compared with a programme of intensive rehabilitation for the management of patients with chronic low back pain: cost utility analysis based on a randomised controlled trial. *BMJ* **330**: 1239.

7. O'Brien, B. and Gafni, A. 1996. When do the 'dollars' make sense? Toward a conceptual framework for contingent valuation studies in health care. *Medical Decision Making* **16**: 288–299.

8. Shackley, P. and Donaldson, C. 2002. Should we use willingness to pay to elicit community preferences for health care? New evidence from using a 'marginal' approach. *Journal of Health Economics* **21**: 971–991.

9. Klose, T. 1999. The contingent valuation method in health care. *Health Policy* **47**: 97–123.

10. Johannesson, M. 1996. *Theory and Methods of Economic Evaluation of Health Care* Dordrecht/Boston/London: Kluwer Academic Publishers.

11. Olsen, J.A. and Smith, R.D. 2001. Theory versus practice: a review of 'willingness-to-pay' in health and health care. *Health Economics* **10**: 39–52.

12. Diener, A., O'Brien, B., and Gafni, A. 1998. Health care contingent valuation studies: a review and classification of the literature. *Health Economics* **7**: 313–326.

13. Olsen, J.A., Kidholm, K., Donaldson, C., and Shackley, P. 2004. Willingness to pay for public health care: a comparison of two approaches. *Health Policy* **70**: 217–228.

14. King, J.T., Jr., Styn, M.A., Tsevat, J., and Roberts, M.S. 2003. 'Perfect health' versus 'disease free': the impact of anchor point choice on the measurement of preferences and the calculation of disease-specific disutilities. *Medical Decision Making* **23**: 212–225.

15. Slothuus, U. and Brooks, R.G. 2000. Willingness to pay in arthritis: a Danish contribution. *Rheumatology (Oxford)* **39**: 791–799.

16. Slothuus, U., Larsen, M.L., and Junker, P. 2000. Willingness to pay for arthritis symptom alleviation. Comparison of closed-ended questions with and without follow-up. *International Journal of Technology Assess Health Care* **16**: 60–72.

17. Ethgen, O., Tancredi, A., Lejeune, E., *et al.* 2003. Do utility values and willingness to pay suitably reflect health outcome in hip and knee osteoarthritis? A comparative analysis with the WOMAC Index. *Journal of Rheumatol* **30**: 2452–2459.

18. Thompson, M.S., Read, J.L., and Liang, M. 1984. Feasibility of willingness-to-pay measurement in chronic arthritis. *Medical Decision Making* **4**: 195–215.

19. Cross, M.J., March, L.M., Lapsley, H.M., *et al.* 2000. Determinants of willingness to pay for hip and knee joint replacement surgery for osteoarthritis. *Rheumatology (Oxford)* **39**: 1242–1248.

20. Andersson, G.B., Brown, M.D., Dvorak, J., *et al.* 1996. Consensus summary of the diagnosis and treatment of lumbar disc herniation. *Spine* **21**(24 Suppl.): S75–S78.

21. Postacchini, F. 1999. Surgical management of lumbar spinal stenosis. *Spine* **24**: 1043–1047.

22. Lipson, S.J. 2004. Spinal-fusion surgery – advances and concerns. *New England Journal Medicine* **350**: 643–644.

23. Ryan, M., Scott, D.A., Reeves, C., *et al.* 2001. Eliciting public preferences for healthcare: a systematic review of techniques. *Health Technology Assess* **5**: 1–186.

24. Evans, C. 1997. The use of consensus methods and expert panels in pharmacoeconomic studies. Practical applications and methodological shortcomings. *Pharmacoeconomics* **12**(2 Pt 1): 121–129.

25. Cohen , J. 1960. A coefficient of agreement for nominal scales. *Educational Psychological Measurement* **20**(1): 37–46.

26. Landis, J.R. and Koch, G.G. 1977. The measurement of observer agreement for categorical data. *Biometrics* **33**: 159–174.

27. Von Korff, M., Jensen, M.P., and Karoly, P. 2000. Assessing global pain severity by self-report in clinical and health services research. *Spine* **25**: 3140–3151.

28. Bolton, J.E. 1999. Accuracy of recall of usual pain intensity in back pain patients. *Pain* **83**: 533–539.

29. Stewart, W.F., Lipton, R.B., Simon, D., *et al.* 1999. Validity of an illness severity measure for headache in a population sample of migraine sufferers. *Pain* **79**: 291–301.

30. Haas, M., Nyiendo, J., and Aickin, M. 2002. One-year trend in pain and disability relief recall in acute and chronic ambulatory low back pain patients. *Pain* **95**: 83–91.

31. Bateman, I. and Carson, R. 2002. *Economic valuation with stated preference techniques: a manual*. Cheltenham: Edward Elgar.

32. Smith, R.D. 2000. The discrete-choice willingness-to-pay question format in health economics: should we adopt environmental guidelines? *Medical Decision Making* **20**: 194–206.

33. Donaldson, C., Shackley, P., Abdalla, M., and Miedzybrodzka, Z. 1995. Willingness to pay for antenatal carrier screening for cystic fibrosis. *Health Economics* **4**: 439–452.

34. Swan, J.S., Fryback, D.G., Lawrence, W.F., *et al.* 1997. MR and conventional angiography: work in progress toward assessing utility in radiology. *Academic Radiology* **4**: 475–482.

35. Pinto-Prades, J., Farreras, V., and Fernandez de Bobadilla, J. 2006. Willingness to pay for a reduction in the mortality risk after a myocardial infarction: an application of the contingent valuation method to the case of eplerenone. In: *Department of Economics*. University Pablo de Olavide.

36. Min-Naing, C., Lertmaharit, S., Kamol-Ratanakil, P., and Saul, A.J. 2000. Ex post and es ante willingness to pay (WTP) for the ICT Malaria Pf/Py test kit in Myanmar. Southeast. *Asian Journal of Tropical Medicine and Public Health* **31**: 104–111.

37. Shackley, P. and Donaldson, C. 2000. Willingness to pay for publicly-financed health care: how should we use the numbers? *Applied Economics* **32**: 2015–2021.

38. Haefeli, M., Elfering, A., McIntosh, E., Gray, A., Sukthankar, A., and Boos, N. 2008. A cost-benefit analysis using contingent valuation techniques: A feasibility study in spinal surgery. *Value in Health* **11**(4): 575–588.

Appendix 8.1 Item characteristics, WTP questions, and reproducibility of WTP survey

Item	Response format	Acceptability	Floor/ceiling effects	Distribution	Reproducibility N = 52	
					ICC	Kappa
Suppose your insurance would not have covered the cost of the surgery. What would be the maximum amount you would have paid for the intervention out of your own pocket?	Absolute value Open-ended	N = 77 73.3%	–	Skewness: 2.453 Kurtosis: 9.401	0.494 C.I.: 0.222–0.696 P < 0.001	–
Would you be willing to take on a loan, if you could not pay for the surgery?	Likert scale (yes, probably yes, probably no, no)	N = 98 93.3%	Ceiling: 50.5% Floor: 15.2%	Skewness: 0.878 Kurtosis: −0.771	–	0.351 P < 0.001
Suppose your household income was €5,769 and your wealth was €128,205. What would be the maximum you would have paid for the intervention out of your own pocket?	Absolute value Open-ended	N = 75 71.4%	–	Skewness: 3.456 Kurtosis: 17.574	0.5916 C.I.: 0.349–0.760 P < 0.001	–
Would you have renounced surgery for money? If yes, for how much?	Dichotomous (yes, no)	N = 96 91.4%	–	Skewness: −5.474 Kurtosis: 28.560	–*	–
Would you recommend your type of surgery to family and friends?	Likert scale (no, probably no, probably yes, yes)	N = 101 96.2%	Ceiling: 71.4% Floor: 1.9%	Skewness: 2.047 Kurtosis: 3.864	–	0.741 P < 0.001
Would you recommend your type of surgery to family and friends, even if they have to pay for it out of their own pocket?	Likert scale (yes, probably yes, probably no, no)	N = 99 94.3%	Ceiling: 58.1% Floor: 3.8%	Skewness: 1.582 Kurtosis: 2.125	–	0.473 P < 0.001

Item	Scale	N / %	Ceiling / Floor	Skewness / Kurtosis		
TIOLI: Imagine the surgery would cost €x. Would you have chosen the operation? (x = 6,410 for discectomy, 12,821 for spinal decompression, 19,231 for spinal fusion)?	Likert scale (yes, probably yes, probably no, no)	N = 99 94.3%	Ceiling: 51.4% Floor: 5.7%	Skewness: 1.105 Kurtosis: 0.210	—	0.413 $P < 0.001$
How much do you estimate the total hospital costs for your intervention?	Absolute value open-ended	N = 91 86.7%	—	Skewness: 1.764 Kurtosis: 2.927	0.811 C.I.: 0.695–0.892 $P < 0.001$	—
What is your monthly gross household income?	Numerical rating scale (NRS)	N = 91 86.7%	—	Skewness: 1.448 Kurtosis: 1.710	–*	—
Do you own real estate?	Dichotomous (yes, no)	N = 97 92.3%	—	Skewness: 0.105 Kurtosis: −2.031	–*	—
Financial solvency: How easy is it for you to gather €32,051 in cash within short-term?	Likert scale (very difficult, difficult, rather difficult, rather easy, easy, very easy)	N = 95 90.5%	Ceiling: 1.0% Floor: 29.5%	Skewness: 0.790 Kurtosis: −0.286	—	0.415 $P < 0.001$

*These items were not included in the test–retest experiment

ICC: Intraclass Correlation Coefficient; PCA: Percent Agreement; C.I.: Confidence Interval

Chapter 9

Using revealed preference methods to value health care: The travel cost approach

Philip M. Clarke

The fact that a patient does not have to pay his GP for a consultation does not mean that consultations are costless to the patient. Visiting a surgery requires the patient to sacrifice time—travelling to and from the surgery, waiting to see the GP, and the time spent in the consultation itself... (If he travels to the surgery by car or by public transport, of if he has to take time off work, the consultation may also involve outlays of money).
(*Robert Sugden and Alan Williams 1978, p. 149*)*

9.1 Introduction

Following on from the stated preference, or direct approaches, outlined in Chapters 6, 7, and 8 indirect or revealed preference (RP) methods are a class of techniques that have been developed to value non-market and unpriced goods. There has been a long tradition of using these methods in the valuation of the health benefits associated with improving the quality of the environment and the value of life, which is implied by the purchase of safety equipment. In contrast, there are very few studies using this method that have valued health care goods. The evaluation of health care in developed countries normally involves goods or services that prevent or treat non-infectious diseases. Government intervention has two dimensions – the regulation of product quality and the regulation of price to ensure that consumers pay only a zero or a nominal price to receive health care. Here we primarily focus on the implications of the latter for economic evaluation.

There are two ways in which RP methods can be applied in the evaluation of health care. One way is to value health care by valuing its outputs. There are however several disadvantages with using this approach. Firstly, for the reasons outlined in Chapter 2, it may be difficult to extend this approach to the valuation of changes in morbidity associated with the consumption of health care. Secondly, it is impossible to value non-health related outcomes, such as the value of information or 'process utility'. Thirdly, the approach does not take into account the possibility that the individual's attitude to risk might differ across different types of goods (1, p. 115). Finally, although safety equipment and averting inputs are exchanged in markets, the market price only reflects the marginal consumer's WTP. All that can be inferred is that the market price represents the lower bound for the value of safety for those who purchase the equipment and an upper bound for those who do not purchase it.

The other approach that has largely been overlooked in the evaluation of health care is the travel cost model. The travel cost model focuses on access cost rather than price because there is likely to be much greater variation in the former. It has been widely used in environmental economics to value recreation areas such as national parks. For an overview of these applications see Ward and Beal (2) or Parsons (3). The remainder of this chapter is devoted to examining the scope for using this method in the evaluation of health care goods and services.

9.2 **Travel cost model**

The travel cost model overcomes the unpriced goods problem by focusing on the individual's outlay on other inputs necessary for the production of health. An individual will seek medical care if the benefit she gains is greater than her total time and travel costs.

9.2.1 **Historical development**

The origins of the travel cost model can be traced back to a letter from Harold Hotelling written in the late 1940s in response to a US National Parks Service solicitation on ways to value the economic benefits of national parks (4, pp. 683–684). National parks are difficult to value using conventional welfare economic analysis, because users are normally charged only nominal amounts to gain entry, and a fixed fee does not generate sufficient price variation to estimate a demand curve for the park. Without a demand curve, it is impossible to estimate the benefit recreationalists derive from using the park. Hotelling's letter contained the insight that it is possible to estimate a demand curve by studying the behaviour of users at various distances from the recreation site.

Hotelling's suggestion was taken up several years later by Clawson in his work on benefits associated with the recreational use of Yosemite and the Grand Canyon National Parks (5). Clawson's approach involved estimating an aggregate demand curve by conducting on-site interviews at each park. Each user was then assigned to a geographic zone depending on the origin of her trip. This information was used to construct a demand curve based on the utilization rate and the average travel cost per zone. The welfare benefits associated with the recreational use of the park are the area under this curve (4).

In recent years, the focus of travel cost research has shifted from zonal utilization rates to individual demand (6). Individual travel cost models come in two forms: (i) a *single-site travel cost model* that focuses on the number of visits an individual makes over a fixed period of time and (ii) a *multi-site travel cost model* that examines the choice of site on a single occasion (7). Both these models are outlined in Section 9.2.2.

9.2.2 **Single-site travel cost models**

The purpose of the traditional recreational travel cost model is to estimate the benefits associated with a single recreation site over a specific time period such as a season. This approach estimates the demand for a site based on the behavioural assumption that users experience diminishing marginal utility each time they re-visit the site within this period of time (8).

The trip demand equation is as follows:

$$x_1^i = \beta_0 + \beta_1 c_1^i + \beta_2 S^i + \varepsilon^i \qquad (9.1)$$

where, x_1^i is the number of trips $(x_1 = 1,2,3..q)$ the ith individual makes to the site; c_1^i is their access cost; S^i is a vector of the characteristics of the individual (e.g. age, income, and whether they are a member of a recreational organization); β_0 is the constant term; β_1 is the coefficient on the cost term and β_2 is a vector of coefficients for variables in S^i; and ε^i is an error term. The compensating variation (CV) of a decline in access costs is:

$$CV = e(c_1^0, U^0) - e(c_1^f, U^0) = \int_{c_1^0}^{c_1^f} x_1^c, \qquad (9.2)$$

where U^0 is the initial level of utility and x_1^c is the Hicksian demand for the site. The CV is often approximated using the Marshallian consumer surplus (i.e. $CS = \int_{c_1^0}^{c_1^f} x_1^m$). This welfare benefit is represented graphically in Figure 9.1.

At the initial access cost c_1^0, users will make x_1^0 visits per year. If the access cost delines to c_1^f the number of visits will increase to x_1^f and so CS will be given by the area to the left of the demand curve between these costs.

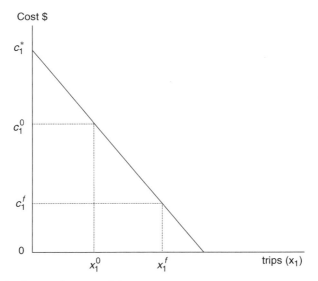

Fig. 9.1 Single-site travel cost model.

The total welfare benefits associated with the site can be estimated by setting c_1^f equal to the cost at which the individual ceases to visit the site and c_1^0 equal to a zero cost in order to capture the entire area under the demand curve:

$$CV_1 = \int_0^{c_1^*} x_1^c dc_1, \tag{9.3}$$

where c_1^* is the 'choke' access cost.

9.2.3 Multi-site models

The travel cost model has also been used to model the demand for different sites. Multi-site studies often apply a random utility model (RUM) and focus on the individual's choice among a set of alternate sites on a single occasion. The RUM involves specifying a utility function to represent the characteristics of each site:

$$U_j^i(z_j, y_j^i, S^i) = W_j^i(z_j, y_j^i, S^i) + \varepsilon_j^i, \tag{9.4}$$

where z_j is a vector of k on-site characteristics (i.e. $z_j = (z_j^0, ..., z_j^k)$) for the jth site; y_j^i is the individual's income; and S^i is a vector representing individual characteristics. If we define one of the alternatives ($j = 0$) to be the individual not attending any site, the access cost associated with each site is the difference in income ($c_j^i = y_0^i - y_j^i$). The main application of this type of model is in the valuation of 'quality' characteristics of differences between sites. To illustrate the welfare measurement of a change in quality, assume there are only two sites and that they differ in only one respect. The welfare benefit/loss associated with the change in quality is:

$$CV_2 = e(c_1, z_1, U^0) - e(c_1, z_2, U^0), \tag{9.5}$$

where $z_1 = (\hat{z}_j^0, z_j^2 .. z_j^k)$ and $z_2 = (\tilde{z}_j^0, z_j^2 .. z_j^k)$. Mäler (9) has shown that this measure of welfare change is the area between the Hicksian demand curves associated with z_1 and z_2 providing the individual only values a site if they use it (i.e. weak complementarity holds). In this case:

$$CV_2 = \int_{c_1^0}^{c_1^*} [x_1^c(c_1, z_2, U^0) - x_1^c(c_1, z_1, U^0)]. \tag{9.6}$$

In practice, the area between the two Hicksian demand curves is often approximated using the area between the Marshallian demand curves.[1]

9.3 The health care travel cost model

There is scope for using the single-site or the multi-site travel cost model in the evaluation of health care. For example, the single-site model could be used to value a treatment which requires the patient to make multiple visits to a single medical facility

---

[1] For a discussion of the issues surrounding the validity of using Marshallian demand curves in this context see (10).

(e.g. a doctor's surgery) over a period of time. Alternatively, a multi-site model could value characteristics of differences between different facilities.

While the single and multi-site travel cost models provide a useful starting point, it is important to stress that some types of health care have several features that may require the development (or adaption) of new types of model. Firstly, health care goods are often homogeneous products that are supplied from different sites. For example, a patient can obtain the same drug from many different pharmacies. Secondly, demand depends on the type of health care a patient requires. Although a single facility might offer a range of health care services, generally we are interested in one type of service – not the demand for the facility as a whole.

These features make it difficult to directly apply either the single-site or multi-site travel cost model in the evaluation of health care. One way of adapting the travel cost model is to focus on the relationship between distance to the *closest* facility and demand for different services (e.g. mammographic screening) rather than the demand for a service at a particular facility. For example, if identical products are offered at different locations, then the characteristics of the site z_j can be ignored, because they do not influence choice (e.g. $z_1 = z_2$). In which case, data on S^i and c_1^i can be collected in different areas and the relationship between the demand for health care and the distance to the *closest* facility can be modelled in order to value care.

Although non-site specific models are likely to be the most common form of health care travel cost model, it should be recognized that health care is not always a homogeneous product. Medical facilities may offer similar, but not identical products (e.g. women might prefer to be treated by a female GP). In this case, the model should be extended to incorporate on-site characteristics (z_j). Such a formulation is similar to the recreational travel cost models discussed above.

Another complicating factor in the valuation of health care is that it is sometimes essential for survival (e.g. insulin for people with Type 1 diabetes). Johansson (11) has explored the conditions under which it is possible to use costs related to the consumption of health care. The key conditions are that the costs must be essential for consumption of heath care, but the care produced must be non-essential for survival in order for there to be finite choke prices for the demand curves.

9.4 Methodological issues with the travel cost approach

Estimation of a travel cost model might appear to be relatively straightforward, because it involves the observed behaviour and thereby avoids many of the difficulties that arise when trying to directly elicit preferences using stated preference methods. In practice, estimation is just as difficult, because it requires the researcher to overcome a different set of problems stemming from the unobserved nature of travel costs. As Randall (12) notes, unlike market prices which can be directly observed, travel costs must be imputed from behaviour. A key issue concerns methods to value a patients time.

9.4.1 The valuation of time

In addition to the out-of-pocket expenses incurred while travelling to a medical facility (e.g. the cost of petrol), patients must also allocate some of their time in order to receive health care. It is generally accepted that the opportunity cost of this time is strictly positive, because the time spent on health care reduces the time available for work or leisure. However, there is little agreement on its method of valuation. Most empirical studies value time as a function of the marginal wage since the labour market is one place where time is traded for money. This is the starting point for the theoretical work presented below.

9.4.1.1 A general framework

The neo-classical model of labour supply assumes that an individual maximizes utility by consuming goods (x_c) and leisure (non-work) time (t_l) subject to an income and a time constraint. The maximization problem is therefore:

$$\max U(x_c, t_l)$$
$$s.t. y_u + t_w w - p_c x_c \geq 0 \qquad (9.7)$$
$$T - t_w - t_l = 0$$

where, y_u is unearned income; t_w is the time spent working; w is the wage rate; p_c is the price of the consumption good; and T is the total time available. Unlike income, all time must be allocated to either labour or leisure and so the time constraint is an equality. The Lagrangian for this model is:

$$\ell = U(x_c, t_l) + \lambda(w t_w + y_u - p_c x_c) + \mu(T - t_w - t_l). \qquad (9.8)$$

Denoting partial derivatives by subscripts (i.e. $U_{x_c} = \dfrac{\partial U}{\partial x_c}$) the solution to the Lagrangian yields:

$$\frac{U_{x_c}}{U_{t_l}} = \frac{\mu}{\lambda} p_c, \qquad (9.9)$$

where, the parameter λ is the marginal utility of money and μ is the marginal value of time. In equilibrium, the 'scarcity value' of time equals the marginal wage:

$$w = \frac{\mu}{\lambda}. \qquad (9.10)$$

In this simple model, only leisure time is a source of utility. It is also possible that individuals derive (dis)utility from the time they spend at work. This can be incorporated into the model by including work time (t_w) as well as leisure time in the utility function (13). If U_{t_w} denotes the (dis)utility associated with time spent at work (9.10) becomes:

$$w = \frac{\mu}{\lambda} - \frac{U_{t_w}}{\lambda}. \qquad (9.11)$$

Equation (9.11) suggests that the marginal wage not only reflects the scarcity value of time, but also the (dis)utility of work time. This latter term has been labelled the 'commodity value' of time (14). If $U_{t_w} < 0$, the wage must compensate for the disutility of undertaking work as well as the sacrifice of time. In these circumstances, the value of non-work time is *less* than the marginal wage rate, because extra compensation is not required for the sacrifice of non-work time.

Activities undertaken in non-work time can also be a source of (dis)utility. For example, Cesario (15) argues that travel time should be valued at less than the marginal wage because the individual enjoys travel. Many environmental travel cost studies adopt this approach and value travel time at 20–50% of the marginal wage (e.g. 15–17).[2] An exception is Larson (18), who assumes that people gain utility from work and so leisure time has a value greater than the marginal wage.

The time involved in the production of health care might also have a commodity value (e.g. waiting for a GP consultation may be a source of great disutility!). Alternatively, a patient might gain utility from the time she spends with a GP if she feels that the quality of treatment is positively correlated with the length of the consultation. If we divide t_l into the time an individual devotes to health care as t_h and other time t_o the maximization problem becomes:

$$\max U(x_c, t_h, t_o)$$
$$s.t. y_u + t_w w - p_c x_c \geq 0 \qquad (9.12)$$
$$T - t_w - t_h - t_o = 0$$

Again solving the Lagrangian, the value of time spent in health care is:

$$w = \frac{\mu}{\lambda} - \frac{U_{t_h}}{\lambda}. \qquad (9.13)$$

If $U_{t_h} < 0$, then (9.13) implies that the value of time is greater than the marginal wage. If the patient reduces t_h it not only allows her to reallocate her time to other activities, but reduces her disutility and so the value of this time should be *greater* than her marginal wage.

9.4.1.2 Labour market constraints and the value of time

The other reason the value of time differs from the marginal wage is that constraints in the labour market prevent the substitution of work time for leisure. The simple labour supply model represented by (9.7.) assumes that individuals have total discretion over their hours of work. Such a highly simplified labour supply model captures none of the institutional constraints that govern modern labour markets. In most labour markets, individuals must choose between a job in which they are required to work minimum number of hours per week, or unemployment. However, even in these circumstances, there is often flexibility, as an employee in a job with fixed hours might have the opportunity to work overtime or take up a second job. Such a situation is illustrated in Figure 9.2.

---

[2] This range reflects the utility an individual gains from driving to a recreation site. A patient travelling to a medical facility is more likely to experience disutility than utility so there is no basis for using these values in a health care travel cost model.

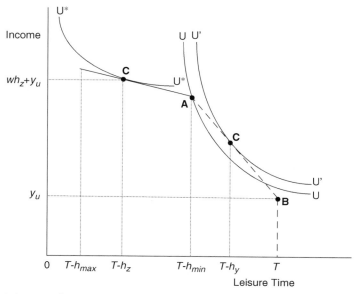

Fig. 9.2 Labour market constraints and the value of time.

Figure 9.2 illustrates a typical labour market situation (19). The discrete nature of the decision to work is represented by the 'hole' in the budget constraint between T and $T - h_{min}$, with h_{min} being the minimum number of hours that the individual can work. Consider an individual with an indifference curve UU, she can gain more utility from working h_{min} hours (at point A) than being unemployed (point B). If she has discretion over her hours of work, she would move to point C on the higher indifference curve (U'U') by working h_y hours. At point A or B the marginal rate of substitution of income for leisure does not equate with the budget line. At either point the value of time is not the marginal wage. It does not even represent the upper or lower bound since the true value depends on the (unobservable) marginal rate of substitution of income for leisure.

Above h_{min}, the individual has discretion over her hours of work and so the budget line is continuous between h_{min} and h_{max}. In this range, the wage is the value of time. For example, an individual will maximize her utility at point C on the indifference curve U^*U^* by working h_z hours, the value of her time is the negative of the slope of the budget line, which is determined by the marginal wage of the second job or the wage paid for working overtime.

9.4.1.3 Health status and the value of time

Health status also places constraints on the allocation of time, because a person in poor health is likely to be unable to work and is restricted in the range of other activities they can undertake. Hence, the scarcity value of time for a seriously ill person might be quite low. The commodity value of time spent in ill health is influenced by two factors – the level of disutility experienced while spending time in a low health state and the marginal utility of money. It is safe to assume that people suffer disutility when they are in ill health, but the effect of health on the marginal utility of money is less clear. Evans and Viscusi (20) suggest poor health has two effects on the marginal utility of money. Initially, reductions in health status are likely to lower the marginal utility of money. At the same time, people who suffer a serious illness are normally unable to work, which results in a reduction in income. This is likely to have the secondary effect of increasing the marginal utility of money. The net impact of these two effects on the marginal utility of money would be an interesting area for future research.

9.4.1.4 The role of time in the household production model

The role of time is central to the household production model (HPM) since it must be combined with other goods to produce non-market commodities such as health. In Becker's original formulation of the HPM, time does not directly enter the utility function and so its value is constant across all activities. This implies time only has a scarcity value. The consumer's problem is to:

$$\max U(H_t, Z_t)$$
$$s.t. y_u + t_w w - p_1 x_1 + p_c x_c \geq 0$$
$$T_t - t_w - t_1 x_1 - t_c x_c = 0 \tag{9.14}$$
$$H_t = f(x_1, t_1)$$
$$Z_t = f(x_c, t_c)$$

Recall that H_t, Z_t are a health commodity and another commodity respectively; x_1 is a health care good; and x_c is a good used in the production of Z_t. The two constraints are not independent if the consumer can freely trade time for money in the labour market. For these individuals, the time constraint can be collapsed into the money constraint by trading time for money at the margin. Thus, the two constraints in (9.14) can be combined to give:

$$y_u + t_w w - (p_1 + wt_1)x_1 - (p_n + wt_c)x_c = 0. \tag{9.15}$$

Alternatively, this can be written as:

$$Y - c_1 x_1 - x_c = 0, \tag{9.15a}$$

where, c_1 is total access cost $(c_1 = p_1 + wt_1)$ and $Y = y_u + t_w w$. This reduces the problem to the conventional single constraint problem where the utility function in (9.14) is maximized subject to (9.15) or (9.15a).

For those individuals working a fixed number of hours, the scarcity value of time is not the marginal wage and so the individual will be subject to separate time and income constraints. In these circumstances, the demand for medical care is a function of both money *and* time. One way of estimating the *monetary* value of time is to observe the rate at which individuals trade time for money in their choice of health care. (i.e. their choice between a high cost/low time medical care and a low cost/high time alternative).[3] If such a trade-off does not exist, time and travel costs are highly correlated and so it is not possible to impute the value of time from behaviour.

9.5 Measuring other types of access cost

In addition to time costs, a user often must travel to a health care facility and may have to pay a user fee to access health care. Ways of obtaining information on each of these costs is discussed below.

Information on travel distance can be obtained through direct questioning (e.g. How far the did you travel to obtain health care?), but this relies on respondents being able to accurately estimate the distance they travelled when they sought care. Previous empirical work suggests that many respondents have difficulty in accurately estimating travel distances (21).

Another way of ascertaining travel distance is to ask respondents for their residential location and destination. The travel distance can then be imputed from the road distance between her place of residence and the medical facility. This method is not free from error, because the respondent might not have taken this route or may have initiated the journey from another location (e.g. from her place of work). Additional questions could be used to reduce measurement error, but this increases the length of the questionnaire and the burden on the respondent.

In order to calculate the travel cost, the distance travelled must be multiplied by a unit cost of travel. Using survey questions to estimate the cost of travelling by a private vehicle is problematic because most people have difficulty assessing vehicle running costs. They seem to pay more attention to routine costs, such as cost of petrol, than the costs which are incurred infrequently (e.g. cost of maintenance and depreciation) (22;23). For this reason, most travel cost studies apply a third party assessment of the running cost such as those produced by motoring organizations.

For those users that travel by public transport, unit travel costs are not meaningful and the total cost of the journey (i.e. ticket price) should be used. The time taken is also likely to be much longer, because public transport routes often require the user to travel to a 'transport hub' and then to their destination (21, p. 25).

In regard to user charges, what is important are the 'out-of-pocket' charges that are not covered by insurance (i.e. the deductable or co-payment). Again this information would need to be obtained through direct questioning, or from administrative information on the standard fee normally levied for the type of health care under evaluation.

---

[3] In fact a utility maximization problem subject to two constraints has two duals, one of which minimizes monetary costs subject to utility and the time constraint the other which minimizes time costs subject to utility and income constraints (19).

9.6 **Health care applications**

The impact that travel distance has on health care utilization has long been recognized. For example, Acton (24) examined the influence of distance on the demand for zero-priced outpatient services in New York. This type of study is often referred to as a 'distance decay' study since it models the relationship between travel distance and health care utilization (25). The travel cost method differs from the distance decay approach in that it converts physical measures of access into a money metric in order to facilitate the measurement of welfare gain (or loss) in monetary terms. A summary of travel cost method applications to value health care are listed in Table 9.1.

One of the earliest health care related applications of the travel cost model is Deyak and Smith (26) who attempted to measure the cost of institutional and legal restrictions in accessing abortion services in the United States prior to the 1973 ruling of the Supreme Court which legalized abortion in all States. Prior to this, legal abortions could only be obtained in a limited number of States such as New York and women living in other States had to travel in order to obtain an abortion. Deyak and Smith (26) used data on the distances travelled by women to New York to estimate a demand curve for abortion services and calculated the consumer surplus associated being able to access these services without having to travel interstate (which was the effect of the Supreme Court's decision). However, as the authors note the consumer surplus associated with improved access is only one potential component of welfare impacts of the abortion reform. Such policies also may have significant non-use costs such as psychological losses of those opposed to abortion which potentially would need to be taken into account in a full CBA.

Both Wang'ombe (27) and Gertler, Locay, and Sanderson (28) and more recently Jeuland *et al.* (29) have used travel costs to estimate demand curves for medicare in developing countries. The first of these estimated the demand curve of the use of community health workers in rural areas of Kenya for two different sites. Using the demand curve, he calculated consumer surplus as a way of evaluating the overall benefits and compared these with the cost of providing these services. Overall the total benefits exceeded the total costs over a wide range of assumptions regarding the discount rate and the value of time.

In developed countries, the applications of the travel cost method can be divided into those concerned with preventative services and those related to treatment. With regard to preventative services, Clarke (30) and Sandstrom (31) used the travel cost method to value mammographic screening in Australia and Sweden, respectively. Both studies used a similar discrete choice framework to examine the probability of being screened as function of access costs which are related to the travel distance for women living in different areas. Welfare benefits were then obtained from the estimated demand curve. Another study that used the travel cost method to evaluate a preventative health care service is Ohshige, Mitzushima, and Tochikubo (32), which used a demand curve for annual health checkups based on access costs (including time and travel costs) for residents in Tokyo, Japan. The visit rate was plotted against the estimated access cost to obtain a demand curve which was used to calculate individual willingness to pay.

Table 9.1 Summary of previous travel cost model studies used to value health care

Publication date	Authors	Country	Type of health care valued	Aim of analysis
1976	Deyak and Smith	United States	Abortion	Estimation of welfare cost associated with legal restriction
1984	Wang'ombe	Kenya	Community-based health care project	Cost–benefit analysis of providing these services
1987	Gertler, Locay, and Sanderson	Peru	Public hospital, public clinic, and private doctor	Examination of the impact of user fees on consumer welfare
1995	Anex	United States	Household hazardous waste collection and disposal services	Zonal travel cost model to estimate consumer surplus associated with provision of the service
1998	Clarke	Australia	Mammographic screening	Cost–benefit analysis of improving access through use of mobile screening units
1999	McNamara	United States	Hospitalizations	Welfare loss from hospital closure
1999	Sandstrom	Sweden	Mammographic screening	Value of a statistical life
2004	Ohshige, Mitzushima, and Tochikubo	Japan	Public health check-up programme	Cost–benefit analysis
2008	Solano and McDuffie	United States	Substance abuse outpatient treatment	Estimate demand and utilization
2009	Jeuland, Lucas, Clemens, and Whittington	Mozambique	Demand for cholera vaccines	Estimate of willingness to pay for a cholera vaccine

With regard to the applications of health care treatments, McNamara (33) has used the travel cost approach to estimate the welfare loss arising from closures of rural hospitals using a discrete choice travel cost framework. More recently, Solano and McDuffie (34) have used variations in access costs to estimate the demand for substance abuse outpatient treatment in Delaware USA, with the intention of evaluating options for decentralized services. Beyond health care, the travel cost method has also been used to value public provision of services that impact risk such as household hazardous waste disposal services (35).

While there have only been a limited number of health-related travel cost studies, the diverse range of applications of those studies contained in this review suggests considerable scope for use of this method in the future evaluations of health care goods and services.

9.7 **The travel cost model in action**

An example of a travel cost model used to value health care is contained in Clarke (30). This study uses CBA to evaluate the provision of mammographic screening in rural areas of Australia, where travel distances represent a significant proportion of the costs incurred by users. The section draws on a contingent valuation study which also attempted to value these screening units (41).

9.7.1 **Background**

In recent years, several developed countries including Australia have set up organized programmes for breast cancer screening by making mammograms available to women in the target age range free of charge. In rural areas, this aim can be achieved by adopting one of two modes of service delivery: (i) 'service to the client' and (ii) 'client to the service'. The first approach involves the use of mobile screening units that visit towns too small to have fixed screening units. The alternative approach is to place fixed units only in major regional centres. Women in smaller towns must travel to these centres in order to have a mammogram. This case study examines how the travel cost method can be used to evaluate whether mobile screening units should be used to screen women in ten different rural towns.

9.7.2 **Benefits of improving access to mammographic screening**

If a mobile unit visits a rural town without a permanent screening facility, women in the area benefit from having to travel a lesser distance to have a mammogram. Clarke (30) derives welfare benefits of reducing time and travel costs. The total cost of travelling to a screening unit is $c_1 = p_1 + wt_1$, where p_1 are *out-of-pocket* travel expenses (e.g. cost of petrol), w is the value of time, and t_1 is the total time required to be screened. Both p_1 and t_1 are in turn functions of the distance women must travel to have a mammogram.

Consider a town in which a woman must incur a cost of c_1^0 to have a mammogram at a permanent facility (fixed site) located outside her town. When a mobile screening unit visits the town, her access cost is reduced to c_1^f. Given the binary nature of the screening decision (i.e. to have a single mammogram or remain unscreened) the population of women eligible for screening can be divided into three groups which are illustrated in Figures 9.3(a)–(c). Each figure illustrates the welfare change resulting from a visit by a mobile unit for women who are willing to pay different amounts for a mammogram (denoted by $c_1^{\#}$, $c_1^{\sim}$, and c_1^{*}). Figure 9.3(a) shows the WTP of a woman who is prepared to travel to a permanent facility because her WTP is greater than the cost of travelling to that site ($c_1^0 < c_1^{\#}$). Her welfare gain, if a mobile unit visits her town of residence is the reduction in access costs (i.e. $c_1^f - c_1^0$) or the shaded area in Figure 9.3(a). Figure 9.3(b) shows the WTP of a woman who chooses not to have a mammogram at the permanent facility ($c_1^0 > c_1^{\sim}$), but has a mammogram at the mobile unit. For this woman, the welfare gain associated with the reduction in access costs from c_1^0 to c_1^f is the shaded area or the difference between the final access cost and her WTP for a mammogram (i.e. $c_1^f - c_1^{\sim}$). The final figure (Figure 9.3(c)) shows the WTP of a woman who chooses not to have a mammogram even when the access costs are reduced (i.e. $c_1^f > c_1^{*}$). She gains no use benefit from visiting of a mobile screening unit.

9.7.3 Specification of the random utility model

Section 9.7.2 illustrates the measure of welfare change associated with a reduction in access costs. In this section, it is reformulated in probabilistic terms using a RUM. In order to make this model operational, an appropriate conditional utility function must be specified to represent a woman's decision on whether to have a mammogram.

The conditional utility function for the ith individual is:

$$V_j(m_j, Y^i, S^i) = W_j(m_j, Y^i, S^i) + \varepsilon_j^i, \qquad (9.16)$$

where W_j is a conditional utility function; m_j denotes whether the individual has a mammogram; Y^i is income; S^i is other characteristics of the consumer; and ε_j^i are

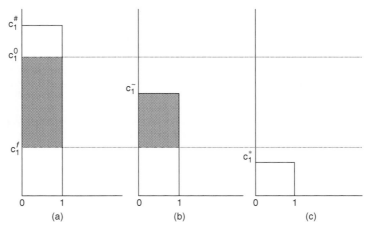

Fig. 9.3 Welfare gains associated with mammographic screening. Reproduced from Clarke, P.M. 2000. Valuing the benefits of mobile mammographic screening units using the contingent valuation method. *Applied Economics* **32**:1647–1655, with permission.

errors of observation. Women must make a dichotomous choice on whether to attend a screening unit. Let $j = 1$ denote the decision to have a mammogram and $j = 0$ not to have a mammogram. From the investigator's point of view, an individual will choose to have a mammogram if:

$$W_1 (1, Y^i - c_1^i, S^i) + \varepsilon_1^i > W_1 (0, Y^i, S^i) + \varepsilon_1^i. \tag{9.17}$$

By assuming a joint probability function on ε_j^i the decision can be reformulated in probabilistic terms:

$$\pi_1^i = \Pr[\varepsilon_0^i - \varepsilon_1^i < W_1 (1, Y^i - c_1^i, S^i) - W_0 (0, Y^i, S^i)], \tag{9.18}$$

where π_1^i is the probability that the individual chooses to have a mammogram, given her access cost, income and other characteristics (36). In order to calculate empirical estimates, it is assumed that a random sample of n individuals ($i = 1..n$) is drawn from the population under study (consisting of N individuals). If a maximum likelihood probit estimator is applied, the probabilities are:

$$\pi_1^i = \Phi(W_1^i - W_0^i), \tag{9.19}$$
$$\pi_0^i = 1 - \pi_1^i,$$

where $\Phi(\cdot)$ is the cumulative density function of the standard normal distribution. The probability π_1^i can be interpreted as the proportion of the ith group that have a mammogram. Small and Rosen (37) show how welfare measures can be calculated, for example the CV is given by:

$$\Delta e^i = -\frac{1}{\gamma^i} \int_{\varpi_1^0}^{\varpi_1^f} \Phi(W_1^i - W_1^f) dW_1, \tag{9.20}$$

where $\varpi_1^0 = W_1^i(Y - c_1^0) - W_0^i$; $\varpi_1^f = W_1^i(Y - c_1^f) - W_0^i$; and γ^i is the marginal utility of income. One way of interpreting (9.20) is through the graphical representation of the cumulative density function is given in Figure 9.4. If access costs fall from c_1^0 to the probability of having a mammogram rises from π_1^0 to π_1^f. The welfare gain is the area under this curve between the transformed initial and final costs. This is converted to a money metric measure of utility by adjusting for the estimated marginal utility of income (γ^i).

To operationalize the travel cost model it requires the empirical estimation of a probit model to estimate the access cost faced by women at different distances from a screening unit.

Following Hanemann (36) one approach to estimate a travel cost model is a log specification where $W_1^i = \alpha_1 + \beta_1 \ln(Y^i - c_1^i) + \gamma_1 S^i + \varepsilon_1$ and $W_0^i = \alpha_0 + \beta_0 \ln(Y^i) + \gamma_0 S^i + \varepsilon_0$. This leads to:

$$W_1^i - W_0^i = (\alpha_1 - \alpha_0) + \beta \log(1 - \frac{c_1^i}{Y}) + (\gamma_1 - \gamma_0)S^i + \varepsilon_1 - \varepsilon_0$$
$$\approx (\alpha_1 - \alpha_0) - \beta \frac{c_1^i}{Y} + (\gamma_1 - \gamma_0)S^i + \varepsilon_1 - \varepsilon_0, \tag{9.21}$$

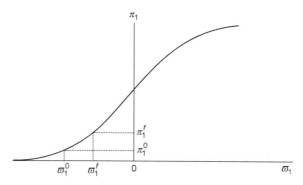

Fig. 9.4 The welfare benefits from a decline in access costs. Reproduced from Clarke, P.M. 1998. Cost-benefit analysis and mammographic screening: A travel cost approach. *Journal of Health Economics* **17**: 767–787, with permission.

where $\dfrac{c_1^i}{Y^i}$ represents the proportion of an individual's income spent on a mammogram. If c_1^i is small relative to Y^i this is approximated by the negative income share $(-\dfrac{c_1^i}{Y^i})$ associated with having a mammogram. The marginal utility of income is given by $\lambda^i = -\dfrac{\beta}{Y^i}$.

However, in order to estimate this model data are needed on the access cost incurred by a woman when having a mammogram. These costs cannot be observed for women who do not have a mammogram. To overcome this problem, a method commonly employed in labour economics is used to fill in the missing data. This involves the use of a two-stage procedure (38). The first stage consists of specifying an access cost or income share equation which is estimated using the sub-set of k individuals that have attended a screening clinic ($k < n$). The reduced form is:

$$\frac{c_1^i}{Y^i} = \Pi_0 + \Pi_1 S^i + \Pi_2 X^i + v^i, \tag{9.22}$$

where X^i is a vector of exogenous variables not included in the random utility function; Π_0, Π_1, and Π_3 are the reduced form coefficients for the constant term, S^i and X^i, respectively; v^i is an error term. The estimated parameters from (9.22) are then used to calculate the *predicted* access cost or income share variable of all n individuals in the sample.

9.7.4 Mammographic screening equation

The random utility function can then be estimated using the maximum likelihood probit model based on the predicted rather than actual access cost or income share:

$$W_1^i - W_0^i(\alpha_1 - \alpha_0) - \beta \frac{\hat{c}_1^i}{y^i} + (\gamma_1 - \gamma_0)S^i + \varepsilon_1^i - \varepsilon_0^i. \tag{9.23}$$

This constitutes the second stage of the two-stage procedure. The coefficient on income share variable (9.23) should have a negative sign since the probability of attending should decline as the access cost increases. The use of $\frac{\hat{c}_1}{Y}$ introduces an additional source of random variation which invalidates the standard asymptotic co-variance matrix of the second stage equation. To take this into account an adjustment procedure is applied to the asymptotic co-variance matrix for a two-equation OLS-Probit model (39, p. 245).

9.8 Empirical application

The remainder of this chapter illustrates the use of the travel cost method by undertaking an indicative CBA of a hypothetical programme to have mobile screening units visit ten randomly selected rural towns in New South Wales. At the time of the evaluation none of the towns had a permanent mammographic screening facility, so the residents of these towns travelled to fixed screening sites located at different distances from these towns.

The study employs data from a random telephone survey of ten rural towns in New South Wales which was collected as part of the *Cancer Action in Rural Towns* (CART) Project. A rural town is defined as any postcode with a population of between 5,001 and 15,000 persons aged 18–70 years, that is more than 50 km from a major city in New South Wales (Sydney, Newcastle, or Wollongong). Several questions relevant to the travel cost model were added to a much larger telephone survey on cancer-related behaviours. Of the women contacted by telephone, the consent rate varied between 85% and 91% across the ten towns. In all, 901 interviews were completed involving women aged between 40 and 70 years.

9.8.1 Variables used in the model

Indicator of attendance at a screening clinic
The dependent variable is set to one if a woman within this age group had a screening mammogram within the last 2 years, and to zero if she had not. Women who had diagnostic mammograms were excluded from the sample (55 observations). After purging 23 incomplete observations, the sample consisted of 645 women. Only 161 of these women had been screened in the last 2 years.

Access cost
The access costs associated with having a mammogram can be divided into three components: medical costs, travel costs, and the opportunity costs of time. The latter two are a function of travel distance. Two questions were asked on travel distance in the survey. The first asked respondents to state the distance they travelled and the second the name of the town where they had their mammogram. The latter was judged to be more reliable because it is often difficult for respondents to recall accurately how far they travelled. The distance was calculated by measuring the shortest road distance between their town of residence and the location where they said they had a mammogram.

The three components of access cost were then calculated as follows:

Medical costs: The medical costs depended on whether women had a mammogram at a public screening centre or through a private radiologist. The former provides the service at no charge to the user, while the Medicare Benefits Schedule fee for the latter was $78.50. However, if the woman was referred by a General Practitioner she is eligible to claim a rebate under Australia's universal public health insurance system of approximately 85%, which would reduce the cost to approximately $13.

Travel costs: More than 93% of the women in the sample who had a mammogram travelled to the screening unit by a private vehicle. In order to simplify the calculations, access costs have been calculated using an estimate of the private vehicle operating cost of $0.50 per km. This estimate was provided by an Australian motoring organization and is based on the cost of running and maintaining a 2-l car.

Time costs: Time is valued at the marginal wage rate. In order to ascertain the total time taken it has been assumed that all travel is undertaken at 90 km per hour and that it takes one hour to be screened.

All three costs are combined to obtain the access cost (c_1) for each woman.

Other explanatory variables
The other explanatory variables included in the model were income share (i.e. the cost divided by imputed income), age, education, marital status, and whether they received advice from a doctor to have a mammogram.

9.8.2 Model estimates

The estimated travel cost models are reported in Table 9.2. The initial specification includes all variables described earlier in this section. Only 'income share' and 'advice' were significant and so all other variables were dropped from the model.

9.9 Cost–benefit analysis

The empirical estimates from the model in Table 9.2 can be used to calculate the benefits of reducing access costs such as a hypothetical programme that introduces mobile mammographic screening units in ten rural areas of New South Wales. It is important to note that this study is *not* a CBA of breast cancer screening *per se*, but an evaluation of the provision of one method of service delivery. A societal perspective is used in the analysis.

The programme evaluated is a one-off visit by a mobile screening unit to each of the ten rural towns. This analysis should be regarded more as a demonstration of the travel cost method than a detailed evaluation of the use of mobile screening units in rural areas. Given the geographic dispersion of the ten rural towns chosen for this study, women in different towns face a large variation in the distance to the nearest fixed screening site and therefore gain different benefits from the introduction of mobile units. In order to determine the access cost in the absence of a mobile unit, it is assumed that all users travel to the nearest fixed screening site. The distance between the nearest

Table 9.2 Empirical estimates of a probit model of the mammographic screening decision

	Initial model	Final model
Constant	−1.255 (2.783)[b]	−0.654 (5.065)[b]
Income share	−47.830 (3.249)[b]	−47.518 (3.421)[b]
GP advice	1.422 (9.933)[b]	1.4286 (10.011)[b]
Education		
Senior high school	0.111 (0.554)	
Technical college	0.073 (0.336)	
University	0.283 (1.413)	
Other variables		
Married	0.172 (1.140)	
Age	0.008 (1.108)	
LLF(β) (full model)	−295.04	−297.06
LLF(0) (intercept only)	−362.43	−362.43
L RI	0.19	0.18
(Homoscedaticity) χ^2	7.4	0.08

[a] Asymptotic *t*-ratios are reported in parentheses.

[b] Significant at 1% level.

[c] Significant at 5% level.

Source: Reproduced from Clarke, P.M. 1998. Cost-benefit analysis and mammographic screening: A travel cost approach. *Journal of Health Economics* **17**: 767–787, with permission.

fixed site and the towns in the sample is reported in the second column of Table 9.3. The towns have been ranked according to this distance. The introduction of mobile screening units does not totally eliminate travel costs since some intra-town travel is required. To account for this, it is assumed that the introduction of a mobile unit reduces the travel distance to a 10-km round trip and the total time taken (waiting and screening time) remains 1 hour.

The data on the cost of providing mobile services is based on estimates from Carter and Cheok (40). The average cost differential between mobile units and fixed units was estimated to be $20.34 per woman screened. The cost of screening 'new' women (i.e. those who would not have been screened if the mobile unit was not available) was $93.40.

The costs and benefits of a one-off visit by a mobile unit are reported in Table 9.3 (for the sake of brevity only estimates based on income share specification are reported). The benefits are calculated for each observation in the sample by numerically integrating the cumulative density function reported in (9.20) between the two access costs and multiplying this by the estimated marginal utility of money (see Figure 9.4. for a graphical illustration of welfare benefits associated with a reduction in costs). The average CV for women in the sample is reported for each town. These ranged from $1.46 for town one (15 km from a fixed screening unit) to $48.20 for

Table 9.3 Benefits and costs of mobile screening

Town		Probability of being screened (average)		Average CV	Total benefits ΣCV	Total costs	Benefit– cost ratio
No	Distance	Fixed unit	Mobile unit				
1	15 km	0.37	0.37	$1.46	$2,521	$12,776	0.2
2	20 km	0.24	0.27	$3.59	$8,743	$18,484	0.5
3	20 km	0.32	0.34	$4.75	$8,346	$14,513	0.6
4	50 km	0.38	0.42	$20.37	$35,803	$19,897	1.8
5	50 km	0.28	0.32	$15.59	$16,516	$9,874	1.7
6	65 km	0.32	0.36	$24.39	$37,546	$15,579	2.4
7	95 km	0.26	0.35	$32.65	$34,503	$14,340	2.4
8	130 km	0.23	0.32	$43.11	$77,144	$23,210	3.3
9	135 km	0.19	0.29	$39.05	$80,024	$26,845	2.9
10	160 km	0.21	0.32	$48.20	$1,20,436	$36,056	3.3

Source: Reproduced from Clarke, P.M. 1998. Cost-benefit analysis and mammographic screening: A travel cost approach. *Journal of Health Economics* **17**: 767–787, with permission.

town ten (160 km from a fixed screening unit). Differences in the average CV between towns at the same travel distance from a fixed screening unit can be attributed to the proportion of women in each town that are given advice to have a mammogram. For example, towns four and five are the same distance from a fixed unit, but town four has a higher average CV, because a higher proportion of women in this town were given advice to have a mammogram.

The average CV was multiplied by the number of women in each town to calculate the total welfare benefits associated with the programme. Similarly, cost estimates of providing mobile units were calculated and the benefit–cost ratio reported in the last column of Table 9.3. The results suggest that the benefits outweigh the costs of providing a mobile unit in towns four to ten.

9.10 **Summary and conclusions**

This chapter has been concerned primarily with the use of revealed preference methods in the evaluation of health care. Revealed preference methods study actual choices concerning goods which in some way affect the individual's health. The overwhelming majority of studies have used averting behaviour as a means of evaluating policies designed to improve the quality of the environment and public safety.

Most of this chapter is devoted to examining the travel cost model which is another revealed preference method that has rarely been used in the evaluation of health care. The travel cost model was originally developed to value recreation areas. The method is based on the premise that observed behaviour at different distances from a recreation site provides an insight into a potential user's valuation of that site. The purpose of the traditional recreational travel cost model is to estimate the benefits associated with a single recreation site over a specific time period. More recently, the approach has been extended to model an individual's choice among a set of alternate sites on a single occasion. Both of these models require some modifications if they are to be used in the valuation of health care.

One of the main challenges for travel cost research is to convert physical measures of access, such as the distance travelled or time taken to receive health care, into monetary costs. This issue is the focus of two sections of this chapter. Section 9.3 examines the method by which time can be valued. Although many studies equate the value of time with the marginal wage, it has been argued that the conditions under which this result holds are quite restrictive. Firstly, it must be assumed that an individual receives no (dis)utility from the time she spends at work relative to the time she spends undertaking leisure activities (15). Secondly, an individual must have flexibility over her hours of work. If either of these conditions is not met the value of time is likely to diverge from the marginal wage. In addition to time, the travel cost model requires estimates of other components of access cost such as the unit cost of travel. Again, there are difficulties with measuring these components, even in physical terms (e.g. travel distance). All these issues provide scope for further work that should be undertaken so that the method can be fully developed as a tool for health care evaluation.

References

* Sugden, R., and Williams, A. 1978. *The principles of practical cost-benefit analysis*. Oxford: Oxford University Press.

1. Pauly, M.V. 1995. Valuing health care benefits in monetary terms. In: Sloan, F.A., editor. *Valuing health care: costs, benefits and effectiveness of pharmaceuticals and other medical technologies.* Cambridge: Cambridge University Press.

2. Ward, F.A. and Beal, D. 2000. *Valuing nature with travel cost models.* Cheltenham: Edward Elgar.

3. Parsons, G.R. 2003. The travel cost model. In: Champ, P.A., Boyle, K.J., and Brown, T.C., editors. *A primer on nonmarket valuation, series: The economics of non-market goods and resources*, Vol. 3, Dordrecht: Kluwer Academic Publishers.

4. McConnell, K.E. 1985. The economics of outdoor recreation. In: Kneese and Sweeney, editors. *Handbook of natural resource and energy economics.* Amsterdam: North-Holland.

5. Clawson, M. 1959. Methods of measuring the demand for and the value of outdoor recreation, Reprint No. 10, Resources for the Future: Washington DC.

6. Willis, K. and Garrod, G. 1991. Valuing open access recreation on inland waterways: On site recreation surveys and selection effects. *Regional Studies* **25**: 511–524.

7. Bockstael, N.E., McConnell, K.E., and Strand, I.E. 1991. Recreation. In: Braden, J.B. and Kolstad, C.D., editors. *Measuring the demand for environmental quality.* Amsterdam: North-Holland.

8. Bockstael, N.E. 1996. Travel cost models. In: Bromley, D.W., editor. *The handbook of environmental economics.* Oxford: Blackwell.

9. Mäler, K.G. 1974. *Environmental economics: A theoretical inquiry*, Resources for the Future, Inc. Baltimore, MD: John Hopkins University Press.

10. Bockstael, N.E. and McConnell, K.E. 1983. Welfare measurement in the household production framework. *American Economic Review* **73**: 806–814.

11. Johansson, P.-O. 1997. On the use of market prices to evaluate medical treatments. *Journal of Health Economics* **16**: 609–615.

12. Randall, A. 1994. A difficulty with the travel cost method. *Land Economics.* **70**: 88–96.

13. Johnson, M.B. 1966. Travel time and the price of leisure. *Western Economic Journal* **4**: 137–150.

14. Chavas, J.P., Stoll, J., and Sellar, C. 1989. On the commodity value of travel time in recreational activities. *Applied Economics* **21**: 711–722.

15. Cesario, F.J. 1976. Value of time in recreational benefit studies. *Land Economics* **52**: 32–41.

16. McConnell, K.E. and Strand I. 1981. Measuring the cost of time in recreation demand for outdoor recreation. *American Journal of Agricultural Economics* **63**: 153–156.

17. Smith, V. K., Desvouges, W.H., and McGivney, M.P. 1983. The opportunity cost of travel time in recreational demand models. *Land Economics* **59**: 259–278.

18. Larson, D.M. 1993. Separability and the shadow value of leisure time. *American Journal of Agricultural Economics* **75**: 572–577.

19. Bockstael, N.E., Strand, I.E., and Hanemann, W.M. 1987. Time and recreation demand model. *American Journal of Agricultural Economics* **69**: 293–302.

20. Evans, W.N. and Viscusi, W.K. 1991. Utility-based measures of health. *American Agricultural Economics Association* **73**: 1422–1427.

21. Ashby, J., Buxton, M., and Gravelle, H. 1989. What costs do women meet for early detection and diagnosis of breast problems?. *HERG Research Report* No. 6.

22. Hensher, D. 1985. An econometric model of vehicle use in the household sector. *Transport Research* **19B**: 303–314.

23. McFadden, D. 1996. Why is natural resource damage assessment so hard? Available at: http://emlab.berkeley.edu/wp/mcfadden0496/hibb_f56.ps

24. Acton, J.P. 1975. Nonmonetary factors in the demand for medical services: Some empirical evidence. *Journal of Political Economy* **83**: 595–613.

25. Oldroyd, L. 1986. Access costs and the demand for primary health care. *Discussion Paper No. 04/86*, Health Economics Research Unit: University of Aberdeen.

26. Deyak, T.A. and Smith, V.K. 1976. The economic value of statute reform: The case of liberalized abortion. *Journal of Political Economy* **84**(1): 83–100.

27. Wang'ombe, J.K. 1984. Economic evaluation in primary health care: The case of western Kenya community based health care project. *Social Science and Medicine* **18**: 375–385.

28. Gertler, P., Locay, L., and Sanderson, W. 1987. Are user fees regressive?: Welfare implications of health care financing proposals in Peru. *Journal of Econometrics* **36**: 67–88.

29. Jeuland, M., Lucas, M., Clemens, J., and Whittington, D. 2009. Estimating the private benefits of vaccination against cholera in Beira, Mozambique: A travel cost approach. *Journal of Development Economics* **91**(2): 310–322.

30. Clarke, P.M. 1998. Cost-benefit analysis and mammographic screening: A travel cost approach. *Journal of Health Economics* **17**: 767–787.

31. Sandstrom, F.M. 1999. Can we use market methods to evaluate health risks. In: *Evaluating the benefits and effectiveness of public policy*, Ph.D. Thesis. Stockholm School of Economics.

32. Ohshige, K., Mizushima, S., and Tochikubo, O. 2004. Willingness to pay for a public health checkup program: assessment by the travel cost method. *Nippon Koshu Eisei Zasshi* Nov; **51**(11): 938–944.

33. McNamara, P.E., 1999. Welfare effects of rural hospital closures: A nested logit analysis of the demand for rural hospital services. *American Journal of Agricultural Economics* **81**(3): 686–691.

34. Solano, P.L. and McDuffie, M.J. 2008. Determination of the demand and utilization of substance abuse outpatient treatment. Working Paper of the Health Services Policy Research Group (HSPRG), Center for Community Research and Service University of Delaware Newark, Delaware.

35. Anex, RP. 1995. A travel-cost method of evaluating household hazardous waste disposal services. *Journal of Environmental Management* **45**(2): 189–198.

36. Hanemann, M.W. 1984. Welfare evaluations in contingent valuation experiments with discrete choice responses. *American Journal of Agricultural Economics* **66**: 332–341.

37. Small, K.A. and Rosen, H.S. 1981. Applied welfare economics with discrete choice models. *Econometrica* **49**: 105–130.

38. Wales, T.J. and Woodland, A.D. 1980. Sample selectivity and the estimation of labour supply functions. *International Economic Review* **21**: 437–468.

39. Maddala, G.S. 1983. *Limited dependent and qualitative variables in econometrics.* Econometrics Society Monographs, Cambridge: Cambridge University Press.

40. Carter, R. and Cheok, F. 1994. Breast cancer screening cost study. *National program for the early detection of breast cancer – evaluation of phase one: 1 July 1991–30 June 1994,* Canberra: Commonwealth Department of Health.

41. Clarke, P.M. 2000. Valuing the benefits of mobile mammographic screening units using the contingent valuation method. *Applied Economics* **32**: 1647–1655.

Chapter 10

Experimental design and the estimation of willingness to pay in choice experiments for health policy evaluation

Richard T. Carson and Jordan J. Louviere

10.1 Introduction

This chapter focuses on stated preferences obtained from discrete choice experiments (DCEs also known as SPDCEs), as opposed to data that reflect real market choices (revealed preferences (RP) as discussed in Chapter 9). DCEs try to simulate the essential elements of real market options that consumers might face in the future. Unlike real market choice data, DCEs rely on constructed markets in which key factors that are hypothesized to drive choices are systematically varied. To the extent that the consumers in a DCE make choices in a manner consistent with the way in which they would actually choose in a real market, one can derive standard welfare estimates for policy changes. The remainder of this chapter is devoted to discussing and illustrating how this can be accomplished with DCEs. More details on DCEs can be found in Louviere, Hensher, and Swait (1).

In order to collect DCE data information from consumers, one must identify factors that drive the choices of interest. These factors are called 'attributes' of the choice options. Once these attributes are identified, one must assign them values, known in experimental design parlance as 'levels'. Taken together, the attributes and levels define and determine possible choice options that can be offered to consumers in a DCE survey. That is, a factorial combination of attribute levels completely defines the possible choice options. So, for example, if there are three attributes, say A(4), B(3), and C(2), with the associated number of levels in parentheses, the factorial combinations, or all possible options are $4 \times 3 \times 2 = 24$. We refer to that factorial combination as a 'full' or 'complete' factorial design. Typically, the number of combinations in a full factorial design is too many to use in practical field applications of DCE surveys, so one has to sample from the full factorial to reduce the size of the problem. There are many ways to sample from full factorials, but a common approach in DCE surveys is to sample based on what is known as a 'fractional factorial design'. We return to these ideas in more detail later in the chapter.

The type of experimental design used to construct a DCE survey is important for three reasons: 1. it determines the economic quantities of potential interest that can be statistically identified from an estimation perspective; 2. it strongly influences confidence intervals associated with these quantities (statistics) given a fixed sample size or equivalently, influences the sample size needed to achieve a given confidence interval or level of precision for a statistic, and so plays a major role in the cost of a project; 3. the attributes/levels can influence the plausibility of questions; and hence, influence the quality of data obtained. The first two issues are largely statistical in nature and are the subject of this chapter.[1] The third issue deals more with issues of survey design and are not considered further here, although it may place constraints on what can be measured in a DCE survey.[2]

This chapter uses examples from health policy research, but these examples also have application in analysing consumer choices in areas like culture, environment, transport, utilities, or more generally where government has a strong role in determining which options are available and/or how they are priced, like health. Overviews of the use of DCE methods to value health issues can be found in various sources (e.g. 8–11).[3]

We begin by considering a single binary choice (SBC) contingent valuation question because many basic issues associated with experimental design can be easily seen in the context of the SBC format (see, e.g. (13)). This question format is popular in the stated preference literature and enjoys a number of desirable incentive properties under certain conditions.[4] This question format also is the simplest example of a more general discrete choice experiment format (see, e.g. (1)). The key properties of the SBC format from our perspective are:

1. Only one choice question [set] is asked;

2. The question asked offers only two alternatives; and,

3. Only one attribute of the scenario, typically cost, is varied across respondents.

For example, consider the following simple proposition. A large university in the USA is considering offering employees the option of purchasing a dental plan. The dental plan covers 80% of normal costs associated with all standard, non-cosmetic dental procedures. The university is interested in what fraction of employees will subscribe to the dental plan at various prices. A DCE for this policy problem would describe the

---

[1] The two key statistical properties of an experimental design are identification and precision. Louviere, Hensher, and Swait (1) note two other properties that can influence the desirability of a design that are not statistical in nature. These are cognitive complexity and market realism. Both considerations can restrict the nature of the attributes and design used.

[2] There are several general books on survey design (e.g. 2–4) but there is a surprising lack of guidance on the issue of SP choice questions in a policy context. Some exceptions are (5;6). A small but growing literature (e.g. (7) looks at the implications of task complexity in choice experiments.

[3] For an overview of different health valuation methods including SP methods with an emphasis on determining the value of a statistical life, see (12).

[4] The SBC question format was recommended by the Arrow *et al.* (14) panel that looked at SP methods for valuing natural resource damages for the U.S. Government. Carson and Groves (15) examined the incentive properties of different types of SP questions in detail.

dental plan in sufficient detail for employees to understand what they would be purchasing, provides the monthly cost associated with the plan and asks the question 'Would you subscribe to this plan if offered to you?'. The employee can choose to accept the plan or reject it (the two options). In this case, a single attribute is varied over a range of levels, namely the cost attribute. This allows the analyst to trace out the fraction of employees who would subscribe at each presented level of cost.

In more general DCE formats, one often sees: (a) more than one choice set asked, (b) more than two alternatives offered, and (c) more than one attribute varied. Frequently, however, only one or two of the three generalizations of the SBC format are used, so it is useful to keep in mind the specific generalization of the SBC format when thinking about issues involving DCEs. The nature and properties of different experimental designs become more important as DCE formats grow more complicated and we systematically illustrate where new issues arise and how the statistical models that can be estimated are tied to the experimental design used to construct a SP survey.[5]

From an applications standpoint, we focus on three cases:

1. A new good may be provided, and if it is provided, the person using it has to pay for it (everyone pays if it is a pure public good provided via coercive taxation). Interest lies in estimating total willingness to pay (WTP) for having the good supplied rather than the current status quo good.

2. One wishes to estimate the WTP to have one or more new alternatives added to a set of choices available to a consumer.

3. One wishes to estimate the WTP for a change in one or more of the attributes of an alternative.

We begin our discussion by laying out the theoretical welfare measures for the three above cases. We then introduce the basic concepts of experimental design in the context of the SBC format. Next, we illustrate the issues involved in moving to different types of DCE formats. Finally, we try to provide guidance to applied researchers who want to conduct a DCE study using reasonably efficient designs where the statistics of primary interest are statistically identified.

10.2 Economic welfare measures for health policy changes

SP surveys analysed from a random utility perspective often aim to produce estimates for policy purposes; hence, we briefly review the theory relating to welfare economic measures of value. Literature on this topic is vast, so to more fully appreciate the issues involved, interested readers may wish to pursue comprehensive treatments in (16–18).

We begin by denoting the item being valued by q and initially treat this as a single item that could be a commodity or a programme involving some mix of commodities

---

[5] There are many other relevant cases for measuring changes in welfare. In particular, there are a set of analogous measures that focus on minimum willingness to accept (WTA) compensation for undesirable changes (see Chapter 6 and 7).

treated as a fixed group – the key feature is that q is a scalar. Later, we will let q consist of a bundle of attributes and we will ask questions about how a change in one attribute influences economic values. The latter does not change the underlying framework as one can define two distinct q's that differ only in a change in one attribute of interest. We assume that a consumer has a utility function defined over quantities of various market commodities, denoted by the vector x, from which a consumer can freely choose and the item q. Thus, the direct utility function is given by $u(x, q)$. Often analysts work with the corresponding indirect utility function, $v(p, q, y)$, where p is the vector of the prices of the market commodities x, and y is the consumer's income.[6] We make the conventional assumption that $u(x, q)$ is increasing and quasi-concave in x, which implies that $v(p, q, y)$ satisfies the standard properties with respect to p and y[7]; but we make no assumptions about q. If the agent regards q as a 'good', $u(x, q)$ and $v(p, q, y)$ both will be increasing in q; if it is regarded as a 'bad', $u(x, q)$ and $v(p, q, y)$ both will be decreasing in q; and if the agent is indifferent to q, $u(x, q)$ and $v(p, q, y)$ both will be independent of q. We make no assumption about quasi-concavity with respect to q.

The act of valuation implies a contrast between two situations: one with item q, and one without q. This is an important concept because economic valuation always involves a comparison/tradeoff between two or more situations where the 'or more' part always can be rewritten as a set of binary comparisons. We interpret what is being valued as a change in q.[8] Specifically, suppose that q changes from q^0 to q^1; the consumer's utility changes from $u^0 \equiv v(p,q^0,y)$ to $u^1 \equiv v(p,q^1,y)$. If she sees this change as positive, $u^1 > u^0$; if she sees it as negative, $u^1 < u^0$; and if she is indifferent, $u^1 = u^0$. The value of the change to her in monetary terms is represented by the Hicksian income compensation measure, C, which is the amount of money that satisfies:

$$v(p,q^1,y-C) = v(p,q^0,y) \,.^9 \tag{10.1}$$

---

[6] The definition of income is always problematic in empirical work. Ideally, it refers to some notion of permanent household supernumerary income, which is disposal permanent income less total expenditure on subsistence minima and previously committed expenditures.

[7] That is, we assume $v(p, q, y)$ is homogeneous of degree zero in p and y, increasing in y, non-increasing in p, and quasiconvex in p.

[8] The alternative is to represent it as a change in p. McConnell (19) adopts this approach for a valuation question of the form 'Would you accept a payment of $A to give up your right to use this commodity for 1 year?' Let $p^\star$ be the choke price vector (i.e. a cost vector such that, at these costs, the individual would choose not to consume the resource), and let p^0 be the baseline price vector. McConnell represents the change as a shift from (p^0, q, y) to $(p^\star, q, y)$.

[9] Note that we also can get the Hicksian equivalence measure, which in this case is WTA for giving up the right to q^1. If the sign of $u^1 - u^0$ is positive then WTP and WTA will both be positive. The Hicksian income compensation function often is formally defined as the difference between two (Hicksian) expenditure functions, another alternative representation of the direct utility function that describes how much income is needed to achieve a specified level of utility given a price vector for marketed goods and the level of q. $C = m(p, q^0, u^0) - m(p, q^1, u^0)$. The first term on the right is simply equal to y.

To emphasize the dependence of the compensating measure on (i) the starting value of q, (ii) the terminal value of q, and (iii) the value of (p, y) at which the change in q occurs, we sometimes write it as:

$$C = C(q^0, q^1, p, y) \,. \tag{10.2}$$

For a desirable change which the consumer does not have the property right to enjoy without paying

$$\text{WTP} = C(q^0, q^1, p, y) \,. \tag{10.3}$$

One can parameterize either the WTP function directly (20) or begin with a parameterization of the underlying utility function (21). Typically, applied researchers fit simple linear or logarithmic functions, but one can fit more complex utility functions, and SP data often is better suited for this than RP data. We illustrate these concepts with a specific example, the Box–Cox indirect utility function:[10]

$$v_q = \alpha_q + \beta_q \left(\frac{y^\lambda - 1}{\lambda} \right), \quad q = 0, 1, \tag{10.4a}$$

where $\alpha_1 \geq \alpha_0$ and $\beta_1 \geq \beta_0$. Equation (10.4a) can be regarded as a form of CES utility function in q and y with λ being the income elasticity of WTP. The corresponding formula for C is

$$C = \left(\frac{\beta_0 y^\lambda}{\beta_1} - \frac{\lambda \alpha}{\beta_1} + \frac{\beta_1 - \beta_0}{\beta_1} \right)^{\frac{1}{\lambda}}, \tag{10.4b}$$

where $\alpha \equiv \alpha_1 - \alpha_0$. McFadden and Leonard (22) employ a restricted version of this model with $\beta_1 = \beta_0 \equiv \beta > 0$, yielding

$$v_q = \alpha_q + \beta \left(\frac{y^\lambda - 1}{\lambda} \right), \quad q = 0, 1, \tag{10.5a}$$

$$C = y - \left(y^\lambda - \frac{\alpha}{b} \right)^{\frac{1}{\lambda}}, \tag{10.5b}$$

where $b \equiv \beta / \lambda$. This specification is somewhat flexible as it permits a variety of income elasticities of WTP; the income elasticity of WTP is negative when $\lambda > 1$, zero when $\lambda = 1$, and positive when $\lambda \leq 0$. It also nests many utility models in the existing literature. For example, if $\lambda = 1$, C equals the familiar ratio of $-\alpha/\beta$ often associated with a measure of mean WTP from a logit or probit model.[11]

Now, consider the case where there is more than one possible alternative to the status quo good. As long as a status quo good will remain available and a consumer

---

[10] For simplicity, we suppress p and write the indirect utility function as a function of q and y; however, α_q and/or β_q are in fact functions of p and z.

[11] Often there are measurement issues with respect to y that play a major role in econometric estimation, pushing empirical researchers to assume that $\lambda = 1$.

will only get utility from at most one good that is an alternative to the status quo good then the economic value of the set of alternatives is simply the maximum WTP defined over all binary paired comparisons involving the status quo good. If the status quo good is chosen in a deterministic setting, WTP equals zero. Otherwise, the economic value equals the maximum amount of money a consumer has to pay for the most preferred of the alternatives relative to being indifferent between choosing the status quo good and the most preferred alternative.[12]

One can make q a function of a bundle of attributes in the sense originally explicated by Lancaster (23). Here α_q is replaced by a function, $g(z)$, where z is a vector of attributes. Typically, $g(z)$ is represented as an additive linear function of the individual attributes some of which are potentially indicator variables, i.e. $\gamma_1 z_1 + \gamma_2 z_2 + \gamma_3 z_3$. In this case, there is nothing particularly special from a welfare economic view from moving from a change in a status quo good versus an alternative good compared to changes in the attributes of goods other than having to choose the functional form that specifies how the attributes enter the utility function.[13] Other common ways to specify the attribute function are: (a) an additive linear function of the logs of the individual attributes, (b) an additive linear function of the individual attributes plus the first-order interactions between the individual z, and (c) an additive linear representation like a Translog utility function that is a second order approximation to an unknown function that include squares of individual attributes and first order interaction terms between attributes. When there are attributes in the model one often is interested in the marginal effect on WTP of a change in z_i, which is simply $\partial C/\partial z_i$, or the relative effect of a marginal change in one attribute relative to another attribute that can be scaled in a comparable way by looking at $(\partial C/\partial z_i)/(\partial C/\partial z_j)$.

10.3 Going from choice to WTP estimates

SP questions measure a consumer's WTP (or WTA) for change in q or a discrete indicator related to WTP. The utility theoretic model of consumer preference outlined above provides a way to interpret responses to these questions. From a statistical modelling viewpoint, the convention is to treat the survey responses as the realization of a random variable. So, it is necessary to recast the deterministic model of WTP outlined above into stochastic models that can generate probability distributions of the survey responses. Mapping from a deterministic WTP model to a probabilistic model of survey responses involves two steps: 1. adding a stochastic component into

---

[12] The case where a consumer would use more than one of the alternatives is beyond the scope of this chapter and rarely is examined in SP choice models. Such cases are often dealt with by going to some type of allocation model or bundling alternatives so that bundles are mutually exclusive.

[13] The only 'attribute' that plays a special role is a good's cost. A consumer does not get utility from the cost of a good per se, but instead via the effect of a good's cost on income. In most empirical work this distinction is ignored or an implicit assumption is made about the marginal utility of income so that the only thing that enters the utility function for two (or more) goods is the difference in the cost of the goods.

the deterministic utility model that leads to what is called a *WTP distribution* and 2. specifying a connection between the WTP distribution and what we will call the *survey response probability distribution* based on the assumption of a utility-maximizing response to the survey question. We denote the WTP cumulative distribution function (cdf) as $G_C(z_p)$; for a given individual it specifies the probability that the individual's WTP for the item in question is less than the cost z_p, and we now use the convention of denoting attributes of the good as z_i and the special attribute of cost as z_p:

$$G_c\left(z_p\right) \equiv Pr\left(C \le z_p\right), \tag{10.6}$$

where the compensating variation, C, is now viewed as a random variable.[14] The corresponding density function is denoted as $g_C(z_p)$.

We illustrate this via a simple example with a *closed-ended, single-bound* discrete choice format. That is, a respondent is asked 'Would you favour a change from q^0 to q^1 if it would cost you z_p?' Suppose the response is 'yes'. This means that the value of C for this individual is some amount more than z_p. In terms of the underlying WTP distribution, the probability of obtaining a 'yes' response is given by

$$Pr\left(\text{Response is 'yes'}\right) = Pr\left(C \ge z_p\right) \equiv 1 - G_c\left(z_p\right). \tag{10.7}$$

Note that a response to this question does not reveal the exact value of C, but instead provides information that C lies in an interval bounded from above or below by z_p.[15]

There are two basic sources of the stochastic component: (a) factors related to the nature of the good or the consumer that influence choice, and are known to the consumer but unknown to the analyst (e.g. 25;26) and (b) a true random component potentially including recording and optimization errors.[16] These two sources effectively are equivalent from the perspective of the simplest statistical estimators, but they have quite different implications for WTP estimates. While source (a) leads to the well-known model of random utility maximization (RUM) in which error components play an integral role in the estimate of summary statistics involving WTP distributions; in contrast, it is desirable to purge source (b) error components from WTP estimates. These two views of error sources also have different implications for what might be observed. Under (a) the probability of picking a dominated alternative should be zero, while under (b) some respondents should pick dominated alternatives with positive probability. For more complex statistical estimators (a) leads one to try

---

[14] For now, we assume the change is regarded as an improvement so that C measures WTP.

[15] Other relevant information may help to more tightly bound the interval in which the consumer's WTP lies. For example, if the alternative cannot be a 'bad', it may be reasonable to assume a distribution for WTP with no support in the negative range. Carson and Jeon (24) look at ways to use constraints on the upper end related to income.

[16] Excellent discussions of the two perspectives are provided by Hanemann (21) and Cameron (20). McConnell (19) lays out the relationship between the two from the perspective of estimating welfare measures. It is important to note that analysts often claim to estimate a RUM model but use measurement error perspectives when calculating WTP measures.

to allow for heteroscedasticity in preference parameters, while (b) leads one to try to model the error term to allow for heteroscedasticity in some fashion.[17]

The RUM approach proceeds by specifying a particular indirect utility function $v(p,q,y;\varepsilon)$ and a particular distribution for ε. An example of a RUM version of the restricted Box–Cox model is

$$u_q = \alpha_q + \beta\left(\frac{y^\lambda - 1}{\lambda}\right) + \varepsilon_q \quad q = 0,1, \tag{10.8a}$$

where ε_0 and ε_1 are random variables with a mean of zero. Consequently,

$$C = y - \left(y^\lambda - \frac{\alpha}{b} - \frac{\eta}{b}\right)^{\frac{1}{\lambda}}, \tag{10.8b}$$

where $\alpha \equiv \alpha_1 - \alpha_0$, $b \equiv \beta/\lambda$, and $\eta \equiv \varepsilon_1 - \varepsilon_0$.

In contrast, if we take the second view and operationalize it with an additive error term, we would have

$$C = C(q^0, q^1, p, y) + \varepsilon. \tag{10.9}$$

In the case of the Box–Cox model (7), for example,

$$C = y - \left(y^\lambda - \frac{\alpha}{b}\right)^{\frac{1}{\lambda}} + \varepsilon. \tag{10.10}$$

Comparison of (10.8b) with (10.10) illustrates the difference between the two approaches to formulating a WTP distribution. Inserting an additive random term in utility function (10.8a) leads to a random term that enters into the formula for C in a *non-additive* manner. Even when both approaches lead to similar estimates for mean and median WTP, the implied pdf's may be quite different, particularly in the tails.

Often there can be substantial problems in empirically estimating WTP measures from discrete choice data from either survey choices or market choices.[18] The problems largely stem from the fact that in all discrete choice models the parameters are identified only up to a scale factor.[19] Because of scale, WTP estimates are a ratio of parameter estimates; hence, they can be ill-behaved even if the individual parameter estimates are normally distributed (as suggested by the theoretical foundation

[17] Under (a) the main source of heterogeneity typically is assumed to be differences in preferences, while under (b) the main source of heterogeneity typically is assumed to be differences in ability to answer questions.

[18] Indeed, it usually is better to work with SP data than RP data because the cost variable typically has a much more limited range and there are high correlations between various attributes.

[19] In the case of binary discrete choice, where only cost is varied, one can use non-parametric techniques to avoid some of the problems associated with the scale issue. However, these techniques give much coarser estimates and have not been generalized to the multinomial choice case. See (18) for a discussion.

underlying maximum likelihood estimation) because the ratio of two normal variables is distributed as a Cauchy distribution (although this can be simulated). Further, there is a very tight relationship between the functional form assumed for the cost (z_p) variable and the assumed distribution of WTP.[20] For example, it is common to specify $ln(z_p)$ in a logit model, which implies that the WTP distribution is log-logistic. Unfortunately, this distribution has an (implausible) infinite mean for a wide range of estimated parameter values, although it typically cannot be distinguished from a log-normal (or a Weibull) that has a finite mean in terms of statistical fit.

The problem is that similarly shaped WTP distributions over a wide range of monetary values may have very different behaviour in the far tails,[21] and using more flexible functional forms to allow heterogeneity in preferences can exacerbate problems. For example, if one specifies a cost variable as a random effect and assumes the effect to be normally distributed, it typically implies that some consumers have a negative WTP even if this is implausible. This may concentrate a large fraction of the distribution near zero, causing traditional formulas for mean WTP to blow up.[22]

Often problems in estimating mean WTP are not reported because the analyst assumes them away by estimating a logit or probit model with a linear specification for the cost variable, forcing mean and median WTP to be equal. A similar problem occurs if one estimates a model with the log of cost as a regressor but mistakenly assumes that the correct formula for mean WTP is $EXP[-\alpha/\beta]$, where α is the constant term (assuming no other attributes) and β is the coefficient on log(cost). This is the correct formula for median WTP but the correct formula for the mean includes a function of the variance, such as the following for a normal distribution: mean WTP $= EXP[-\alpha/\beta]EXP[1/2\beta^2]$. Often a better solution to this problem is to recognize that percentiles of the distribution, including the median, usually can be reliably estimated far out in the tails. Traditional welfare economics focuses on mean WTP but policymakers typically care about more than one summary statistic of the WTP distribution.

10.4 Experimental design for a single binary discrete choice question

The simplest case for experimental design of a choice experiment occurs when one asks a single binary discrete choice CV question of each respondent and only one attribute (typically cost (z_p)) is varied, as earlier noted. Collection of discrete choice

---

[20] Typically, analysts use the cost of the alternative instead of the more theoretically suitable income minus cost, which is justified by particular assumptions about marginal utility of income. A large amount of measurement error in income also may offset the theoretically desirable properties.

[21] Cost amounts in the far tails are rarely if ever observed in market data and it may be implausible to ask respondents about them in SP surveys.

[22] The key issue is that a non-trivial fraction of consumers may be indifferent to the introduction of any of the alternatives to the status quo, leading to a spike at zero that formally can be modelled as a mixture distribution (27).

data requires the use of a set of design points that represent the cost to agents who are then randomly assigned to those design points. Choice of these design points can greatly influence how many observations are required for a given level of statistical efficiency, which is often referred to as the precision of the estimate.[23]

We begin by considering a linear regression model measuring WTP as a function of changes in a single design factor, say the number of treatments an insurance plan would pay for, z_i, where the line goes through the origin if the value of the design factor is zero. Now, we ask the question 'if you have n observations and can run the experiment at two values of the factor, what values would you chose and how many observations should you allocate to each to minimize the confidence interval of the WTP estimate at a particular level of the factor' (i.e. the estimated slope parameter times the factor level of interest)? In this case, the confidence interval for WTP is simply a function of the confidence interval for the slope parameter, so one should choose two values of the factor that are as far apart as feasible. In the case of DCEs, the two values should be chosen to be as far apart as is plausible to respondents. One should allocate half the sample to each of these two values; and it is straightforward to show that this minimizes the confidence interval on the slope parameter.[24] This is a desirable property of a simple DCE because in cases where the expected response to cost is linear, one only needs two levels of cost to accurately estimate the slope. The trick is to ensure that the two points are placed sufficiently far apart to cover much of the response distribution, but not so far into the tails of the distribution that one observes only a few choices.

For example, consider a plan where as before WTP for the plan varies with the number of treatments paid for, but the plan also has other fixed benefits (e.g. information, access to other services at discounts) that do not vary with the number of treatments. Let us represent the WTP for a plan with no treatments by α. Now, WTP for a plan is represented by $\alpha + \beta z_i$, and the objective is to minimize the confidence interval around this quantity for a particular z_i. One can do this by choosing two values for z_i that are as far apart as possible because the confidence interval for α also is minimized by this choice.

Much of this basic intuition extends to binary discrete choice models with a single factor, typically cost. DCEs for these models are analogues of dose–response experiments in medical and related applications; For example, instead of 'cost', experimenters vary the magnitude of a dose of – say – an insecticide, and analytical interest focuses on the percent of the sample population alive falls as dose amount increases. In the case of a DCE for – say – a dental insurance plan, the 'dose' is the levels of cost, and analytical interest focuses on the fraction still in 'favour' as cost increases. Different choice models

---

[23] Like survey design, experimental design is not generally taught in economics departments. A classic text is (28). A more modern, comprehensive reference is (29) or (30).

[24] The slope parameter is proportionate to the reciprocal of the square root of $\Sigma_i(z_i - E(z_i))^2$. Given any finite constraint on how far apart the two values of z_i can be from each other, it is possible to show that this quantity is maximized by placing half of the z_i at each end of the constrained distance.

have different likelihood functions and most are non-linear in the model parameters, which has four major implications:

1. The curvature of the likelihood function for most commonly used choice models suggests that the design points should be closer together than in a traditional linear model, but the general principle that they should not be very close remains. The main caveat is not to place the design points too far in the tails because there is too little density to accurately measure the choice probabilities in samples of reasonable size.

2. The optimal design will depend on the number of parameters in the underlying distribution.

3. The optimal design also will depend on the values of those parameters. Generally, one does not need more design points than parameters, but to be able to test more general distributions than one assumes, more design points are needed. Yet, the general principle is that if one fits a parametric distribution characterized by a small number of parameters, one should have relatively few design points so the distribution can be estimated with reasonable precision at a small number of places.

4. The choice of z_i that minimizes the confidence interval on β in non-linear models generally is not the one that minimizes confidence intervals on functions of α and β, and hence, the confidence interval for WTP.

As noted earlier, in the simplest case, estimates of mean (and median) WTP are a ratio of two parameters $(-\alpha/\beta)$, where α is the estimate of the constant from a logit or probit model and β is the estimate of the cost parameter. Two basic criteria are used in the stated preference literature for this case: 1. directly minimize the confidence interval around the mean WTP estimate and 2. maximize the determinant of the information matrix for the estimated parameters. Statistical designs that minimize confidence intervals around mean WTP are known as C-optimal designs. Alberini and Carson (31) and Alberini (32) show that C-optimality can be substantially more efficient (on the order of 50%) than maximizing the determinant of the information matrix (D-optimality) under conditions relevant to DCE studies.[25] Both the C- and D-optimality criteria lead to choosing only two design points if the underlying distribution can be fully characterized by two parameters and the design is not constrained to have more design points.[26] C- and D-optimal designs differ in where the points are placed, with D-optimal designs generally placing them further in the tails of the distribution.

---

[25] C-optimal designs are closely related to fiducial designs popular in biometrics.

[26] A design can be constrained to have more design points, but forcing a design to have four design points results in two design points being replicates, or being arbitrarily close to the two original points if they are forced to be distinct. If the distribution is assumed symmetric, equal numbers of observations generally are assigned to design points on either side of the median; asymmetric distributions can result in an asymmetric assignment of observations being optimal.

D-optimal designs are popular even in binary discrete choice cases with one z_p as a regressor, as it is natural to think in terms of maximum likelihood estimation; they also are easier to construct than C-optimal designs. D-optimal designs become more compelling in cases where goods are bundles of attributes and interest lies not in a single WTP estimate but in WTP estimates for a sizeable number of marginal tradeoffs. In this case, D-optimal designs effectively strike a balance in estimating all the marginal effects with reasonable precision for a given sample size. Much of the rest of this chapter is devoted to D-optimal designs when there are multiple attributes of interest.

Generally speaking, a D-optimal design is one that minimizes the determinant of the Fisher Information Matrix associated with a particular class of designs. The best D-optimal design is the one with the largest determinant. Street and Burgess (33) show that such designs exhibit level balance (each level of each attribute occurs equally often), and the differences in the attribute levels are orthogonal. It is difficult to generalize beyond this description because designs for non-linear models like choice models depend on the particular problem specification, namely the number of attributes, the number of levels associated with each attribute, the indirect utility specification associated with the problem, and the form of the underlying choice process model.

Both C- and D-optimality rely on certain knowledge of the model parameters, but this is never satisfied in practice because if the parameters were known there would be no need to do an experiment. Yet, one usually has at least some knowledge of the likely parameter values, so a good way to begin is to ask if theory can bound the parameter space, with inequality constraints being quite useful. Additionally, does existing literature on related goods help to bound the likely estimate of mean/median WTP? An obvious next step is to use data from pre-test and pilot studies to assist with this. Such a process is better thought of as 'sequential design', and Kanninen (34) discusses issues related to such a sequential design process. In general, the more uncertainty about the nature of the underlying WTP distribution, the more design points one should use, which can be shown using a formal Bayesian approach to design problems. Yet, one needs to recognize that there is a clear tradeoff between the precision at which the distribution is pinned down at individual design points and the number of design points.[27]

10.5 Generalizing attributes of binary discrete choice questions

Now, we consider what happens if an attribute is not continuous, but instead categorical, with greater than two levels. For example, an attribute of a GP practice might

---

[27] Alberini and Carson (31) suggest it is hard to justify more than eight design points, and show that four to six design points spanning the expected quartiles of the expected WTP give estimates that are reasonably efficient and robust to fairly large deviations in expected and observed WTP distributions, as long as the presumed distribution of WTP is of low dimensionality. McFadden (35) shows that a very different design is required if one wants to be able to consistently estimate mean WTP without making parametric assumptions about the nature of the distribution; this design involves spacing a large number of design points over the support of the WTP distribution.

be opening hours, such as 9–5, 9–7 and 9–9. If only this attribute is presented and the respondent's response options are to keep the status quo or choose the new opening hours, the theory and analysis are the same as in Section 10.4. Now, consider the case of adding a cost attribute with three discrete levels that cover the possible range of costs to opening hours. Now, we have a case where we must jointly vary two attributes each having three levels. The design involves both attributes; all combinations of them represent a 3×3 factorial design (= 9 combinations).

The implied DCE involves offering a respondent nine (or fewer) combinations of opening hours and costs. For each of the nine combinations that we will call 'scenarios', a respondent is asked whether they will stay with the status quo or switch to the new health service represented by a particular level of opening hours and a level of cost. Any design that uses less than all nine combinations will have some parameters that are not statistically identified without some identifying assumption/restriction for the underlying utility function.

If one believes that the true relationship between utility and cost is linear, the proper way to design this experiment is to only use two levels for the cost attribute, as discussed in Section 10.4. Thus, this DCE would have only six combinations. On the other hand, if one does not know the true relationship, and it is possible, perhaps likely, that it is non-linear, then one needs to assign *at least* three levels to the cost attribute. Typically, one would assign four levels to the cost attribute to be able to visualize relationships between utility and cost and rule out a quadratic polynomial if it is inappropriate. For example, if the true relationship is S-shaped, one needs at least four levels to visualize and test this.

The previous theoretical insights also apply to this case. That is, one may wish to value a change in opening hours from 9–5 to 9–9. This requires one to estimate the value of the utility difference between the two levels of opening hours, and if the relationship between utility and cost is linear, one would divide this utility difference by β, the estimate of the cost effect. If the status quo option varies across consumers, one must calculate the difference between the status quo and the proposed change in opening hours for each consumer and use the method of sample enumeration (36) to calculate the implied WTP. As before, if cost is treated as a random effect, one needs to calculate statistics for the WTP distribution, and one may need to simulate the WTP distribution in the case of complex models that allow random effects and covariances among effects and/or non-constant diagonal error variances and covariances.

Lancsar and Savage (42) discuss calculation of WTP for cases involving forced choice of one or more of the alternatives compared with the status quo, relying heavily on Hanemann's (21) discussion of issues involved in applying welfare ideas to discrete choice problems. For example, in the case of a simple binary choice model where the choice is between a constant status quo and a series of one-at-a-time designed choice options, one needs to examine the utility of each alternative and the probability of each alternative being chosen using 'expected utility'. The WTP expression for this case is

$$\frac{1}{\beta(cost)}\left[\ln \sum_{i=1}^{n} e^{V_i^0} - \ln \sum_{i=1}^{n} e^{V_i^1} \right], \tag{10.11}$$

where the cost effect is as previously defined, and $\ln \sum_{i=1}^{n} e^{V_i}$ is the so-called 'inclusive value', or expected maximum utility for the status quo (superscript 0) and the alternative of interest (superscript 1). So, (10.11) tells us that in cases where consumers can choose two or more alternatives one must evaluate the difference in expected utility between two options divided by the cost effect to calculate WTP. If the cost effect is non-linear, a more complicated expression is required but the concept is the same. If both cost and attribute are random effects, one must simulate the distribution.

Including more attributes is a direct extension of the above discussion. In general, for attributes $X_1(l_1), X_2(l_2), ..., X_k(l_k)$, the total number of combinations is given by the full factorial expansion $X_1(l_1) \times X_2(l_2) \times ... \times X_k(l_k)$, where X_k is the kth attribute and l_k is the number of levels of that attribute. Thus, a DCE that involves asking a sample of respondents to compare a status quo option with some number of designed options one-at-a-time can be designed by (a) constructing the full factorial, and if sufficiently small, assigning all respondents to it, or if too large to do that, blocking the factorial into subsets (typically, randomly assigning sets without replacement) and assigning respondents randomly to each block (version); (b) using a fractional factorial design to sample from the full factorial and assigning all respondents to the scenarios given by the fraction, or blocking the fraction as described for the factorial, and randomly assigning respondents to one of the blocks (versions).

Random utility again underpins the specification of statistical models used to describe the choice process of respondents who participate in such DCEs. That is, as before we think of an indirect utility function with systematic and random components. Respondents seek to maximize their utility in their choices, but the analyst fails to include all factors known to the respondent and/or the respondent makes choices imperfectly, giving rise to the random utility case. Appropriate statistical models of the choice process for this case include (a) fixed effects for the attributes with additional terms that represent interactions of observable covariates with the intercept that reflects the propensity to choose the status quo versus the other options and/or interactions with the attributes or (b) random effects for the intercept and/or attributes to capture unobserved, latent differences in preferences (or, possibly a hybrid of a and b). Currently, random effects models are popular with academics and practitioners, but it remains unclear how to use such models to forecast choices and/or evaluate policies that will occur in the future and/or in other locations unless one assumes that random components are stable over time and/or space.

10.6 **Multinomial alternatives**

This case has two different versions: 1. there are multiple alternatives but all alternatives are generic and 2. at least one of the multiple alternatives differs in some significant way that requires the analyst to view this as 'non-generic' (or, 'alternative-specific'). For example, suppose a person's GP asks them to have a particular diagnostic test, and informs them that the test service is provided by (a) several named hospitals, (b) several named clinics, and (c) several named stand-alone testing services. Suppose further that the testing options can be described by (i) waiting time to be tested, (ii) locational convenience to the person, and (iii) cost.

If the objective is to understand and model the *type of service* that will be chosen by people facing this decision, or the *particular named option* within each type of service that will be chosen, then the problem is alternative-specific. If, on the other hand, the objective is to understand people's decisions/preferences for types or services and features of these services, where particular manifestations of the service options available for each type are examples, then the problem is generic. That is, alternative-specific problems arise when one wants to model the choices of particular named options that are members of a general class of options; generic options arise when one wants to model the choices of non-named options that lie within the general class. The former provides very specific information about the choices of particular options that would be of interest to – say – the owners of each type of option (e.g. owners of testing clinics); the latter provides very general information about the entire class of possible options. Tables 10.1a and b illustrate two possible choice tasks for these cases using the testing example.

These cases are treated at length in (1), Louviere, Hensher, and Swait (hereafter 'LHS') as 'generic' and 'alternative-specific' DCEs. For generic DCEs, designs discussed and illustrated in LHS are obsolete because optimal design theory developed by Deborah Street, Leonie Burgess and colleagues (e.g. (33)) provides the theory and methods to construct optimal designs for this case. For 'alternative-specific' DCEs, the design theory originally proposed by Louviere and Woodworth (37) remains the primary way to construct such experiments. It is important to note that in the latter case, identification issues are well-understood and typically can be satisfied in virtually all

Table 10.1a An alternative-specific task

Features	Hospital	Clinic	Stand-alone
Wait time for testing	Same day	1 week	Next day
Locational convenience	15 min away	1 hour away	2 hours away
Cost	$75	$50	$100
I most likely will choose:	❏	❏	❏

Table 10.1b A generic task

Features	Option A	Option B
Type of test service	Hospital	Clinic
Wait time for testing	1 week	Next day
Locational convenience	2 hours away	15 min away
Cost	$100	$50
I most likely will choose:	❏	❏

applications but the efficiency of the designs relative to an optimal design is unknown.

Those who wish to construct optimally efficient designs for the generic case should consult Street and Burgess (33), which provides software to help analysts implement the design theory. In the case of alternative-specific designs, the theory detailed in LHS (1) or Louviere and Woodworth (37) provide the way to construct the designs. In the case of generic designs, attribute parameters specified in indirect utility functions are the same for all choice options, whether specified as fixed or random. In the case of alternative-specific designs, attribute parameters can be specified to be the same for some, but not all effects. That is, at least one attribute effect must differ for at least one alternative, regardless of whether the effects are specified as fixed or random.

Generic DCEs and associated models are consistent with the previous discussion of the theory that underlies calculation of WTP. If some model effects are alternative-specific, this implies that WTP will differ by (at least one) alternative. If cost effects are alternative-specific, this raises interesting issues over which cost effects to use in WTP calculations, as different cost effects imply different values of marginal values for income. Our position is that one generally should use cost effects associated with a given option to calculate the WTP associated with changes for that option, particularly when the cost for the base option is known. Comparisons between multiple pro-grammes are more complicated and, for this reason, researchers often try to use only one cost parameter unless there is clear evidence to the contrary.

A variation on the above theme is a DCE that presents respondents with multiple choice options, where one of these options is a constant option. To this point, the constant option has always implicitly been the status quo, but when multiple choice options are offered to respondents, a logical choice often is to choose none of the options, which is feasible since it involves zero cost. In the case of a constant status quo option, one can choose to incorporate the attribute levels of the status quo option in the estimation matrix or treat it as a fixed or random effect. In the case of the 'choose none' option, there are no associated attributes, and hence, one must be care-ful about how to specify this option. For example, as before, one can choose to allow it to be a fixed or random effect and/or one can allow the variance of the random component associated with this option to differ from the other options (as in nested or tree logit models).

10.7 **Common designs**

Two good sources of information about designs used in SP studies are LHS (1) and Street and Burgess (33). As these sources are available, our focus here will be on briefly describing the options and their advantages and disadvantages.

10.7.1 **Ad hoc designs**

From time-to-time one sees ad hoc designs used in SP studies. By 'ad hoc' we mean a design that is constructed without reliance on formal statistical design theory. Basically, one should **NEVER** do this, primarily because the properties of such designs are rarely known in advance, and it is likely that they are (a) statistically inefficient relative to an optimal design and/or (b) poorly conditioned, including the possibility of identification issues. Because applied economists rarely receive training in experimental design, and because econometrics historically has had to deal with 'messy' data, there is a tendency for applied economists to think that 'any design will do'. The sooner this notion is dispelled, the better.

10.7.2 Full-factorial designs

These designs may not be practical because the number of combinations of attribute levels can be very large. That said, let us distinguish two types of applications: 1. a design administered to everyone in a sample and 2. a design blocked into 'versions' with respondents randomly assigned to a particular version without replacement. Type 1 designs typically are used when one wants to be able to compare individuals and/or if one wants to estimate a model for each individual. For example, one type of comparison that often arises in practice is to group the individuals into segments based on their choices. The latter application is well beyond the scope of this chapter. Interested readers may wish to consult reference works on taxonomic methods such as cluster analysis or latent class methods. Type 2 designs typically are used when the design of interest has more than 16 or 32 attribute level combinations or choice sets and one does not want to compare individuals' choices directly.

Full factorials can be used as both type 1 and type 2 designs. In the case of type 1 designs, the class of factorials probably is restricted to those designs that have 32 choice sets or fewer, although it may be possible to use larger designs in certain cases where the incentives are sufficiently high, such as paying physicians enough to motivate them to 'do' perhaps 64 or more scenarios. In the case of multiple choice response tasks, however, only very small factorials are possible for type 1 applications. Researchers interested in such applications should consult Street and Burgess (33). In the case of type 2 applications, it is likely that full factorials can be practical for many cases because the factorial can be blocked into versions. For example, suppose that a researcher wished to design an experiment for ten attributes, each with two levels (2^{10}). The full factorial has 1,024 attribute level combinations, and if the researcher is confident that each respondent can and will 'do' 16 scenarios, the design can be blocked into 64 versions, with each respondent randomly assigned to one version. So, a full factorial of this size would be practical with samples of 400–800 people, which are not uncommon in SP applications. In our experience, many researchers rule out full factorials due to their size without realizing that they could have been used.

The major advantage of full factorials is that they allow one to estimate and test all possible main and interaction effects. In type 1 applications, there typically is a lot of statistical power to conduct these tests, and to the extent that one takes differences in individuals into account (e.g. preference heterogeneity), one can estimate and test these effects allowing for differences. The primary advantage of being able to estimate and test interaction effects is that one does not have to assume strictly additive indirect utility functions but instead can allow for more complex forms. The disadvantage, of course, is that there are typically many more effects to estimate, so analyses are more complicated. The advantage that is associated with type 1 applications does not necessarily apply to type 2 applications because (a) the power of the tests will be less due to smaller sample sizes associated with interaction effects, (b) it may not be possible to take individual differences into account as easily or as thoroughly as one can with type 1 applications because versions may be confounded with differences, and (c) it is unrealistic to rely on assumptions that all respondents have exactly the same indirect utility function.

In summary, full factorials probably can be used in many more applications than most SP researchers think, although their use in multiple choice response tasks is likely to be limited only to very small problems.

10.7.3 Orthogonal main effects plans

Orthogonal main effects plans (OMEPs) are a sample of attribute level combinations from the full factorial that have the property that all main effects are independent of one another. The advantage of OMEPs is that they typically are smaller than other designs. The disadvantage, however, is that one must assume that the indirect utility function is strictly additive for all respondents. Worse yet, if this assumption is false, one cannot test and reject it. It probably is fair to say that OMEPs are used much more often than they should, particularly in so far as they are the most widely used designs in SP research. If one has a type 1 design application, it may be that OMEPs are the only feasible option to allow rigorous comparisons of individuals. However, for type 2 design applications, it rarely would be the case that one would need to use an OMEP, and so researchers should consider other options discussed below.

10.7.4 Designs that allow estimation of main and interaction effects

Readers who want to construct and apply these designs should consult reference works in the design literature, although a good starting place is LHS (1). These types of designs are distinguished by what can be estimated and what must be assumed about omitted effects:

1. Main effects are orthogonal to one another, and are also orthogonal to unobserved but potentially significant two-way interactions. These designs protect estimates of main effects from two-way interaction effects that cannot be estimated. Their advantage is that they typically are relatively small(er), and hence, can be used in many applications. Two-way interactions are the most likely interactions to be significant and large, and so should be considered a key potential source of bias in main effects when they are omitted. Another disadvantage is that one must assume that all interactions of higher order than two-way are not significant, and that one cannot test this assumption to determine whether it is false. These designs typically need to be blocked into versions, but for smaller designs, it may be possible to use them in type 1 design applications.

2. One also can construct designs for problems that involve estimation of all main effects and a subset of the two-way interactions (known as 'selected two-way interactions'). It is hard to generalize about these designs because they typically are constructed on a case-by-case basis, but sources of these designs exist, as noted in Street and Burgess (33). The advantage of these designs is that they are smaller than

the design discussed below. The disadvantage is that designs for the exact subset that a particular researcher is interested in may not exist, and one must assume that all unobserved interactions are not significant, leaving one open to bias from unobserved two-way interactions that are significant.

3. Main effects and two-way interactions are orthogonal to one another, and both types of effects can be simultaneously estimated. These designs often are large, especially if the number of attributes and levels is greater than 8–10. However, for smaller problems, these designs have the advantage that they allow estimation of both main and two-way interaction effects, but at the cost of assuming that all other unobserved interaction effects are not significant. It rarely will be the case that one can use these designs in a type 1 design application, so the vast majority of applications of these designs will be for type 2 design problems.

4. One also can construct designs that allow one to orthogonalize the main effects and two-way interactions to unobserved and potentially significant three-way interactions. One also can construct designs that allow independent estimation of all main, two-way and three-way interactions. These types of designs are rarely used because they typically are fairly large, and require considerable design skill.

10.7.5 **D-optimal designs**

As previously noted, these designs optimize the determinant of the Fisher Information Matrix for the design. D-optimal designs for the case of all effects equal to zero have been developed by Street and Burgess (33), and readers should consult this reference for construction methods. What appears to be widely misunderstood about these designs is the fact that Monte Carlo simulations show that these designs are optimally efficient for choice probabilities that are not extreme and that they remain reasonably efficient for very large and very small choice probabilities. So, they are a good choice for almost all DCE problems. It also is worth noting that if one observes choice probabilities in the far tails in a DCE, this implies a very poor choice of the attribute levels or that the underlying process is almost deterministic. In addition to the Street and Burgess designs, designs can be constructed using SAS macros developed by Kufeld (38). Comparisons with Street and Burgess designs, however, suggests that the SAS designs sometimes do not have diagonal information matrices and can require substantial computation time to construct a highly efficient design.

10.7.7 **Random designs**

A number of SP researchers use what we call 'random designs'. These designs are constructed in various ways, but typically one or more sets of starting designs are constructed or one randomly samples from the complete set of all possible choice sets. If one uses a set of starting designs, say m of them, one typically randomly selects an attribute level combination from each of the m simultaneously to create an m-tuple that represents an m-element choice set. This design procedure was discussed by Louviere and Woodworth (37), but modern advances in optimal design of DCEs has made them obsolete. Similarly, some commercial DCE software creates choice sets by drawing them randomly from the entire set of possible choice sets, which typically is very large. Neither way of designing DCEs is a good idea since one cannot determine *a priori* which effects can be estimated with any precision, nor can one identify *a priori* what will be identified.[28] This approach also has the disadvantage that differences in individuals may be confounded with differences in the choice sets faced. Our advice is not to use this approach since better alternatives are available.

10.8 **Using prior information**

Naturally, it is always better to use whatever prior information one has available to construct designs, as noted earlier. So, if one has theoretical or empirical reasons to impose sign restrictions on the attribute effects, this will (a) restrict the classes of designs to consider and (b) will restrict the indirect utility functions to be estimated. For example, suppose there are three two-level attributes, and each has a known sign for the main effects. If the indirect utility function is strictly additive, only four scenarios are required to estimate the model in a binary discrete choice task. There are 16 possible binary response patterns that could be observed because each of the four scenarios can receive either of the two binary responses (2^4). Of these 16 patterns, only seven are consistent with additivity and sign restrictions, assuming that basing responses on only a single attribute or a pair of attributes is acceptable.

If the utility function is not additive, one must use the full factorial ($2 \times 2 \times 2 = 8$ attribute level combinations), which greatly increases the allowable response patterns to nearly 128, again assuming that one can base one's choices on one or a pair of attributes as well as all three attributes. It should be obvious that as the number of attributes and/or the number of response categories increase, the number of possible response patterns that can be consistent with a particular set of sign restrictions grows exponentially. Thus, as the number of attributes and/or the number of levels increases, sign restrictions may not help bound the problem in any practical sense. As such, sign restrictions are most useful for smaller problems.[29]

Finally, one can use a sequential design approach. In this approach, one uses experiments on small(er) samples to explore as much of the design space as possible. This approach can be viewed as a type of model selection problem where the objective is to identify as many possible significant and meaningful effects as possible *a priori*, while at the same time eliminating as many non-significant and non-meaningful effects as possible. In this way, one can bound the problem, which may allow one to use a smaller, special purpose design to identify and estimate the effects that one has *a priori* reason to believe will be significant and meaningful.

---

[28] Use of random design is often believed to identify all of the parameters of a model. That is true, however, only asymptotically as the design drawn approaches the full factorial. In the typical application, many parameters will not be statistically identified and other very poorly identified if subsamples receiving particular attribute combinations is small.

[29] One also can impose informative priors on the parameters of the utility function. This takes one in the direction of Bayesian designs if uncertainty around the priors is formally quantified. If one is prepared to assume that the parameters are known with certainty, it is possible to determine the design that maximizes D-optimality.

10.9 **Desirability and implications of common design criteria**

In this section, we review several design criteria that are frequently discussed in the various DCE literatures.[30]

10.9.1 **Orthogonality**

Orthogonality of the effects to be estimated means that the information matrix is block diagonal, and hence, all effects of interest can be estimated independently of one another. This is a desirable but not essential criterion. What is essential is that the degree of shared covariance between effects to be estimated is low.

10.9.2 **Level-balance**

This means that each level of an attribute occurs equally often, and more generally, this should hold for all attributes. This criterion is associated with the precision of the estimate of the attribute levels, such that if level balance holds, the model parameters associated with each level will be estimated with equal precision. Again, this criterion is desirable, but not essential. However, unless one has good reasons for not satisfying level balance, such as one of three levels being far more important to the work than the other two, it is desirable to satisfy this criterion. A similar criterion is a balanced level co-occurrence. That is, if a design is orthogonal, it will be the case that the levels of each pair of attributes will co-occur equally often. This criterion insures minimal shared covariances.

10.9.3 **Attribute overlap**

This refers to correlations among two or more attributes, such that it may not be possible to vary them independently. This leads to what are called 'nested' factors/attributes because the way to deal with these problems is to combine the attribute levels into a single attribute that can be varied independently. For example, if a particular health service attribute is the amount of use of the system, and a second is the cost of using the system, it is likely to be the case that higher levels of use will covary with cost, so one would want to combine these two attributes into one.

10.9.4 **Elimination of dominated/infeasible alternatives**

If all the attributes are numerical and their signs are known *a priori*, any of the standard design constructions will lead to dominated and/or infeasible options. However, while this happens in practice, our experience suggests that there is far too much concern about this criterion than should be the case.[31] The first thing a researcher should

---

[30] Viney, Savage, and Louviere (39) look at these concepts in the context of a specific empirical example.

[31] In empirical applications, the more serious problem is likely to be that particular attributes are known to have sufficiently high correlation so that the absence of this correlation in attribute bundles is noticeable.

do is to determine whether it is reasonable to expect the respondent sample to actually know which attribute level combinations are infeasible. Typically, the sample does not know this; but the experts, such as doctors or medical researchers do. If the sample cannot tell if a scenario or an option is infeasible, a researcher may want to proceed to use standard design construction methods as these will provide significantly better statistical properties than alternative methods.

If many respondents in fact know that something is infeasible and/or there can be dominant options in choice sets, then one typically must modify the standard construction methods to deal with this. For example, one way to deal with dominance is to randomly replace one or more levels with levels that are non-dominant. Ideally, one should test various random replacements, using those that minimally modify the statistical properties of the design. Infeasible options are a different problem as they have to be eliminated from the design. One way to do this is to construct the full factorial of possible options that can be created from the attributes and levels of each choice option (if the options are not generic), then eliminate all the infeasible combinations and check the statistical properties of the remaining combinations. If the shared covariances are not large and the inverse of the information matrix is well-conditioned, then use that design. If the statistical properties are poor, then one could try to select combinations from the feasible pool with the objective being to select a sample that has the best properties.

10.9.5 Utility balance

It is not clear why this criterion is considered important, although it has achieved considerable prominence in the marketing literature. Put simply, this criterion means that one should try to construct choice sets in such a way that the options in each set are as close in utility as possible. While this may seem like an intuitive criterion, if one could achieve this objective, there would be *NO* useful statistical information provided by the choices. That is, satisfying this criterion is equivalent to making all the choice options equally probable because if the option utilities are perfectly balanced, the respondents should be totally indifferent to all of them, and so should choose randomly. Thus, this criterion should not be used in the design of DCEs.

10.10 Concluding remarks

Experimental design is a key component of a successful choice experiment to help evaluate health policy alternatives. It is all too easy to construct and implement designs that do not statistically identify the parameters of interest or that greatly diminish the precision of the estimates relative to what could have been achieved with an efficient design. The underlying statistical theory for generic choice experiments is now well-understood (33), and software for producing reasonably high quality designs is now available (e.g. Street and Burgess design software that comes with their book); so, there is little justification for choosing and using the poor quality designs that appear all too often in the current literature.

Applied researchers need to think seriously about the attributes of the programs they wish to compare and the class of underlying utility functions they wish to estimate.

Invest time upfront in extensive qualitative work of the type illustrated by the ICEPOP Program (31;41), where extensive and iterative qualitative work was used to understand not only attributes, but also key words and phrases. Also plan time for elaborate and extensive pre-testing to identify tasks and associated survey instruments that 'work'. By 'work' we mean that (a) will be understood by all respondents, (b) will be meaningful to them, and (c) will simulate the actual choices one wants to observe as closely as possible. Often it makes sense to ask more choice questions rather than more complicated choice questions, or to ask more questions about the options in each choice set instead of more choice sets. Make reasonable restrictions on the nature of the utility function to reduce the size of the model space. Fix the attribute levels that are relatively unimportant to the policy issues being evaluated to further reduce the size of the model space and the task. More generally, one should avoid complex models and designs unless the project budget allows for extensive pretesting and large sample sizes.

Spend time observing the actual choices made by the population(s) of interest. Interview these populations and ask them how they make the choices, what are the pros and cons of each choice, and whether they feel like they have sufficient and/ or 'the right' information to make the right decision(s); if they do not have sufficient or 'right' information, what would assist them? Relying on experts to tell you how consumers make decisions rarely is a good idea because few of them actually know this. If, in fact, the expert is the one who makes the decision for the consumer, then model the expert; yet, even here, one may want to understand and model how the expert's decision(s) impact(s) the consumer.

Finally, there is a great deal of misinformation and misunderstanding about the design of DCEs in the applied health economics literature. The literature on the optimal design of DCEs is highly technical, and it is easy to make mistakes as noted by (33;43). There are no quick fixes and no easy routes; the literature on the design of experiments for linear models has evolved over more than 80 years, with some problems yet to be resolved. So, beware those who claim to have answers for all DCE design problems. Currently, we barely understand the generic design case for conditional logit models, and while designs for the alternative-specific case have been around since Louviere and Woodworth (37), few formal proofs of the properties of these designs exist even for conditional logit models. Furthermore, there are virtually no results available to guide those who want to estimate more general choice models than conditional logit, although mixed logit models at least should be identified with current generic and alternative-specific designs (each person is represented by a conditional logit model; only the parameters of that model differ across people).

It also is worth noting that this chapter has had little to say about types of tasks, task context, task complexity, methods of survey administration, survey length, incentive compatibility, sampling strategies, and a host of other issues relevant to whether any given stated preference DCE survey is reliable and valid. Similarly, we have said nothing about validating SP model predictions, pooling data from various sources, taking account of observable and unobservable heterogeneity and many other issues that are germane to particular applications. The choice modelling and SP literatures are now extensive on each of these topics, and interested readers should consult the workshop reports from the triennial Invitational Choice Symposia published in special issues of the journal *Marketing Letters* (e.g. *Marketing Letters* 1991, 1993, 1996, 1999, 2002, 2005, 2008), as well as standard reference sources like (1;44) for guidance.

References

1. Louviere, J.J., Hensher, D.A., and Swait, J.D. 2000. *Stated choice methods: analysis and application.* New York: Cambridge University Press.
2. Bradburn, N.M., Sudman, S., and Wansink, B. 2004. *Asking questions: The definitive guide to questionnaire design—for market research, political polls, and social and health questionnaires.* San Francisco, CA: Jossey-Bass.
3. Presser, S., Rothgeb, J.M., Couper, M.P., Lessler, J.T., Martin, E., Martin, J., and Singer, E. 2004. *Methods for testing and evaluating survey questionnaires.* New York: Wiley.
4. Tourangeau, R., Rips, L.J., and Rasinski, K. 2000. *The psychology of survey response.* New York: Cambridge University Press.
5. Mitchell, R.C. 2002. On designing constructed markets in valuation surveys. *Environmental and Resource Economics* **22**: 297–321.
6. Kaplowitz, M.D., Lupi, F., and Hoehn, J.P. 2004. Multiple methods for developing and evaluating a stated choice questionnaire to value wetlands. In: Presser, S., Rothgeb, J.M., Couper, M.P., Lessler, J.T., Martin, E., Martin, J., and Singer, E., editors. *Methods for testing and evaluating survey questionnaires.* New York: Wiley.
7. Swait, J. and Adamowicz, W. 2001. The influence of task complexity on consumer choice: A latent class model of decision strategy switching. *Journal of Consumer Research* **28**: 135–148.
8. Viney, R., Lanscar, E., and Louviere, J. 2002. Discrete choice experiments to measure consumer preferences for health and healthcare. *Expert Review of Pharmaco-economics and Outcomes Research* **2**: 319–326.
9. Ryan M. and Gerard, K. 2003. Using discrete choice experiments to value health care: current practice and future prospects. *Applied Health Economic Policy Analysis* **2**: 55–64.
10. Bryan, S. and Dolan, P. 2004. Discrete choice experiments in health economics: for better or worse. *European Journal of Health Economics* **5**: 199–2002.
11. Lancsar, E. and Donaldson, C. 2005. Discrete choice experiments in health economics: distinguishing between the method and its applications. *European Journal of Health Economics* **6**: 314–316.
12. Viscusi, W.K. and Gayer, T. 2005. Quantifying and valuing environmental health risks. In: Karl-Göran, M. and Jeffrey R.V., editors. *Handbook of Environmental Economics,* vol. 2, Amsterdam: North-Holland.
13. Mitchell, R.C. and Richard, T.C. 1989. *Using surveys to value public goods: The contingent valuation method.* Baltimore, MD: Johns Hopkins University.
14. Arrow, K., Solow, R., Portney, P.R., Leamer, E.E., Radner, R., and Schuman, H. 1993. Report of the NOAA Panel on Contingent Valuation. *Federal Register* **58**: 4601–4614.
15. Carson, R.T. and Groves, T. 2007. Incentive and information properties of preference questions. *Environmental and Resource Economics* **37**: 181–210.
16. Just, R.E., Darrell, L.H., and Andrew, S. 2005. *The welfare economics of public policy: A practical approach to project and policy evaluation.* Northampton, MA: Edward Elgar.

17. Bockstael, N.E. and Freeman, A.M. 2005. Welfare theory and valuation. In: Karl-Göran, M. and Jeffrey, R.V., editors. *Handbook of environmental economics*. vol. 2, Amsterdam: North-Holland.

18. Carson, R.T. and Hanemann, W.M. 2005. Contingent valuation. In: Karl-Göran, M. and Jeffrey, R.V., editors. *Handbook of environmental economics,* vol. 2, Amsterdam: North-Holland.

19. McConnell, K.E. 1990. Models for referendum data: the structure of discrete choice models for contingent valuation. *Journal of Environmental Economics and Management* **18**: 19–34.

20. Cameron, T.A. 1988. A new paradigm for valuing non-market goods using referendum data: maximum likelihood estimation by censored logistic regression. *Journal of Environmental Economics and Management* **15**: 355–379.

21. Hanemann, W.M. 1984. Welfare evaluations in contingent valuation experiments with discrete responses. *American Journal of Agricultural Economics* **66**: 332–341.

22. McFadden, D.L. and Gregory, K.L. 1993. Issues in the contingent valuation of environmental goods: methodologies for data collection and analysis. In: Jerry, A.H., editor. *Contingent valuation: A critical assessment*, pp. 165–216. Amsterdam: North-Holland.

23. Lancaster, K. 1966. A New Approach to Consumer Theory. *Journal of Political Economy* **84**: 132–157.

24. Carson, R.T. and Yongil, J. 2000. On overcoming informational deficiencies in estimating willingness to pay distributions, paper presented at the American Agricultural Economics Association Meeting, Tampa, FL. Chilton, S.M., and W.G. Hutchinson (1999), Do focus groups contribute anything to the contingent valuation process? *Journal of Economic Psychology* **20**: 465–483.

25. McFadden, D.L. 1974. Conditional logit analysis of qualitative choice behavior. In: Zarembka, P. editor. *Frontiers in econometrics*, pp. 105–142. New York: Academic.

26. Manski, C. 1977. The structure of random utility models. *Theory and Decision* **8**: 229–254.

27. Kriström, B. 1997. Spike models in contingent valuation. *American Journal of Agricultural Economics* **79**: 1013–1023.

28. Box, G.E.P., Hunter, W.G., and Hunter, J.S. 1978. *Statistics for experimenters: An introduction to design, data analysis, and model building.* New York: Wiley.

29. Atkinson, AC. and Donev, A.N. 1992. *Optimum experimental designs.* New York: Oxford University Press.

30. Wu, C.F.J. and Hamada, M. 2000. *Experiments: planning, analysis, and parameter design optimization.* New York: Wiley.

31. Alberini, A. and Richard, T.C. 1990. Choice of thresholds for efficient binary discrete choice estimation. Discussion Paper 90-34. San Diego: Department of Economics. University of California, San Diego.

32. Alberini, A. 1995. Optimal designs for discrete choice contingent valuation surveys: Single-bound, double-bound, and bivariate models. *Journal of Environmental Economics and Management* **28**: 287–306.

33. Street, D.J. and Burgess, L. 2007. *The construction of optimal stated choice experiments: theory and methods.* New York: Wiley.

34. Kanninen, B.J. 1993. Design of sequential experiments for contingent valuation studies. *Journal of Environmental Economics and Management* **25**: S1–S11.

35. McFadden, D.L. 1999. Computing willingness-to-pay in random utility models. In: Moore, J., Riezman, R., and Melvin, J., editors. *Trade, theory, and econometrics: essays in honor of John S. Chipman.* London: Routledge.

36. Ben-Akiva, M. and Lerman, S. 1985. *Discrete choice analysis: theory and application to travel demand.* Cambridge: MIT.

37. Louviere, J.J. and Woodward, G. 1983. Design and analysis of simulated consumer choice or allocation experiments: An approach based on aggregate data. *Journal of Marketing Research* **20**: 350–367.

38. Kufeld, W. 2005. Experimental design and choice modeling macros. Technical Report TS722I, Cary, NC: SAS Institute.

39. Viney, R.,Savage, E., and Louviere, J. 2005. Empirical investigation of experimental design properties of discrete choice experiments in health care. *Health Economics* **14**: 349–362.

40. Coast, J., Flynn, T.N., Natarajan, L., Sproston, K., Lewis, J., Louviere, J.J., and Peters, T.J. 2008. Valuing the ICECAP capability index for older people. *Social Science and Medicine* **67**(5): 874–882.

41. Coast, J., Flynn, T.N, Sutton, E., Al-Janabi , H., Vosper, J., Lavender, S., Louviere, J.J., and Peters, T.J. 2008. Investigating choice experiments for preferences of older people (ICEPOP): evaluative spaces in health economics. *Journal of Health Services Research & Policy* **13**(3): 31–37.

42. Lancsar , E. and Savage, E. 2004. Deriving welfare measures from discrete choice experiments: inconsistency between current methods and random utility and welfare theory. *Health Economic Letters* **13**: 901–907.

43. Street, D.J., Burgess, L., and Louviere, J.J. 2005. Quick and easy choice sets: constructing optimal and nearly optimal choice experiments. *International Journal of Research in Marketing* **22**: 459–470.

44. Train, K. 2003. *Discrete choice methods with simulation.* New York: Cambridge Economic Press.

Chapter 11

Benefit assessment for cost–benefit analysis studies in health care using discrete choice experiments: Estimating welfare in a health care setting

Jordan J. Louviere and Denzil G. Fiebig

11.1 Introduction

The purpose of this chapter is to introduce the idea of using stated preference discrete choice experiments (SPDCEs) for valuation and welfare estimation. We begin by discussing SPDCEs and the random utility theory-based choice models that underlie their analysis. Given the purpose of this handbook, this naturally then leads to a discussion of how to use choice models estimated from SPDCEs to carry out valuation and welfare analysis.

As noted in Chapter 10, the random utility model (RUM) provides a sound, behavioural-theoretic basis for many forms of preference-elicitation procedures, and provides theory to combine, compare, and test various forms of data and preference-elicitation procedures. Thus, RUM provides a theoretical basis for SPDCEs, as well as other forms of non-experimental preference data like direct observations of choices in real or hypothetical markets, ranking multiattribute choice options, and so forth. Here, we focus on specific considerations related to the estimation of welfare in health care using SPDCEs, which includes designs appropriate for economic welfare measurement (state of the world models and multiple choice models); issues of dynamic aspects of choice; and policy analysis using SPDCEs drawn from environmental economics (modelling results and mapping into policy relevant health care scenarios).

Interest in stated preference (SP) elicitation methods in health is growing, with discrete choice workshops at Odense, Denmark (2002), the University of Oxford (2003), and Universidad de Las Palmas (2005), as well as SP courses (Odense, 2002; Oxford 2003), tutorials (iHEA, 2003) and special sessions (iHEA, 2005, 2007). Interest in SP theory and methods by economists is relatively new, although there has long been interest in Contingent Valuation (CV) theory and methods in environmental and resource economics (see Chapters 5–9). Work on other SP methods was encouraged by the Arrow-Solow Committee's review of CV (1), and since then SP research has steadily grown (see, e.g. 2).

We now briefly describe the state of practice of DCEs in health care, building on the survey of Ryan and Gerard (3). We focus on two key components of SPDCEs: 1. experimental design and construction of choice data and 2. statistical methods used to analyse the data. We describe current practice and suggest ways forward to improve the state of the art. Following this overview, we discuss several serious, unresolved issues with SPDCEs and the formulation and estimation of discrete choice models. We then link these issues to empirical generalizations and reliability and validity of choice model results in health. We close with suggestions for further research and ways to potentially resolve some of the unresolved issues.

11.2 **Background**

11.2.1 **Random utility model**

The RUM provides a behavioural-theoretic basis by which one can formulate and test many statistical preference models; we focus on families of probabilistic discrete choice models. Consider the basic axiom of the RUM:

$$U_{ij} = V_{ij} + \varepsilon_{ij}, \tag{11.1}$$

where U_{ij} is the latent utility individual i associates with choice option j, V_{ij} the observable component of utility, and ε_{ij} is the unobservable (unexplainable) component.

We assume individuals are utility maximizers and they compare utilities associated with each of J possible options. Utilities are random, so the choice problem is stochastic. Analysts observe choices, not utilities; so, if we let Y_i be a random variable denoting the choice outcome, the probability that individual i chooses j is given by:

$$P(Y_i = j) = P(V_{ij} + \varepsilon_{ij} > V_{ih} + \varepsilon_{ih}) \text{ for all } h = 1,\ldots,J; h \neq j. \tag{11.2}$$

To move from a probabilistic choice model to an econometric choice model, one must specify the systematic component of utility. For example, a linear in parameters form:

$$V_{ij} = X'_{ij}\beta, \tag{11.3}$$

where X_{ij} is a vector of variables representing observed attributes of option j and β is a conformable vector of preference parameters to be estimated. In practice, V_{ij} can depend on individual-specific characteristics, interacted with attributes of options; we ignore this to simplify the initial discussion.

The popular multinomial logit (MNL) model results from assuming the random terms, ε_{ij}, are distributed as independent and identically distributed (IID) extreme value random variates. This gives a computationally tractable model where the probability that individual i chooses j is given by:

$$P(Y_i = j \mid X) = \frac{\exp(X'_{ij}\beta)}{\sum_h \exp(X'_{ih}\beta)}. \tag{11.4}$$

A disadvantage of MNL arises from assuming IID errors, which in turn results in the Independence of Irrelevant Alternatives (IIA) property. Much work has focused on specifications that relax this assumption like nested logit, multinomial probit (MNP), and random parameter or mixed logit (MXL) models.

The RUM provides a theoretically sound way to compare and test many forms of preference-elicitation procedures, such as SPDCEs (e.g. 4) and/or revealed-preference (RP) observations from choices in real markets. Ben-Akiva and Morikawa (5) provide the theory to compare different elicitation procedures by showing that if the underlying preferences are the same, and both procedures satisfy the RUM, then any common vector of preference parameters estimated from the two sets of data must be proportional.

For example, if one elicits preferences for health care attributes in an SPDCE and a contingent ranking task, vectors of preference parameters estimated from both procedures must be proportional if the underlying preference processes are the same. Likewise, if one observes choices of health options in real markets from the same or independent samples of individuals, and a common subset of attributes is present in both SPDCE and RP market choices, the two vectors of preference estimates must be proportional if the underlying preferences are the same and both procedures satisfy the RUM (6). Louviere, Hensher, and Swait (7) review many comparisons of RP and SP sources, and report that the majority of cases support common preferences. McFadden (8) also cites evidence of common preferences in RP and SP data and for an example in health economics, see Mark and Swait (9). More recently, Louviere (10) notes the continuing consistency of evidence. Thus, one can pool RP and SP data to improve efficiency of estimation results.

11.2.2 Design of discrete choice experiments

Louviere and Woodworth (4) discussed ways to integrate the RUM with statistical design theory for discrete choices. That is, discrete multivariate statistics provides theory and models for analysing crosstab tables that are isomorphic to choice models (11), with crosstab tables being analogues of factorial designs. Louviere and Woodworth (4) proposed designing DCEs that can be viewed as systematically incomplete crosstab tables. Viewed this way, one can simulate many real market choice situations and insure satisfaction of key statistical properties of choice models.

Let there be $k = 1,\ldots, K$ attributes, and let each have L_k levels. All goods that can be described by these K attributes are given by the factorial of their levels; that is, $\prod_k(L_k) = T$, where T is the number of combinations of attribute levels. Let C be the number of possible choice sets of the T goods; this is given by a 2^T factorial where each good is in or out of a set. 'Designs' are systematic ways of sampling from C to satisfy optimality for statistical criteria like efficiency and identification of model effects. There are many ways to optimize designs, but a useful and widely used criterion is D-optimality, which refers to maximizing the determinant of the information matrix; see Chapter 10, Section 10.4 and references 12–14.

DCEs can mimic real markets to an arbitrary degree of accuracy limited only by time and resources, such that almost all real markets can be simulated by DCEs. Two key statistical properties of DCEs are identification and efficiency. Identification refers to the range of utility specifications that can be estimated from DCEs given particular choice model specifications. DCEs also involve humans suggesting other criteria that should be satisfied like task complexity and realism. DCE tasks should be no more complex than a real market task, and the closer the DCE simulates what humans do, the more face validity.

11.3 **Deriving welfare measures from DCEs**

Once estimated, the indirect utility function (IUF) represented by (11.3) provides the basis for welfare analysis whereby we can measure the economic impact of changing existing products or programmes or of introducing new ones.

SPDCE data sources analysed with various forms of probabilistic discrete choice models yield utility estimates for each level of each attribute varied in the DCE (assuming good design of SPDCEs, as later discussed). The utility estimates are measured on interval scales that have the property that the origin (zero point) is arbitrary and the unit of measurement also is arbitrary. Each attribute is therefore measured on a different interval scale, with the consequence that one cannot compare these quantities directly. Instead, one needs a common denominator. For example, the attributes can be compared in terms of choice probabilities associated with each level, and they also can be compared with respect to partial log-likelihoods associated with each level, although one rarely sees this in health (see 15;16 for discussions of these issues).

In economic terms, the valuation problem is known as welfare measurement. Welfare measures are used to compare the effects of attribute utilities and the utilities of goods. The common denominator typically is money, but other numeraires such as time also can be used. In practice, we need to value a product or programme or a specific feature or attribute of such products or programmes. What are people willing to pay for quantity or quality changes in the alternatives on offer? (see Chapters 5–9). We consider the following evaluation cases:

1. A change in utility due to a change in an attribute level of a currently chosen good or service
2. A change in utility due to changes in more than one attribute level of a currently chosen good or service
3. A difference in utility due to changes in attribute levels when there is uncertainty about which alternative is chosen and
4. A difference in utility when a new good or service is provided

Consider Case 1 where a particular attribute is being valued, and rewrite (11.3) as follows:

$$V_{ij} = X'_{ij}\beta = X_{1ij}\beta_1 + p_{ij}\beta_p + \tilde{X}'_{ij}\tilde{\beta}, \tag{11.5}$$

where X_1 is the attribute to be valued, p the price of alternative j, $\tilde{X}$ represents all remaining attributes, and β_1, β_p, and $\tilde{\beta}$ represent the associated parameters to be estimated.

Now, consider an individual who chooses alternative j both before and after a change in attribute 1 that we denote by Δ_1. Then, the change in utility will be given by $\Delta_1\beta_1$ and the price variation required to leave the level of utility unchanged can easily be calculated. Expressed in terms of offsetting income this compensating variation (CV) is given by:

$$CV = \Delta_1 \frac{\beta_1}{\beta_p}. \tag{11.6}$$

If the change represents an improvement then $\Delta_1\beta_1 > 0$ and as $\beta_p < 0$, the resultant CV will be negative indicating the individual is willing to accept a reduction in income (or increase in cost) in order to be indifferent after this particular change in the attribute.

Alternatively, the marginal willingness to pay (MWTP) for X_1 (or the marginal rate of substitution between the attribute and price) measures the change in income people are willing to accept in exchange for small changes in the attribute X_1. This is defined as:

$$MWTP = \frac{\partial V/\partial X_1}{\partial V/\partial p} = \frac{\beta_1}{\beta_p}. \tag{11.7}$$

While providing measures that are easily computed, the exchange between Lancsar and Savage (17;18), Ryan (19), and Santos-Silva (20) emphasizes that some care needs to be taken in interpreting these quantities as welfare measures. In particular, (11.6) will be an appropriate measure if we know that alternative j will definitely be chosen. If instead it is the quality of alternative h that is improved, then this change yields no gain to the individual who chooses alternative j both before and after the improvement. When there is uncertainty regarding which alternative will be chosen, the CV as modified for discrete choice problems by Small and Rosen (21) is the appropriate framework to use.

In the special case of a logit model, the formula for expected CV (ECV) is given by:

$$ECV = \frac{1}{\lambda}\left[\ln \sum_{j=1}^{J} e^{V_j^0} - \ln \sum_{j=1}^{J} e^{V_j^1} \right], \tag{11.8}$$

where the subscripts 0 and 1 refer to before and after the change being considered and λ is the marginal utility of money. This formula is very general and can be used to derive welfare measures arising from each of the four evaluation situations that have been identified.

In ECV calculations, λ is typically set equal to the negative of the coefficient on the price or cost variable that is invariably included in the indirect utility specification, i.e. $\lambda = -\beta_p$. As stressed by Train (22), a key assumption in deriving (11.8) is that the marginal utility of income is independent of income. This is typically what is assumed, but see Morey, Sharma, and Mills (23) for an example involving choice of malaria treatments where this assumption was successfully relaxed.

In order to illustrate the four cases noted above, we use a hypothetical example of a treatment with the following attributes:

– Health benefit with two levels (a little and a lot)
– Number of treatments required (one, every 5 years)
– Who can administer the treatment (GP, specialist)
– Monetary cost ($25, $50).

For ease of exposition, we assume that a properly designed SPDCE was conducted (see Chapter 10) and that a conditional logit model was estimated from the choice data and that the choice involved a status quo (SQ) alternative. The estimated utilities (parentheses) and the implied (additive) indirect utility function are shown below.

Table 11.1 Hypothetical example

Benefit	How many times	Who administers	Cost
Little (-1.50)	Once (0.75)	GP (0.50)	$25 (1.25)
Lot (1.50)	Every 5 years (-0.75)	Specialist (-0.50)	$50 ($-1.25$)

The implied indirect utility function (IUF) using-1, $+1$ effects codes for the attributes and 25, 50 coding for cost:

$$V_{iSQ} = -2.0$$
$$V_{ij} = -0.1(\text{cost}_{ij}) + 1.5(\text{benefit}_{ij}) - 0.75\ (\text{times}_{ij}) - 0.5(\text{who}_{ij}). \qquad (11.9)$$

Case 1: A change in utility due to a change in an attribute level of a currently chosen good

The above IUF implies that the CV for benefit is as follows:

$$\Delta_1 \beta_1 / \beta_p = 2 \times 1.5/(-0.1) = -30.$$

Specifically, this implies that consumers are WTP $30 more for an improved treatment that has a lot of the benefit compared to a little. In a similar manner, we calculate that they are WTP $15 more for a treatment that is administered only once compared to every 5 years, and are WTP $10 more for a treatment that can be administered by a GP compared to a Specialist.

Case 2: A change in utility due to changes in more than one attribute level of a currently chosen good

This case represents a natural extension of Case 1. Now, suppose the treatment is planned to change from being administered every 5 years by a GP to being administered only once by a Specialist. To calculate the implied willingness to pay in this case, we have to calculate the difference in utility of the two treatments and divide by the cost estimate. So, from Table 11.1 this difference will be $0.25 - (-0.25)$ and a difference in utility of 0.5 (all else equal). Now, the calculation is 0.5/–0.1 = –5 implying consumers are willing to forgo $5 in income for a change which represents a net benefit because they value the improvement in time administered more than the unfavourable change in who administers.

Case 3: A difference in utility due to changes in attribute levels when there is uncertainty about which alternative is chosen

Here, we reconsider the Case 2 example but with uncertainty in consumer choices. Suppose the initial choice is between the status quo and a treatment administered every 5 years by a GP that would cost $25 and would deliver little benefit. Now, improve the treatment as in Case 2 so that it is administered once by a Specialist and all other attribute levels remain unchanged. The before change utility levels are:

$$V^0{}_{iSQ} = -2.0$$
$$V^0{}_{i1} = -0.1\times25 + 1.5\times(-1) - 0.75\times1 - 0.5\times(-1) = -4.25$$

while after the change the utility for treatment 1 becomes:

$$V^1{}_{i1} = -0.1 \times 25 + 1.5 \times (-1) - 0.75 \times (-1) - 0.5 \times 1 = -3.75$$

and hence the ECV calculation is:

$$\textbf{ECV} = \{\ln[\exp(-2) + \exp(-4.25)] - \ln[\exp(-2) + \exp(-3.75)]\}/\ 0.1 = -0.6.$$

Thus, the net benefit here is valued at only $0.6 which is much less than the Case 2 valuation of $5 for the same change. The difference now is that the ECV accounts for the uncertainty associated with the choice of alternatives both before and after the change. In this example, treatment 1 is not very attractive relative to the status quo and hence the improvement is valued but would only benefit a relatively small number of people as most would still continue to use the status quo treatment.

Case 4: A difference in utility when a new good is provided

In this case, rather than improving the treatment as in Case 3, a new treatment is added to the choice set. Take as the base the, before change, situation in Case 3 where the choice is between the status quo and a treatment administered every 5 years by a GP that would cost $25 and would deliver little benefit. Now, suppose a new treatment is introduced so that there is a choice between three treatments. This new treatment is the same as the existing treatment but delivers a lot of benefit but will cost $30 rather than $25. The utility calculation for the status quo and treatment 1 are unchanged from Case 3. The utility level for the new treatment 2 is:

$$V^1{}_{i2} = -0.1 \times 30 + 1.5 \times 1 - 0.75 \times 1 - 0.5 \times (-1) = -1.75.$$

Thus, the ECV calculation to value the introduction of the new treatment is:

$$\textbf{ECV} = \{\ln[\exp(-2) + \exp(-4.25)] - \ln[\exp(-2) + \exp(-3.75) + \exp(-1.75)]\}/0.1 = -8.0.$$

Treatment 2 has higher utility than either the status quo or treatment 1 and hence its introduction is highly valued by people. The benefit associated with its introduction is estimated to be $8.

We now turn our attention to reviewing the state of practice of using SPDCEs in health care to provide a frame of reference for appropriate use of welfare analysis. It is important to know how the basic ingredients in the welfare analysis were generated.

11.4 State of practice in health

Ryan and Gerard (3) provide a useful starting point for reviewing SPDCEs in health. They surveyed only studies in English applied to health care based on the RUM that used choice responses, identifying 34 studies from 1990 to 2000. We now briefly update their survey (for more detail see (24)). We identified 25 more studies from 2001 to 2004 and a further 80 until July 2007, which clearly indicates rapid growth in DCEs in health, reflecting similar growth in other areas (see also downloadable Table 12.1 in Chapter 12 for examples of the types of attributes used in discrete choice studies in health care www.herc.ox.ac.uk/books/cba/support). We assess and evaluate studies from 1990 to 2007 with regard to key DCE properties like experimental design, preference elicitation method, estimation procedure, and validity.

11.4.1 Background

Almost all studies were conducted in the UK, Australia, and the USA, with the UK exhibiting the most SPDCE studies. However, over time there has been considerable growth in studies conducted in other countries; Ryan and Gerard (3) reported only one such study in the period 1990–2000 but since then countries other than the UK, Australia, and USA accounted for 33% of all SPDCE studies. A large majority focussed on economic evaluation of health care products. The largest group of people studied were patients, but an increasing number of studies compared preferences of groups of people (e.g. Bishop *et al.* (25) compared professionals' and patients' preferences for screening tests; Bech (26) compared politicians' and hospital managers' preferences for reimbursement schemes; Ubach *et al.* (27) compared preferences of pharmacists and general practitioners for alternative electronic prescribing systems and Hall *et al.* (28) compared preferences for genetic screening for the general population and a high risk sub-population).

11.4.2 Experimental design and choice sets

Of the studies that reported design types, almost all used fractional factorial designs. Most designs were constructed with commercial software; most commonly, SPEED. More than 50% used orthogonal main effects plans (OMEPs) although inclusion of at least some interactions appears to be increasing. Typically, choice sets involved pairs of options. One common way to allocate options to choice sets is random pairing, resulting in respondents being asked to choose between two different, randomly paired options in each choice set. Another popular format involved using binary choice sets where respondents made yes/no decisions about options one-at-a-time, or where one option was fixed for all choice sets. When one option was fixed for all sets, several ways were used to choose it such as using one designed option selected randomly or a status quo option. Few studies used more than two options per choice set and when they did these typically were two hypothetical options plus an opt-out option (i.e. choose between A, B or neither and/or cannot choose) per choice set.

11.4.3 Measurement of preferences, response rate, and comprehension

We observed a trend for fewer choice sets in SPDCEs over the period. We also observed many studies using eight choice sets, which seemed to be associated with reducing designs to 16 options, then pairing them randomly. Self-completion surveys predominated, with little use of computer- or online-administration, even in recent years. Only one computer-assisted study included visual aids to aid interpretation and understanding.

11.4.4 Estimation and validity

Recall that almost all SPDCEs used binary choices. The statistical model of choice was probit instead of logit, more particularly; random effects probit predominated as a way to model multiple responses (i.e. multiple choice sets) of study participants. We were encouraged to see a trend in recent years to include face validity tests, which involved conducting pilot work prior to the SPDCE and modifying scenarios based on that. The vast majority of studies we reviewed ensured validity by checking expected signs after model estimation. Many studies tested for dominance and non-trading behaviour, but relatively few studies tested convergence with other preference elicitation methods and studies testing reliability (i.e. repeating tests over a time period) were rare.

11.5 State of art in SPDCEs and choice modelling

We found great similarities in methods and designs, which allowed us to form some stylized facts from Section 11.4. Most studies used OMEPs based on commercial software to conduct economic evaluations. Most presented respondents with eight pairs of hypothetical options using questionnaires or interviews. Attributes typically were chosen based on consultation and literature review, with pilot work used to refine surveys. Random effects probit was used to estimate and compare the signs of estimates against a priori expectations as a way to validate results.

11.5.1 Design issues

The most popular way to design SPDCEs in health was to use some type of random assignment procedure to construct pairs, triples, etc., of designed attribute level combinations that describe different hypothetical goods. For example, a common method was to randomly assign T total treatment combinations/attribute descriptions generated from an OMEP to pairs. That is, if a particular design generates T total treatments, there are $T(T-1)/2$ total possible pairs. If T is small, the number of pairs is small (e.g. for $T = 9$, there are 36 pairs); but as T increases the number of pairs increases geometrically, rendering such methods infeasible for larger T. So, one must find a way to sample from all the pairs to reduce the size of the problem.

Justifications for keeping T small (e.g. <32) typically were based on concerns with 'overburdening respondents' and/or small design practices typical in transportation research and marketing were uncritically adopted. In particular, the set of all possible pairs satisfies the necessary and sufficient conditions for estimating MNL models (4), but it is not clear that any particular subset sampled from T has suitable statistical properties, and one clearly can generate random or purposive samples that have identification problems (see (14)).

More generally, subsets of pairs from T are unlikely to be very statistically efficient, with many samples having very low efficiency (i.e. less than 40% efficient). Thus, Louviere, Hensher, and Swait (7) note that it rarely makes sense not to use the proper design theory to construct choice sets to insure satisfaction of statistical properties. Moreover, now that design theory is available to construct optimally efficient designs (14), there is no reason to use ad hoc methods like random pairing to construct DCEs.

We found the number of choice sets respondents faced ranged from 1 to 28, with a mode of 8. We suspect that the use of such small numbers of sets is associated with the adoption of conjoint analysis practices in marketing and transport where small designs dominate. Such practices are historical artefacts carried-over from when researchers estimated models for single persons, typically based on rating scale responses (e.g. see (15)). It is worth noting that designs used for conjoint analysis methods that try to model individuals are almost always inappropriate for modelling the choice behaviour of populations of individuals. Using small designs confuses individual-level 'conjoint analysis' with SPDCEs, and perpetuates the illusion that SPDCEs are simply 'another type of conjoint analysis'. Small designs are appropriate if one wants precise estimates of choices for *only* the particular subset of T treatments in a particular design; yet, researchers typically want to generalize to a larger response surface spanning a range of options in T. Moreover, it is not enough to design T; one also has to design ways to assign the T treatments to compete with one another (choice sets).

In summary, therefore, if one wants to model choices of populations of individuals represented by a sample of that population, one typically needs a sufficiently large random sample of individuals to give particular levels of precision for the sample statistics of interest at particular levels of confidence, but one also wants a sufficiently large sample of treatments and/or choice sets to give satisfactory levels of precision for the model parameter estimates and associated standard errors. So, the practice of using small numbers of treatments/choice sets while at the same time assigning them to large samples of people makes little statistical sense. That is, one should use a small sample of treatments/choice sets only if one wants to obtain precise estimates of the choice probabilities for *that particular set* of treatments and/or choice sets. Otherwise, one should use the largest number of treatments one's resources allow and expose those treatments/choice sets to the largest possible sample of people.

We found many studies that tested dominance and non-trading. Dominance arises if all attributes are numerical and/or if the signs on the attribute levels are known a priori for all individuals. Dominance is less serious in larger designs because such designs can be modified with little loss in statistical efficiency; modifications in small designs can have serious consequences for statistical properties. No definitive approach is available for dominance; one often can swap levels or reverse design codes in columns to eliminate virtually all dominance, and this always should be tried first.

Non-trading is rationally consistent, so it is surprising that it has received so much attention. Indeed, Lancsar and Louviere (46) note that many unobserved processes consistent with rationality and economic theory can seem to be non-trading, but are instead a result of design choice. Other cases of non-trading can be due to poor design or experimental practice. Generally speaking, one cannot conclusively test non-trading unless one uses a complete factorial and/or all possible choice sets. We found no uses of these designs in our review; hence, there is little basis for conclusions about irrational behaviour in the health economics literature.

11.5.2 Estimation issues

Ryan and Gerard (3) suggested several future SPDCE research questions, such as what is a manageable number of attributes and choice options. As noted by Louviere, Hensher, and Swait (7) and Louviere and Eagle (29), there is little real evidence regarding the effects of numbers of attributes or options, and what evidence there is suggests that one can use more of both than one typically sees in health applications.

Extensions beyond two choices are required to simulate real market choices in many cases. So, it is surprising that so much work involves a forced choice of two options; that is, respondents could not exercise the option not to choose. Opt-out or no-choice options commonly occur in real markets, such that a respondent can choose 'none of the above', or in other cases, they may choose to stay with a current choice or status quo ('I'd choose my current treatment/GP/etc.'). In some cases, both of these options might be indicated. Indeed, if a current choice is available one often can pool RP and SP data. Instead of mere face validity, such pooling allows tests of external validity. That is, recalling that Ben-Akiva and Morikawa (5) and Swait and Louviere (6) noted that if two elicitation procedures satisfy the RUM, any common vector of preference parameters estimated from the two data sources must be proportional (see also (29)). Unfortunately, this remains very much a missed opportunity in health applications that we hope will improve in future work. Of course, participation cannot be estimated without a status quo option, but the MWTP for any attribute can be estimated if income (minus cost) is included in the vector of choice attributes.

Our survey found that health applications have not yet embraced richer specifications of preference heterogeneity, but instead have relied on fairly simple representations, such as allowing only the intercept to be random in a random coefficients probit. An obstacle to the routine use of new estimation methods is availability of software. In the case of the McFadden and Train (30) mixed logit model (MXL), LIMDEP was quick to offer software support; similarly STATA now incorporates an MXL estimation procedure; and special purpose GAUSS programs written by Kenneth Train (31) are available and used extensively. So, there does not seem to be a reason why extensions beyond binary choice with more complex specifications of heterogeneity cannot be entertained in health applications.

11.6 **Unresolved issues and research opportunities**

11.6.1 **Optimal design**

Recent developments in optimal design theory provide ways to construct efficient designs for many SPDCE design problems (14). So, we now know how to design optimally efficient SPDCEs for many problems, which in turn makes some previous design construction methods for generic problems obsolete like those in Louviere, Hensher and Swait (7). For more general alternative-specific designs (so-called 'labelled' designs), we do not yet know how to construct optimally efficient designs; and as noted by Burgess, Street, and Louviere (12), some constructions can lead to identification problems. So, one should be careful about constructing SPDCEs using the L^{MA} design approach, and one should test every effect before implementing the design to ensure all components of main effects and interactions that one thinks can be estimated from the design, in fact can be estimated.

Slow, but steady progress will continue on various unresolved design problems; new developments will be posted on the website of the Centre for the Study of Choice (http://www.business.uts.edu.au/censoc/) at the University of Technology, Sydney. We also note that CenSoC design research teams have tested commercial software used by health economists and others to construct SPDCEs, and have found that very few designs produced by the options that we tested are optimally efficient, and many have low statistical efficiency (40% or less). To put this in perspective, a design that is 40% efficient effectively reduces one's sample size to 40% of the number of observations. Similarly, ad hoc methods of design construction like random pairings or combinations typically are not very efficient. So, researchers should be cautious in using them (e.g. see (32;14)).

Finally, we found that the vast majority of SPDCEs we reviewed were small, and had high ratios of estimated parameters to observations. This reflects poor design practice that once again seems to stem from confusing designs commonly used in conjoint analysis with designs for SPDCEs. As previously noted, one should not try to minimize designs when one models a population of individuals; rather, one should try to construct and implement designs where the ratio of number of parameters to be estimated relative to the number of observations is low. Thus, for a fixed sample size, a design with twice as many choice sets will be more efficient than the one with less.

11.6.2 **Sample size calculations in SPDCEs**

Generally speaking, one needs to know the true model form and parameters *before* one can calculate the desired sample sizes because choice models are non-linear. Of course, if each individual completes all the choice sets in the SPDCE, one can calculate the desired sample sizes for a particular level of confidence in the observed choice proportions associated with each choice outcome in each choice set. If one does not know the true model and parameters, one can assume that the choice proportions are binomial (multinomial) and use the usual formulas for calculating confidence intervals for binomial (multinomial) random variates. As usual, confidence intervals depend on a researcher's risk with respect to the probability that a particular observations will fall outside the desired confidence interval. So, at present there is no general solution to this problem, and a computationally straightforward way to do this in general would be desirable. Moreover, in most cases, researchers want to be able to estimate covariate effects and/or identify segments/latent classes and estimate models for them. In such cases, it is virtually impossible to anticipate sample sizes in advance without a great deal of a priori knowledge that researchers almost never have. Thus, the best we can do at present is to recommend the largest sample that resources allow.

11.6.3 Variance-scale confounds in discrete choice models

Estimation using discrete choice data, involves a fundamental identification problem. All choice models specify a structural relationship between a categorical indicator variable (response) and a latent variable like utility. One must specify the origin and variance or scale (inverse of the error standard deviation) of the latent variable to identify the parameters in the utility function. For example, standard probit models assume a threshold of zero and variance of one. There is an important link between confounding of scale and preference weights and moving to more complex specifications of heterogeneity in SPDCEs, with MXL models focusing on differences in ways respondents trade off and value attributes. Yet, preference heterogeneity is only one source of heterogeneity, and while random parameter models have implications for the structure of the variance in choice models this is not their focus. So, the field needs to recognize that other sources of unobserved variability in choices also exist and need to be taken into account. Failure to take into account systematic differences in error variances across choice sets and/or people can result in serious bias in estimated parameters, and misinferences about attribute effects. So, while the consequences of such confounds can be quite significant, current choice models cannot distinguish between individuals with different tastes from those with identical tastes but different scales. Also, policy implications can differ for models that separate variance sources and those that do not. For example, if individuals have different tastes, but different intercepts, one can try to change basic predispositions and/or initiate new programmes by targeting tastes because all individuals make similar tradeoffs. If individuals have similar tastes but unequal error variances, one can also try these strategies, or one can try to change individual variances. However, more generally, the scale/model estimate confound is likely to be lead one to infer that tradeoffs differ in the latter case, when they do not – the variances differ.

This problem arises because different underlying processes lead to observationally equivalent outcomes (utilities and choice probabilities), even if the process underlying the outcomes differ. In an important paper, de Palma, Myers, and Papageorgiou (33) prove profound theoretical consequences if individuals differ in their ability to make decisions due to differences in the number of errors they make. Despite this theoretical advance, much more work is needed empirically to understand how and why individuals differ in choice variability.

There are currently several ways that one can try to deal with this confound. One way suggested by Louviere (34;35) and Louviere *et al.* (36) is to estimate choice models for single persons. If one can estimate models for individuals, there is no need to make potentially incorrect assumptions about the joint multivariate distribution of tastes in random parameter models as one (by definition) has an empirical estimate of the distribution from the sample estimates. Thus, if one can estimate models for single individuals, one can directly estimate the mean of the distribution and any other moments that are of interest, such as the variance in the mean estimates. Louviere and Eagle (29) and Meyer and Louviere (37) discuss ways to do this, and discuss the results of several projects. Additional discussion is in the workshop report of the 2007 Choice Symposium 'Putting more behaviour into choice models' (38).

A second way to capture the scale differences is to specify heteroskedastic error variance models. Several authors in environmental and resource economics and marketing proposed and estimated models of this type for DCEs, such as Swait and Adamowicz (39;40), DeShazo and Fermo (41), Dellaert, Brazell, and Louviere (42), and Islam, Louviere, and Burke (43). The Islam, Louviere, and Burke paper is particularly interesting because it shows how to specify error variances as a function of a variety of factors related to response tasks and experimental conditions. The paper also uses a monte-carlo simulation experiment to show that these models fit in-sample choices much less well than random coefficient models, but either beat random coefficient models or do no worse than them in out-of-sample fits. Their simulation experiment results were confirmed by a large empirical study involving over 40 experimental conditions. Although not illustrated in their paper, one also can specify the error variance to be a function of individual covariates, allowing one to capture a wide array of potentially significant and interesting variance components.

11.7 Implications of the review for welfare evaluation

Here, we focus on two types of implications, one associated with the design of SPDCEs and the second associated with modelling data produced by SPDCEs and the interpretation of subsequent results. As noted earlier, a large proportion of SPDCEs previously used in health can be described as binary discrete choice tasks (see Chapter 10) that are analysed with some form of probit model. Tasks can be (a) 'accept/reject' several designed options presented one-at-a-time, (b) choice between a constant, fixed option like the status quo and several designed options presented one-at-a-time, or (c) choice between two designed options. Thus, virtually all previous SPDCEs in health were generic, meaning that the options being chosen did not have specific labels, with the possible exception of task type 'b' above. A small number of tasks involved choice between two generic options or the choice not to choose either, which also can be construed to be labelled or 'alternative-specific'.

Generic SPDCEs and associated tasks imply choice models that specify all the attribute effects as generic. That is, the effects of a particular attribute are the same for all choice options. Generic choice model specifications are particularly easy to estimate and to apply to policy analyses, although more complicated random effects forms require simulation methods to estimate welfare measures and to predict policy outcomes. These types of tasks and models are suitable for the following cases: (a) there is no current option of the type being studied, and only one option will be introduced if the number who will takeup the new option is sufficient to justify this; (b) there is a current option (i.e. status quo), and interest centres on whether enough people will switch to a new option if introduced to justify the switch. These tasks should not be used for other choice modelling projects. It is worth noting that tasks that ask respondents to choose between a status quo and more than one option at a time are technically unnecessary because case 'b' above provides all the information needed to make decisions. This illustrates why it is important to carefully conceptualize the actual decision that people will face, and use that as a basis to design the SPDCE task.

As noted earlier, we were surprised that there were few alternative-specific, multiple choice tasks applied in health care. A little thought suggests that there are many such tasks possible. Here are several examples:

1. Patients can choose between being treated by an individually owned, single-practice GP (one GP), a multiply-owned, multiple GP practice (more than one GP), a private company-owned GP practice with other medical services, a publicly listed company-owned, multiple GP practice with other medical services, a hospital-owned/associated multiple GP practice/emergency room, etc. These choice options potentially differ in quality and personal service, locational convenience and costs, among other attributes. Patient sensitivity to the attributes of these services may depend on the type of service, leading to the potential to observe alternative-specific attribute effects (effects that differ by option).

   There also may be issues related to what we call 'availability', which means that all options may not always be available for choice in particular areas because they do not exist in some areas, they have yet to be introduced, or a combination of the two. Suitable designs for this case include the L^{MA} designs discussed earlier (7), or a design that treats each type of practice option as an independent attribute, and allows one to estimate all main effects and all two-way interactions that the practice option attribute (at a minimum). The latter design approach works because it effectively allows one to estimate separate effects for each attribute *within* each practice option. One important caveat arises if one needs to model availability. Only an L^{MA} design can handle this type of problem, and such of designs can be very complex (7). A second caveat arises if one believes that substitution effects between options are not merely due to heterogeneity in tastes. In the latter case, one must use an L^{MA} design for this type of problem because it allows one to estimate differential substitution effects that are not captured by taste heterogeneity.

2. A doctor offers a patient a choice among four treatment options for treating an early-detected cancer, such as (a) watchful waiting to see if it spreads, and if so, how fast and to where, (b) chemotherapy, (c) radiation, (d) surgery, or (e) a new procedure that can identify the exact location and extent of the cancer, allowing one to see if less aggressive treatments will work. Each option has associated risks and benefits and costs. There likely will be large differences in sensitivity to the attributes of each option within and between patients. As in the first example, this problem requires one to use L^{MA} designs because there are likely to be substitution effects not captured by taste difference alone, and because it is likely that a patient will not be offered all these options simultaneously, and one may wish to model the choices conditional on whether the sets of options differ systematically (i.e. one needs to vary the presence/absence of options).

3. Consider the cervical screening choices of women. At a visit to their GP, they may be offered a standard Pap test or a new liquid-based test. The second test offers potential benefits in terms of increased accuracy, but comes at an increased cost. However, the woman also has the option of not testing and this could very well be determined by the time since her last test and the recommended screening interval. While cost and accuracy will be traded off in choosing between the two tests the context variables, here the time since last test and the recommended screening interval, will only impact on whether to test or not.

The third example is based on the SPDCE documented in Fiebig and Hall (43). Table 11.2 provides a partial listing of the MNL results reported in Fiebig and Hall (43) where for simplicity only the estimated coefficients for price (in Australian (A) dollars), probability of false negatives and probability of false positives have been included. Using these results the MWTP (or CV with $\Delta_1 = 1$) indicate a willingness to pay for improved test accuracy of Pap tests; $A 1.22 for a 1 percentage point improvement in false negative accuracy and $A 11.32 for a 1 percentage point improvement in false negative accuracy.

When more complicated model specifications are used, these calculations become more involved. For example, in MXL models where the attributes are specified with random coefficients varying over respondents, the MWTP will also vary. In such cases, it is often argued that the price coefficient should remain fixed so that the MWTP will have a distribution corresponding to the distribution assumed for β_{1i}. Otherwise one has to deal with a MWTP given in (11.7) that is a ratio of the distributions assumed for the two random parameters. An alternative approach investigated by Train and Weeks (45) is to directly parametrize the model in terms of MWTP and to then directly specify the willingness to pay distribution via a mixed logit model. How best to proceed in such circumstances remains an ongoing research topic.

11.8 Conclusion

Our review of issues associated with the use of choice models suggests that there are a number of serious unresolved issues that can impact the interpretation and use of SPDCE models in a health care setting. Challenges remain in the optimal design of choice experiments and in the specification and estimation of behavioural models incorporating flexible error covariance structures and representing preference heterogeneity. Advances in these areas are also likely to produce challenges for how welfare changes are estimated.

Table 11.2 Estimation results for cervical screening DCE*

Attribute	Estimate	MWTP
Cost	−0.0142	
False negative	−0.0172	1.22
False positive	−0.1606	11.32

* This is only a partial listing of results. See (44) for further details of the DCE study and Table 6.1 for a full listing of results.

Acknowledgement

Some of the material for this paper was initially presented as Jordan J. Louviere's keynote address at the Conference of the Australian Health Economics Society held in Canberra, October 2003. The authors thank the participants and especially Cam Donaldson and Rosalie Viney for their comments and Rochelle Belkar and Ryan Castle for their excellent research assistance. This research was supported by the NHMRC through a Program Grant.

References

1. Arrow, K., Solow, R., Portney, P., Leaner, E., Radner, R., and Schuman, H. 1993. Report of the NOAA panel on contingent valuation. *Federal Register* **58**: 4601–4614.

2. Adamowicz, W., Louviere, J.J., and Williams, M. 1994. Combining revealed and stated preference methods for valuing environmental amenities. *Journal of Environmental Economics and Management* **26**: 271–292.

3. Ryan, M. and Gerard, K. 2003. Using discrete choice experiments to value health care programmes: current practice and future research reflections. *Applied Health Economics and Health Policy* **2**(1): 55–64.

4. Louviere, J.J. and Woodworth, G. 1983. Design and analysis of simulated consumer choice or allocation experiments: An approach based on aggregate data. *Journal of Marketing Research* **20**: 350–367.

5. Ben-Akiva, M. and Morikawa, T. 1990. Estimation of switching models from revealed preferences and stated intentions. *Transportation Research A* **24A**: 485–495.

6. Swait, J.D. and Louviere, J.J. 1993. The role of the scale parameter in the estimation and comparison of multinomial logit models. *Journal of Marketing Research* **30**: 305–314.

7. Louviere, J.J., Hensher, D.A., and Swait, J.D. 2000. *Stated choice methods: analysis and applications.* Cambridge: Cambridge University Press.

8. McFadden, D. 2001. Disaggregate behavioural travel demand's RUM side: A 30-year retrospective. In: Hensher, D.A., editor. *Travel behavioural research: The leading edge,* Amsterdam: Pergamon, pp. 17–64.

9. Mark, T.L. and Swait, J. 2004. Using stated preference and revealed preference modeling to evaluate prescribing decisions. *Health Economics* **13**: 563–573.

10. Louviere, J.J. 2006. What you don't know might hurt you: some unresolved issues in the design and analysis of discrete choice experiments. *Environmental and Resource Economics* **34**(1): 173–188 (Special Issue on *Frontiers in stated preferences methods.* Adamowicz, W. and Deshazo, J.R., editors).

11. Bishop, Y.M.M., Feinberg, S.E., and Holland, P.W. 1975. *Discrete multivariate analysis: theory and practice.* Cambridge, MA: MIT.

12. Burgess, L., Street, D., and Louviere, J.J. 2005. Quick and easy choice sets: Constructing optimal and nearly optimal stated choice experiments. *International Journal of Research in Marketing* **22**: 459–470.

13. Burgess, L., Street, D., Viney, R., and Louviere, J.J. 2006. Design of choice experiments in health economics. In: A. Jones, editor. *Companion to health economics.* Cheltenham: Edward Elgar.

14. Street, D. and Burgess, L. 2007. *The construction of optimal stated choice experiments: Theory and methods.* Hoboken, NJ: Wiley.

15. Louviere, J.J. 1988. *Analyzing decision making: metric conjoint analysis.* Sage University Papers Series Number 67. Newbury Park, CA: Sage.

16. Lancsar, E. Louviere, J.J., and Flynn, T. 2007, Several methods to investigate relative attribute impact in stated preference experiments. *Social Science and Medicine* **64**: 1738–1753.

17. Lancsar, E. and Savage, E. 2004a. Deriving welfare measures from discrete choice experiments: Inconsistency between current methods and random utility and welfare theory. *Health Economics Letters* **13**: 901–907.

18. Lancsar, E. and Savage, E. 2004b. Deriving welfare measures from discrete choice experiments: A response to Ryan and Santos Silva. *Health Economics Letters* **13**: 919–924.

19. Ryan, M. 2004. Deriving welfare measures from discrete choice experiments: A comment to Lancsar and Savage (1). *Health Economics Letters* **13**: 909–912.

20. Santos-Silva, J.M.C. 2004. Deriving welfare measures from discrete choice experiments: A comment to Lancsar and Savage (2). *Health Economics Letters* **13**: 913–918.

21. Small, K.A. and Rosen, H.S. 1981. Applied welfare economics with discret choice models. *Econometrica* **49**: 105–130.

22. Train, K.E. 2003. *Discrete choice methods with simulation.* Cambridge: Cambridge University Press.

23. Morey, E.R., Sharma, V.R., and Mills, A. 2003. Willingness to pay and determinants of choice for improved malaria treatment in rural Nepal. *Social Science and Medicine* **57**: 155–165.

24. Fiebig, D.G., Louviere, J.J., and Waldman, D. 2007. CHERE Working Paper, 2007, CHERE, Sydney.

25. Bishop, A.J., Marteau, T.M., Armstrong, D., Chitty, L.S., Longworth L., Buxton, M.J., *et al.* 2004. Women and health care professionals' preferences for Down's Syndrome screening tests: A conjoint analysis study. *BJOG – An International Journal of Obstetrics and Gynaecology* **111**: 775–779.

26. Bech, M. 2003. Politicians' and hospital managers' trade-offs in the choice of reimbursement scheme: a discrete choice experiment *Health Policy* **66**(3): 261–275.

27. Ubach, C., Scott, A., French, F., Awramenko, M., and Needham, G. 2003. What do hospital consultants value about their jobs? A discrete choice experiment. *British Medical Journal* **326**(7404): 1432–1437.

28. Hall, J.P. Fiebig, D.G., King, M., Hossain, I., and Louviere, J.J. 2006. What influences participation in genetic carrier testing? Results from a discrete choice experiment. *Journal of Health Economics* **25**: 520–537.

29. Louviere, J.J. and Eagle, T.C. 2006, Confound it! That pesky little sclare constant messes up. *CenSoC Working Paper No. 06-002.*

30. McFadden, D. and Train, K. 2000. Mixed MNL models for discrete response. *Journal of Applied Econometrics* **15**: 447–470.

31. Train, K.E. 2004. Mixed logit estimation for panel data using maximum simulated likelihood. http://elsa.berkeley.edu/Software/abstracts/train0296.html [Accessed: December 15, 2004].

32. Viney, R., Savage, E., and Louviere, J.J. 2005. Empirical investigation of experimental design properties of discrete choice experiments in health care. *Health Economics* **14**: 349–362.

33. de Palma, A., Myers, G.M., and Papageorgiou, Y.Y. 1994. Rational choice under an imperfect ability to choose. *American Economic Review* **84**: 419–440.

34. Louviere, J.J. 2004a. Random utility theory-based stated preference elicitation methods: Applications in health economics with special reference to combining sources of preference data. *CenSoC Working Paper No. 04-001.*

35. Louviere, J.J. 2004b. Complex statistical choice models: Are the assumptions true, and if not, what are the consequences?. *CenSoC Working Paper No. 04-002*.

36. Louviere, J.J., Burgess, L., Street, D., and Marley, A.A.J. 2004, Modeling the choice of single individuals by combining efficient choice experiment designs with extra preference information, *CenSoC Working Paper No. 04-005*.

37. Meyer, R.J., and Louviere, J.J. 2007. Formal choice models of informal choices: What choice modelling research can (and can't) learn from behavioural theory. *Review of Marketing Research* **4**:1.

38. Adamowicz, W., Bunch, D., Cameron, T., Dellaert, B., Hanneman, M., Keane, M., *et al.* 2008. Behavioral frontiers in choice modeling. *Marketing Letters* **19**(3): 215–228.

39. Swait, J.D. and Adamowicz, W. 2001a. The influence of task complexity on consumer choice: A latent class model of decision strategy switching. *Journal of Consumer Research* **28**: 135–148.

40. Swait, J.D. and Adamowicz, W. 2001b. Incorporating the effect of choice environment and complexity into random utility models. *Organizational Behavior and Human Decision Processes* **86**: 141–167.

41. DeShazo, J.R. and Fermo, G. 2004. Implications of rationally adaptive pre-choice behaviour for the design and estimation of choice models, working paper, School of Public Policy and Social Research, UCLA.

42. Dellaert, B., Brazell, J.D., and Louviere J.J. 1999. The effect of attribute variation on consumer choice consistency. *Marketing Letters* **10**: 139–147.

43. Islam, T., Louviere, J.J., and Burke, P. 2007. Modeling the effects of including/excluding attributes in choice experiments on systematic and random components. *International Journal of Research in Marketing* **24**(4): 289–300.

44. Fiebig, D.G. and Hall, J. 2005. Discrete choice experiments in the analysis of health policy. *Productivity Commission Conference, November 2004: Quantitative Tools for Microeconomic Policy Analysis*, Chapter 6, pp. 119–136.

45. Train, K.E. and Weeks, M. 2005. Discrete choice models in preference space and willingness-to-pay space. In: Alberini, A. and Scarpa, R., editors. *Applications of simulation methods in environmental resource economics*. Dordrecht: Kluwer Academic Publisher.

46. Lancsar, E. and Louviere, J.J. 2006. Deleting 'irrational' responses from discrete choice experiments: A case of investigating or imposing preferences? *Health Economics* **15**(8): 797–811.

Chapter 12

A practical guide to reporting and presenting stated preference discrete choice experiment results in cost–benefit analysis studies in health care[1]

Emma McIntosh

12.1 Introduction

While CBA is a common form of economic evaluation across other sections of the economy such as the environment (see Chapter 5), other than methodological contributions in the area of benefit assessment such as WTP studies (see Chapters 6–8) the application of the CBA methodology in the health care sector has been notably limited with a widespread reluctance to use CBA for health care evaluations (1;2). As pointed out by Borghi (3), most CBAs in the health care sector have in fact used resource savings or productivity gains as a measure of benefit. Resource savings simply reflect a 'negative' cost and productivity is not consistent with the theoretical basis of utility. However, neither of these are valid measures of economic 'benefit' since there is no attempt to value, in monetary terms, the health or non-health consequences. As outlined in earlier chapters, WTP and SPDCEs offer a means of valuing benefits which is consistent with welfare theory. Even given these theoretically sound approaches however very few WTP studies in health care have gone on to use their results within a formal CBA. Until now, this book has concentrated on the valuation of benefits in monetary terms using standard welfare economic theory, and other than Chapters 9 and 10 outlining the CBAs of spinal surgery and mobile breast cancer screening little has been said regarding the practical side of bringing together costs and benefits within a CBA in health care. Chapters 10 and 11 introduced the concept of using SPDCEs for benefit assessment for use within CBAs. Following a brief introduction to the standard methods of economic evaluation in health care, this chapter will then introduce some more practical guidance for bringing costs and benefits together within health care CBAs using the methodology of SPDCE and building on the material introduced in Chapters 10 and 11.

---

[1] This chapter has been reproduced with permission from Wolters Kluwer Health | Adis (see McIntosh, E. (2006). Using stated preference discrete choice experiments in cost-benefit analysis: some considerations. *Pharmacoeconomics*, **24**(9), 855–69 for the final published version.). Adis Data Information Bv 2006. All rights reserved.

12.2 **Economic evaluation in health care**

As discussed briefly in Chapter 1, there are essentially two main types of economic evaluation used in health economics: CBA and CEA (of which CUA is a form). The key feature that distinguishes among techniques of economic evaluation is the way the consequences of health care programmes are valued (4). The conventional economics approach has been used to show that the amount people are willing to pay in terms of money is an indicator of their strength of preference for a good or characteristic of a good. As was outlined in Chapters 10 and 11, WTP values in SPDCEs are obtained by estimating the compensating variation (CV) measure of welfare, i.e. observing the reduction/increase in income levels people are prepared to accept for improvements/reductions in levels of attributes of a good. For a number of reasons, not least the fact that people often find valuing health related benefits in monetary terms objectionable, it is the case in health care that other economic evaluation techniques for combining costs with non-monetary benefits have been developed. These techniques form the basis of the majority of economic evaluations carried out in this area. These CEA and CUA approaches are well documented in many texts including Drummond *et al.* (4).

The subject of measuring health and measuring disease is the concern of many disciplines beyond health economics (5;6), including public health, epidemiology, and statistics. In health economics, it is widely accepted that it is theoretically possible to use numeraires, other than money, such as health state utility (7–10). Culyer (11) argued for an 'extra welfarist' approach to health, instead of attempting to devise measures of changes in utility the task of measuring changes in 'health' was advocated with the quality adjusted life year (QALY) the instrument of choice (11;12). As a consequence, much of the health economics literature in recent years has concentrated on the issues around measuring and valuing preferences for health care in non-monetary mediums, i.e. quality of life (13–17). This has led to the development of health state valuation measures including QALYs, and healthy years equivalents (HYEs). The following sections introduce some practical suggestions for the application of SPDCEs and WTP in health care.

12.3 **Using SPDCEs in CBA in health care**

There have been a large number of SPDCE and conjoint analysis benefit studies carried out in health care to date, see downloadable Table 12.1 for a comprehensive literature review of these studies (www.herc.ox.ac.uk/books/cba/support). Following on from Chapters 10 and 11 where Carson, Louviere, and Fiebig outlined the key components of design and analysis of SPDCEs for estimating welfare in a health care setting with particular emphasis on statistical designs appropriate for economic welfare measurement and health policy evaluation this section discusses some further practical issues on using SPDCEs in applied CBAs. The aim of this chapter is to discuss how best to report and present the resulting WTP values within a contemporary CBA framework. The potential advantage of using SPDCEs within formal CBA studies in health care is vast, yet so far, surprisingly underdeveloped in the literature (18). To date, whilst there has been much methodological work on the estimation of welfare using SPDCE methods (19–25), apart from work by Clarke (26) using a travel cost approach (see Chapter 9) and recent work by Haefeli *et al.* (27) (see Chapter 8), Borghi (3), and Nocera (28) it is difficult to clearly identify any full CBA studies carried out in health care combining the costs of an intervention formally with the welfare valuations from SPDCEs, or WTP directly for that matter, as the measure of benefit. As Drummond *et al.* note, 'most of the published health care contingent valuation studies are experimental in nature, attempting to explore measurement feasibility issues rather than being full programme evaluations using CBA'(29). A recent published article stated that economic evaluation within the health care field remains dominated by CEA and CUA and that health care payers have been reluctant to embrace CBA (30). Other reviews go so far as to say that lack of consideration of CBA and concentration on CEA by institutions such as the UK's National Institute for Health and Clinical Excellence (NICE) might inadvertently cause allocative inefficiency (31). An editorial recommended that NICE should consider using SPDCEs for patient-centered evaluations of technologies (32).

In light of these recent views, the two main objectives of this chapter are to outline some practical considerations for the advancement of CBAs in health care specifically using SPDCEs and WTP as the tools for benefit estimation (33). This chapter aims to firstly outline explicitly the challenges involved in such an exercise then provide some practical guidance for combining costs and SPDCE-derived benefits within a CBA. The chapter will also outline methods currently used in CEA and highlight how these can be employed to enhance the usefulness of CBAs for policy makers in health care (18).

As outlined in Chapters 10 and 11, to estimate WTP values, the SPDCE should ideally be designed with a cost payment vehicle as an attribute; the methods for estimating welfare within SPDCEs are well documented (19;23;34–38). By including cost as an attribute or having valid income data, marginal WTP values can be estimated for each attribute and combinations of attributes. As noted in the introduction, one of the advantages of SPDCE-derived marginal valuations of attributes is their immense flexibility within welfare analysis (39). That is, once marginal valuations for attributes are identified, total welfare values can be estimated for any possible configuration of attributes and levels (contained in the design) for the aggregate sample and for subgroups depending upon characteristics. An obvious next stage is to then estimate the costs (using resource use data) involved to obtain these alternative configurations and formally combine these costs with the welfare values within a full CBA. However, whilst this may sound a relatively straightforward task, this is not common practice in the applied health economics literature.

12.4 Practical challenges to using SPDCEs in health care CBA studies

Practical challenges to the use of SPDCEs within CBA relate to the methodological barriers to estimating WTP, the design of welfare studies, identifying appropriate methods for eliciting values, timing of preference-related events, and aggregation of costs and benefits. For practical reasons and to adhere to current health economic development these challenges can be categorized as falling into the following three broad categories: adapting cost-effectiveness analysis methodology to develop SPDCEs in a CBA framework; measurement issues specific to SPDCEs and finally: broader SPDCE measurement issues in CBA.

12.5 **Adapting cost-effectiveness analysis methodology to develop SPDCEs in a CBA framework**

12.5.1 **Development of an explicit CBA plane**

The concept of plotting costs and effects on a plane to aid decision making is not new and matrices of costs and effects combined have been around for years, more recently developing into the more familiar cost-effectiveness plane with its cost-effectiveness frontiers, scatter plots, and incremental cost-effectiveness ratios (ICERs) (40–42). There have been some concerns regarding the use of ICERs, associated with the theoretical basis of CEA and the type of efficiency they are addressing (43). However, the use of the ICER along with its technical advantages in reporting and presenting CEA results has achieved widespread acceptance among health economists (29). A potential way forward, addressing the theoretical concerns with ICERS, is to develop CBA methods alongside ICER methodology such that the advantages of the ICER statistical methods can be combined with the theoretical advantages of CBA. An obvious development therefore is a cost–benefit plane (18).

One key advantage of CBA is that both costs and benefits are in the same units so the estimation of net-benefit (monetary benefit minus monetary cost) is straightforward. However, using this simple method in CBA produces a point estimate with no consideration of variation of costs or effects (or covariance of costs and effects) around the point estimate. Hence, estimation of cost–benefit planes, ellipses, and confidence boxes (44) treating the monetary benefit estimate in the same manner as a standard effectiveness or utility estimate would permit the variation in cost–benefit pairings to be reported and presented more effectively. Further, not only would this 'incremental cost benefit ratio' be reported with appropriate measures of variance, but this ratio may be theoretically superior to standard ICERs because any resulting incremental shift outside a fixed budget would be directly comparable with the benefits so facilitate the addressing of allocative efficiency questions. This incremental cost–benefit ratio method would however benefit from the estimation of individual-specific SPDCE estimates (45) (i.e. individual specific coefficients and hence individual-specific WTP values as opposed to mean sample values) so as to aid pairing up with individual cost estimates and standard bootstrapping methods could then be used to generate preference distributions from available preference data. In addition to this, and in line with the ease of working with net present values, a net benefit approach could also be used.

The net benefit approach is simply the incremental difference in effect multiplied by the WTP for that difference minus the cost of achieving the difference. Since the cost–benefit decision rule is as follows: ΔCosts/ΔBenefits $< R_c$ (where R_c is the ceiling ratio), rearranging this expression effectively linearizes the ratio by using the value of R_c to generate the maximum WTP in monetary terms for the effect gain. Once the incremental cost of the intervention is subtracted we are left with the net-benefit of the intervention. This gives the net-benefit equation:

$$NB = R_c{}^* \Delta B - \Delta C. \tag{12.1}$$

If one intervention is both more costly and more beneficial (NE & SW quadrants of the cost–benefit plane, see Figure 12.1) then a trade-off between costs and effects has to be made in deciding which treatment to employ. In a standard CEA, an estimate of the maximum WTP by decision-makers for an additional unit of effect is used as the ceiling ratio (R_c) to make this trade-off. Unlike using a hypothetical decision makers R_c as is commonly carried out in the CEA literature the advantage of the CBA approach is that WTP values are those of the population of interest. Figures 12.1–12.3 provide an example of such a cost–benefit plane, a hypothetical example of a cost–benefit plane incorporating methods of presenting CBA uncertainty using the confidence box and ellipse methods, and a net benefit acceptability curve example.

Figure 12.1 shows a hypothetical example of a cost–benefit plane akin to the cost-effectiveness plane commonly being used in economic evaluations (44). If we represent the relevant decision rule on the plane by a line with positive slope equal to the R_c (traditionally defined as the maximum cost per unit of effect that a *decision-maker* is prepared to pay) then we have effectively divided the plane into two halves. Interventions with a cost/benefit pairing falling to the left of the line are deemed cost-dis-beneficial, while interventions with a cost–benefit pairing falling to the right of the line are cost-beneficial. The only difference is that the CBA plane uses WTP as its measure of benefit and the ceiling ratio, R_c, is not a decision makers WTP but a measure of population WTP values. We can represent this decision rule on the CE plane by a line passing through the origin with positive slope equal to the R_c.

The ellipse and confidence box shown in Figure 12.2 show how the CBA plane could represent the uncertainty in both costs and benefits akin to those presented on the CEA plane.

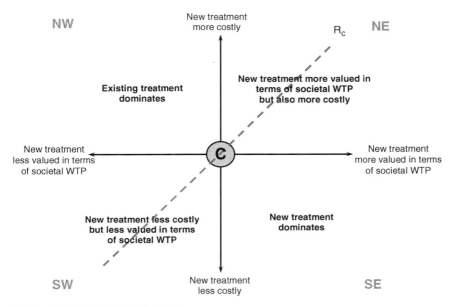

C=Comparator treatment (or status quo)

Fig. 12.1 The cost–benefit plane.

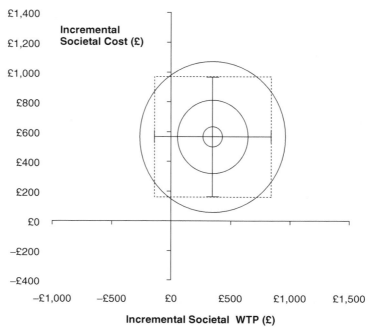

Fig. 12.2 Hypothetical example of cost–benefit plane presenting cost/benefit uncertainty using the confidence box and ellipse methods.

Figure 12.3 shows a hypothetical net benefit acceptability curve akin to those used in standard CEA studies (46). This figure shows the net-benefit results being employed to calculate a net-benefit acceptability curve by plotting the proportion of the estimated net-benefit density that is associated with positive values. Hypothetically, there is no reason why SPDCE methods cannot be used to identify a population R_c for any given configuration of attributes and levels.

Perhaps more importantly, as identified in Section 12.3, SPDCE offers the advantage in that it explicitly estimates the valuation of different levels of different attributes of a health care programme separately. This is in direct contrast to the CEA net-benefit approach and the corresponding CBA net-benefit formula of equation 12.1, which is based on collapsing the measure of outcome to a single dimension before estimating a single WTP value, R_c, for that measure of outcome. That is, instead of $R^c \times \Delta B$ as the monetarized measure of benefit in the net-benefit equation 12.1, we have instead:

$$\sum_{p=1}^{P} k_p \Delta A_p, \tag{12.2}$$

where k is the WTP for each unit of attribute p and ΔA represents the change in the (continuous) attribute p.

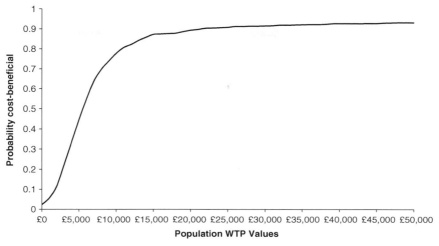

Fig. 12.3 Hypothetical net-benefit acceptability curve.

12.5.2 **Accounting for uncertainty in SPDCE derived CBAs**

There has been recent interest in the estimation of confidence intervals around ICERs (44;47), this is an important consideration when estimating welfare values using marginal rates of substitution (MRS). See also Chapter 10 for guidance on statistical designs that minimize confidence intervals around mean WTP in SPDCEs and Risa Hole (48) for a comparison of approaches to estimating confidence intervals around WTP measures (48). The MRS of good X for good Y is the amount of good Y that a person is willing to give up to obtain one additional unit of good X. The MRS measures the value that the consumer places on one extra unit of a good, where the opportunity cost is quantified by the amount of another good sacrificed. The consideration of appropriate variance around ratios when estimating MRS between attributes and the cost attribute, as well as between the welfare and cost values if estimating CBA ratios and not net-benefit values is important when reporting and presenting the results of CBA (also see Section 12.7.4). Hence, the appropriate method for this purpose should be given some consideration. Methods include the use of Fieller's theorem (49), Taylor's series expansion (50), and bootstrapping methods (47;51). The formula for calculating confidence intervals around SPDCE derived WTP estimates using the variance co-variance matrix required for Fieller's theorem is shown in Box 12.1.

In Box 12.1, *A* is the coefficient on the attribute of interest, *B* is the cost coefficient, and 'cov' relates to the covariance between *A* and *B* which is obtained from the variance co-variance matrix from the SPDCE output file.

Further to this, and related to the issue of generating confidence intervals around the welfare estimates, are issues of measures of variance around the *preferences* for attributes themselves and the impact this has on the CBA ratio using standard sensitivity analysis methods.

Box 12.1 Calculating confidence intervals using Fieller's theorem

$$\frac{\left[A \cdot B - z_{\alpha/2}^2 \, \text{cov}\left(A,B\right)\right]}{B^2 - z_{\alpha/2}^2 \, \text{var}\left(B\right)}$$

$$\pm \frac{\sqrt{\left[A \cdot B - z_{\alpha/2}^2 \, \text{cov}\left(A,B\right)\right]^2 - \left[B^2 - z_{\alpha/2}^2 \, \text{var}\left(B\right)\right] \cdot \left[A^2 - z_{\alpha/2}^2 \, \text{var}\left(A\right)\right]}}{B^2 - z_{\alpha/2}^2 \, \text{var}\left(B\right)}$$

At a more applied level, when carrying out an exploration of how the cost–benefit result is affected by using alternative scenarios, assumptions are required about the levels for the 'actual' policy relevant scenarios. For example, waiting time and duration of consultation may have been included in the SPDCE design as 3, 6, and 12 months and 20, 30, and 40 min, respectively however the actual scenario at a particular hospital may be 7.5 months' waiting time and a duration of 50 min. Defining these scenarios in health care, especially for health status, can be problematic and subject to debate, especially when the net-benefit result is sensitive to changes in the scenarios. Identifying scenarios (or parameters) for such an exercise should be no different to the methods used to identify parameters for a decision analytic model and should include methods such as literature review, expert opinion or in some cases use of a pre-defined policy question (52). Consideration of methods to explore the uncertainty around such scenarios, as well as uncertainty within the original preference distributions, is advised.

Methods such as probabilistic sensitivity analysis (PSA) (53), widely used in decision analytic modelling studies (29), using pre-defined ranges for the parameters could be a new consideration for strengthening CBAs using SPDCEs. Such an approach, using Monte Carlo simulation methods, would provide a means for practical estimation of uncertainty in the input parameter weights. PSA requires that all input parameters of a model be specified as a full probability distribution rather than point estimates, to represent the uncertainty surrounding their values. The choice of distribution to describe the uncertainty in parameters is not arbitrary and should be guided by the form of the data, the type of parameter, and the estimation process (53). With SPDCE and WTP welfare distributions it is likely that distributions similar to those of income data may be relevant, i.e. a Gamma distribution, where the data are positive, continuous, and possibly skewed; however, the distribution of the data should be considered on an individual basis (for example spiked data would require special distributional consideration). It could be argued that the use of PSA to estimate acceptability curves is a reason why we do not need to generate welfare estimates because acceptability curves provide the probability that an intervention is cost-effective over a broad range of hypothetical decision makers WTP values. It could however also be argued that these acceptability curves using hypothetical values of R_c are merely implicit and a poor substitute for preference-based welfare measures of the kind generated by SPDCE and

WTP studies. Indeed, the potential to use separate WTP values for each attribute as presented in equation 12.2 is a major potential advantage of the SPDCE methodology.

The use of SPDCE and WTP welfare measures within CBA models is an area ripe for expansion given the advantages of Bayesian methods. It is hoped that the pursuit of greater methodological consistency in SPDCE and WTP welfare measures will further permit the synthesis of costs and benefits within CBA decision models.

12.5.3 Carrying out a CBA using SPDCE data from clinical trials

One use of SPDCEs in health economic evaluations is to complement effectiveness and utility values measured within clinical trials. Since the outcome measures (attributes) are often clearly defined within trials, this could provide an ideal basis for the estimation of SPDCE-derived welfare values. By devising attributes and levels in line with trial outcomes then the resulting marginal welfare values could be mapped onto any differences arising in the trial outcome and the incremental welfare change estimated. Further to this, the marginal welfare values elicited would then have to be aligned with the resource use required to achieve such gains (losses); hence, the costs being identified and measured within the trial would also have to be collected in line with the anticipated outcome of the SPDCE. For example, if attributes in a SPDCE included: staff time; duration of hospital stay; complication rate; and recurrence rate then the resource use incurred related to these attributes will have to be collected in line with these units. In addition, however, if there were outcomes beyond those capable of being measured using standard outcome instruments then SPDCEs are an ideal way to identify, measure, and value such outcomes. Examples of this may include: attributes for the process of care such as a preferences for laparoscopic over open procedures; attributes to accommodate preferences for say, type of staff seen, waiting times, location, and duration of consultation; and valuing attributes traditionally difficult to measure and value such as the 'stigma' associated with tremor in Parkinson's disease.

It is also highly likely in health care given the *dynamic* nature of health status that some attempt would have to be made to model such complex and ever-changing health states over time within the SPDCE exercise to make the exercise realistic and generalizable. For example, within a trial where patients are receiving an intervention then health status will generally be measured say at baseline then every 3 months up to a year. During this time, the intervention may impact upon a number of attributes of health status including say: pain; nausea; depression; general activity; hospital stay; and so on, all of whose levels will possibly change throughout the follow-up assessments. By measuring the changing attribute levels the values from the SPDCE can be adjusted accordingly for the CBA. Such an exercise would have implications for the handling and analysis of the resource use data. Where it has been possible to design a SPDCE exercise alongside a clinical trial with the aim of supplementing the CEA and CUA data with information on patients' welfare values or preferences, or indeed to carry out a formal CBA, a number of specific, technical issues should be considered at the outset. These include devising the SPDCE attributes in alignment with the trial outcomes and levels if the aim is to 'map' welfare values onto differences between the arms of a trial to produce evidence of welfare shifts. The cost data from the cost-effectiveness exercise could also be used in a CBA and direct comparisons could then be drawn between the results from the two approaches.

12.6 Applied example – SPDCE alongside a clinical trial of miscarriage management

(This section is reproduced from (55) with kind permission from ISPOR.)

12.6.1 Study background

A SPDCE was conducted among 1,200 women with a confirmed pregnancy of less than 13 weeks' gestation, who had been diagnosed with either an incomplete miscarriage or missed miscarriage/early fetal demise and who had been recruited as part of a randomized controlled trial (MIST trial) (54) comparing expectant, medical, and surgical miscarriage. Six attributes each with three levels were used in the statistical design. An orthogonal main effects design was generated and the choice sets devised according to the principles of minimum overlap and level balance. A cost attribute was included to allow estimation of WTP. In order to minimize bias, three different questionnaires were designed such that women were asked their preference for the two management options they had not been allocated to in the trial. For further information about the trial see (54). Figure 12.4 shows an example of a choice set included in the SPDCE (54;55).

Table 12.2 presents the results from the random effects probit models for women allocated to surgical management. The models appear to fit the data well, with more than 75% of observations correctly predicted. The statistical significance of $p < 0.001$ in all three models supports the use of this approach. The estimated coefficients for the attributes included in the SPDCE design are all of the theoretically anticipated sign and are all statistically significant. Women in all three arms of the trial, therefore, expressed a clear preference for decreased levels of time spent in hospital receiving treatment, pain, number of days of bleeding following treatment, time taken to return to normal activities after treatment, personal cost, and chance of complications.

Scenario 1	Surgical Treatment	Expectant Treatment
Time spent at the hospital receiving treatment	1 day	½ day
Level of pain experienced	Low	Moderate
Number of days of bleeding following treatment	3 days	8 days
Time taken to return to normal activities after treatment	3–4 days	5–6 days
Cost to you of treatment (if you were paying)	£150	£50
Chance of complications requiring more time or readmission to hospital	Very unlikely (about 5 in 100)	Quite unlikely (about 10 in 100)

	Prefer Surgical	Prefer Expectant
For scenario 1, which treatment would you prefer?	☐	☐

Fig. 12.4 An example of a choice set included in the miscarriage SPDCE.

Table 12.2 Random effects probit, baseline model for women allocated to surgical management

Variable	Unit	Coefficient	SE	p-value	WTP (£) per unit decrement (95% CI's)*
Constant	/	0.0021	0.1228	0.98	/
Time spent at hospital receiving treatment	Days	−0.033	0.0047	<0.001	£14.02 (£13.95, £14.08)
Number of days of bleeding following treatment	Days	−0.0957	0.0089	<0.001	£40.62 (£40.26, £40.99)
Time taken to return to normal activities following treatment	Days	−0.211	0.0179	<0.001	£89.74 (£88.13, £91.34)
Cost to woman of treatment	£	−0.0023	0.0004	<0.001	/
Chance of complications requiring more time or readmission to hospital	%	−0.062	0.0073	<0.001	£26.52 (£26.32, £26.71)
Level of pain experienced (ref=low)					
– Moderate	Category	−0.463	0.0975	<0.001	£196.89 (£177.69, £216.09)
– Severe	Category	−1.869	0.107	<0.001	£793.50 (£707.94, £879.06)

Number of observations: 2,711
Unbalanced panel: 218 individuals
Log likelihood function: −967.03
Restricted log-likelihood: −1247.86
Chi squared: 524.9
Significance level: <0.001
Hosmer–Lemeshow chi squared: 9.44
% Correct Predictions: 79%
Choice probabilities: Medical: 75.5%; Expectant: 24.5%

* WTP denotes willingness to pay.

These results support the theoretical validity of the study design. The effects are broadly similar across the three management methods of allocation. In none of the models was the alternative-specific constant term a significant predictor of choice at the 5% significance level. This latter result implies that women's preferences were a function of the attributes and levels provided - and not driven by underlying preferences for attributes excluded from the study.

Finally, Table 12.3 shows estimates of women's WTP for unit decreases in the non-cost attributes segmented by each management method (expectant, medical or surgical). The WTP estimates are derived by taking the ratio of the estimated coefficient for each non-cost attribute to that of the cost coefficient. These results help to assess the relative valuation of different attributes depending upon which arm of the trial the respondents were allocated to and also as a function of the management options being offered for preference elicitation in the SPDCE. The highest WTP estimate is for a reduction in the pain experienced; estimated at £182.89 (95% CI: £160.67, £205.11), £189.39 (95% CI: £167.80, £210.99), and £196.89 (95% CI: £177.69, £216.09) for a reduction from moderate to low pain among women allocated to expectant, medical, and surgical management, respectively, and at £548.51 (95% CI: £478.75, £618.26), £763.40 (95% CI: £682.25, £844.55), and £793.50 (95% CI: £707.94, £879.06) for a reduction from severe to low pain among women allocated to expectant, medical and surgical management, respectively. The second most important attribute, as imputed by women's WTP, is time taken to return to normal activities after treatment, followed by number of days of bleeding following treatment, chance of complications requiring more time or readmission to hospital and time spent at hospital receiving treatment. The WTP values for unit changes in the synthesized WTP analysis shown in Table 12.3 differed significantly between women allocated to the three management methods. The WTP values were highest among women allocated to surgical management for the attributes related to the number of days of bleeding, time taken to return to normal activities, chance of complications and level of pain, and highest among women allocated to medical management for the 'time spent at hospital' attribute. As well as demonstrating the potential importance of patient experience of the interventions under study, the results in Table 12.3 demonstrates the potential for WTP to vary as a function of patient characteristics. In principle, therefore, the SPDCE approach is capable both of giving separate WTP values for each attribute, while also allowing for individual responder characteristics to influence the WTP values.

Finally, in a bid to produce estimates for use within a CBA, synthesizing the marginal WTP values summarized in Table 12.3 with the descriptions of the management options in the pre-trial designed SPDCE scenarios generated overall monetary estimates of welfare shifts between one set of attributes to another representing management options. These WTP values are stratified by trial allocation and hence the values represent only those values of the women in a particular trial allocation for the alternative management scenarios as defined by the attributes and levels in the design. These were estimated at £354.82 (95% CI: £330.89 - £378.76) for a shift from medical to surgical management (expectant trial women's preferences), £485.76 (95% CI: £461.37 – £510.20) for a shift from expectant to surgical management (medical trial women's preferences), and £111.15 (95% CI: £109.96 – £112.39) for a shift from expectant to

Tabble 12.3 Comparison of WTP values across the three management methods of allocation

Attribute	Unit	WTP* (£) per unit decrement (95% CIs†)		
		Expectant arm	Medical arm	Surgical arm
Time spent at hospital receiving treatment	Days	£13.74 (£13.66, £13.81)	£14.64 (£14.56, £14.73)	£14.02 (£13.95, £14.08)
Number of days of bleeding following treatment	Days	£17.30 (£17.12, £17.48)	£27.61 (£27.35, £27.87)	£40.62 (£40.26, £40.99)
Time taken to return to normal activities following treatment	Days	£52.25 (£51.15, £53.35)	£72.34 (£70.79, £73.89)	£89.74 (£88.13, £91.34)
Chance of complications requiring more time or readmission to hospital	%	£18.46 (£18.29, £18.63)	£11.34 (£11.24, £11.43)	£26.52 (£26.32, £26.71)
Level of pain experienced (ref=low)				
– Moderate	Category	£182.89 (£160.67, £205.11)	£189.39 (£167.80, £210.99)	£196.89 (£177.69, £216.09)
– Severe	Category	£548.51 (£478.75, £618.26)	£763.40 (£682.25, £844.55)	£793.50 (£707.94, £879.06)

* WTP denotes willingness to pay.
† Derived from the variance co-variance matrix.

medical management (surgical trial women's preferences). The overall monetary estimates of welfare shifts that were calculated using *actual* mean MIST trial data for each attribute observed were more conservative however at £36.31 (95% CI: £35.94 – £36.71) for a shift from medical to surgical management (expectant trial women's preferences), £161.04 (95% CI: £158.70 – £163.40) for a shift from expectant to surgical management medical trial women's preferences), and £131.08 (95% CI: £129.16 – £133.01) for a shift from expectant to medical management (surgical trial women's preferences). See Appendix 12.1 for the pre- and post-trial attribute levels.

Finally on this topic, additional issues for deliberation include: the special consideration of preferences of subgroups and the extent to which this affects the CBA; the discounting of costs and benefits arising in the future; the role of modelling in longer term extrapolation; and the comparison with CEA analyses, i.e. how much weight should be given to the CBA results. Where the trials under consideration are drug trials, attributes and levels can be devised according to the attributes and levels of alternative drug products.

Decision making in health care is increasingly being informed by economic decision models drawing data from a wide range of sources rather than from economic evaluation alongside clinical trials. Following the discussion of the role of PSA in CBA above it is clear that there is a potential role for increased use of SPDCE results in providing parameter information for use within economic models generating CBA results.

12.7 Measurement issues specific to SPDCEs

12.7.1 The nature of health care attributes

Paying particular attention to the 'nature' of health care attributes is a key consideration for any planned CBA using SPDCE-derived benefits. The nature of attributes will influence the validity and generalizability of the resulting CBA depending upon: how they are defined; the context within which they are defined; the timescale associated with the health state or effect; the unit in which the attribute is defined; and whether the attribute is static or dynamic. Dynamic health care attributes may be associated with differing time periods; for instance, particular diseases will be associated with differing health states over time. This then leads to the challenges associated with adjusting for differential timing of costs and benefits, as well as consideration of the context within which preferences for the health states were elicited and the validity of results when used in differing time periods.

Where the intervention (or health state) being evaluated lasts into the future then discounting of resource use costs and 'preferences' should also be considered. Some assumptions will have to be made regarding the time period over which SPDCE-derived preferences are valid. It will also be important to ensure that the resource use required/removed achieving the given welfare gain/loss are also measured and valued in line with the valid time period. It is recommended that explicit 'time periods' be incorporated directly into the context setting of the SPDCE survey to improve the validity of preferences over the time period of interest. It may even be worthwhile incorporating explicit 'reminder' prompts throughout the SPDCE survey itself to ensure validity of time-dependent preferences. These prompts would simply serve as a reminder for the time period for which preferences were being considered. An alternative approach is to incorporate 'time' or 'duration' as attributes themselves within a SPDCE, akin to the time trade off method. It is also worth considering whether preferences have a 'shelf life' at which point they should be re-elicited, this may be due to changes in attitude as a result of say a new development in technology. Once attributes and levels for the SPDCE design have been decided upon, it is a worthwhile exercise to carry out a 'mock welfare analysis', i.e. devising the scenarios of interest for the CBA prior to finalization of the attributes and levels will help to identify any problematic health care attributes prior to statistical and experimental design of the SPDCE.

12.7.2 Elicitation format

A number of different elicitation formats have been used in the literature, these include: a discrete choice binary format (34;36;52;56); multiple choice formats (57); options allowing for an 'opt-out' option; graded pair (58–60) (or strength of preference) elicitation format; closed-ended discrete choice methods (34); best attribute scaling (or maximum difference) formats (61;62); rating scales (63–65); and ranking scales (66;67). All have advantages and disadvantages, and some research has compared alternative formats (66;68) however, the extent to which they all adhere to the theoretical requirements and can validly be combined with costs within a CBA framework is debatable and, as such, consideration should be given to the choice of elicitation format at the outset, see Chapter 10 for further discussion on this topic. Theoretically, any method involving a trade-off is preferred, hence this would exclude methods such as ranking and rating.

Morey et al. (69) noted that contingent valuation estimates are sensitive to the valuation model employed and that modelling the 'participation' decision, i.e. the initial decision by a consumer as to whether to participate in the activity for which there are choices, is critical in obtaining accurate welfare estimates. Mitchell and Carson (70) also noted that *not* including a non-participation alternative and forcing a respondent to make a choice they would not normally make lowers their initial level of utility (i.e. starting level of utility or 'status quo') thus violating the assumption underlying Hicksian compensating measures, i.e. that the welfare gain/loss is obtained by analysing shifts from their initial level of utility (70). Related to this, and of relevance in health care is that we may not even know, or be able to identify, the initial levels of utility. The extent to which the initial level of utility is identifiable is thus an empirical question. The extent to which it is possible to identify and measure the non-participation level of utility is a further consideration. Two key issues are thus the identification and measurement of both the status quo and non-participation utility levels (69). See later sections on '*modelling the participation decision*' and '*reference dependent preferences*'.

A recent review of DCEs in health care showed that the majority of SPDCE applications did not include 'opt-out' alternatives (71). As noted by Ruby et al. (72), the format of the opt-out option is usually the 'no purchase' and 'my current brand'. In health care, however such 'commercial' definitions for opting out are not realistic.

The 'no purchase' option is equivalent to 'I will not consume this health care' and the 'my current brand' is equivalent to 'my current health status'. These two health care formats could be equivalent if the 'I will not have this health care' option leads to no further consumption as that automatically implies 'current health status'. However, it may be the case that rather than having an operation say, the consumer decides to consume an alternative treatment not on offer by the choice scenario, i.e. not-participate. The format 'my current health status' may also be difficult to identify within an SPDCE. This would be the case for example, if the 'current health status' is say, a degenerative health state and without consuming the hypothetical interventions the 'current health status' is not a static alternative but a dynamic event. Modelling this within a choice experiment would be complex and require additional modelling of the transitional health states beyond that possible within the choice experiment context. As noted by Ruby *et al.* (72), one challenge with modelling the opt-out alternative is the identification of what is meant by consumers when they choose this option (72). This is one of the key issues that needs to be explored in SPDCE experiments in health care if the welfare measures are to be used within CBAs. Further to this, the statistical and econometric methods required to handle the differing elicitation formats vary widely and may also affect the ability to estimate welfare values, hence consideration of appropriate analytical methods should also be made at the design stage.

12.7.3 **Modelling the participation decision**

Related to the elicitation format, consideration should be given to whether SPDCE-derived preference data have been elicited from a group of 'demanders' or not, i.e. people consuming the health care of interest (73). Morey *et al.* (69) noted that SPDCE welfare values are sensitive to the valuation model employed and that modelling the participation decision is crucial in obtaining accurate estimates. If the sample are not identified demanders then the welfare values may need to account for this by re-weighting the welfare values accordingly (19;73;74). The implications of this for CBA results are that if the participation decision has not been modelled appropriately and *inaccurate* welfare measures are combined with the resource use data, then the CBA ratio may be invalid and incorrect policy conclusions drawn. This is dealt with in more detail in Section 12.7.4.

12.7.4 **Consideration of the payment vehicle and income effects**

As outlined in Chapters 10 and 11 much of the fundamental theory behind welfare measurement in discrete choice models has been developed by Small and Rosen (74) and Hanemann (75). For a detailed discussion of such theory also see Freeman (76) and more recently for applications of the estimation of welfare within SPDCEs, see Lancsar (19;20), Ryan (21), McIntosh (52), Santos Silva (25), and Hanson (77). One approach to estimating welfare is by calculating the MRS between the attributes and price, i.e. '*state of the world*' models (21;25) (when only one alternative is on offer and the individuals take up the good/service with certainty), as follows:

$$\text{Marginal WTP} = \beta_x/\beta_p, \tag{12.3}$$

where β_x is the attribute coefficient and β_p is the coefficient on the price attribute (payment vehicle). Alternatively, and appropriate when estimating '*multiple alternative models*' (where welfare values must be weighted by the probability of choosing a particular option) is the formula recommended by Small and Rosen (74) to estimate compensating variation and more recently by Lancsar and Savage (19):

$$CV = \frac{1}{\lambda}\left[\ln \sum_{i=1}^{I} e^{V^0}i - \ln \sum_{i=1}^{I} e^{V^1}i \right], \tag{12.4}$$

where λ is the marginal utility of income, V^0i and V^1i are the values for the good or service for each choice option i before and after the change, respectively, and I is the number of options in the choice set. Note this formula relies on the marginal utility of income to estimate WTP values; however, since such information is often unavailable the coefficient on the price attribute (the marginal disutility of price) is often used as a substitute. Hence, the welfare estimation method used depends upon the design of the SPDCE and whether there are reliable data on income levels available. All have implications for the final welfare estimate and the CBA result.

Assuming a payment vehicle is included and data on income levels are not available then the cost attribute (i.e. the 'payment vehicle') plays a key role in the estimation of WTP. The importance of the 'cost attribute' or 'payment vehicle' has been the subject of a small number of methodological papers (22;23), however it is an area where further research is required such that the resulting welfare estimates can be validly married with the resource use required to estimate the welfare gain/loss within a CBA framework. The key areas for consideration are: the type of payment vehicle used (e.g. cost to you, travel cost, donation, tax); the extent to which it is a realistic and plausible attribute (e.g. in a publicly funded health care system); the ability of the payment vehicle to obtain respondent 'values' and not 'anticipated cost', i.e. where the WTP 'value' reflects what they believe the good at stake costs; the functional form of the cost attribute, i.e. whether it is say, linear or diminishing, and the methods from which welfare are estimated, e.g. *state of the world* models or *multiple alternative models* (19;21;25;74).

Given that it is highly likely that correlation exists between income groups, preferences, and health status then SPDCE preferences should be tailored to account for this. Where it is possible to collect valid and reliable income data, analysis should allow for interactions with income groups, i.e. where those with higher incomes are seen to be willing to pay more. Standard SPDCE interaction analysis will permit this however there is little guidance available on what to do with values once they are shown to be different (as theory predicts), although Oliver *et al.* (31) suggest the use of equity weights (31).

12.8 Broader SPDCE measurement issues in CBA

12.8.1 Reference-dependent preferences

In the contingent valuation literature a commonly cited limitation of standard theory are the disparities between WTP and willingness to accept (WTA) values. In this context, the most prominent alternative theory is that proposed by Tversky and Kahneman, in which preferences are reference dependant (78). The idea is that an individuals' preferences are defined in relation to that individuals *reference point*, normally the *status quo* (i.e. original level of utility). This observation ties in very well with the literature in economics which states that to estimate the appropriate measure of welfare compensating variation (CV measure) evaluating a shift from the *status quo* to the alternative is the theoretically correct approach, as discussed earlier (see sections on 'elicitation format' and 'modelling the participation decision'). Hence, the theoretically correct approach to obtain the CV measure in SPDCEs is to identify the '*current*' scenario then compare all the alternatives to this (79;80). This approach however is not always the most practical and may give rise to a large number of scenarios for respondents to value and may be cognitively burdensome (81). If the scenarios are randomly paired (i.e. no fixed status quo) or a foldover design is used (34), this may give rise to less choices having to be made. However, one concern with estimating welfare values from within SPDCEs is that the desired CV measure may not be 'elicited' using such designs since the design structure may not be conducive to allow welfare to be derived from the original level of utility. Roe *et al.* (80) and Bateman *et al.* (79) recommended the inclusion of the status quo within each choice pair in order to derive the compensating measure of welfare, however, it has been suggested that choice sets need not be constrained by the requirement of the status quo in each alternative (82). Carson *et al.* (83) discussed the question of including a constant reference alternative in the context of choice experiments. They noted there are conceptual and empirical advantages and disadvantages of this approach and they concluded that this is 'an open research issue'. Whilst often used in environmental economics because of the ease of defining individuals 'status quo', such scenarios are often not routinely used as a basis from which to elicit preferences in health care. The reason for this is that defining the status quo/current health scenario for individuals in a health context can be complex, often due to the special nature of health care attributes (see Section 12.7.1) as well as their, often dynamic nature and issues around duration of effects.

The issue of reference-dependent preferences is important for the derivation of CBAs. The complexity arises where the status quo for each individual *differs*. Where the current provision is the same for everyone and the attributes and levels for the status quo scenario are fixed for all then it is simpler. If values were being elicited for attributes of say, a drug or health status, then this is more likely to require the identification of each individual's status quo scenario, with which individual cost data would have to be identified and combined with the welfare shift values. Collecting data on individuals' status quo and then modelling the resulting choice will introduce complexities for the statistical design of SPDCEs. Further research is required into the experimental design requirements when status quo's differ at an individual level.

A final point about reference-dependent preferences is that while preferences can be defined with respect to the status quo – the utility of benefits is not equivalent to the disutility of an equal loss. Essentially, losses loom larger than gains, which may represent a further challenge for estimating health care benefits using SPDCE (as well as direct WTP measures). However, one advantage with SPDCEs is that empirical tests can be set up to measure this disparity as a function of the difference in marginal values per individual attribute.

12.8.2 **Time frame and habituation effects**

Identifying the relevant costs and benefits over the relevant time period is an obvious consideration for any CBA; however, the estimation of values based upon SPDCE-elicited preferences will *also* be restricted by the time frame imposed within the *context* of the SPDCE, in addition to the definition of attributes and levels. For example, the context for an SPDCE may be a short-term operative setting and the attributes and levels for say pain, infection, and recurrence may be defined with specific reference to this short time period. It would therefore be invalid to use the resulting WTP values to estimate welfare shifts for a long-term chronic condition where the context was different even though the attributes of pain, infection, and recurrence are the same. Further to this, preferences may change over time as well as being influenced by the impact of habituation (or wearing in) upon preferences (84); hence, some attempt should be made to identify this phenomenon and accommodate it when it occurs. One potential way of avoiding habituation effects is to use society's values within CBAs. However in health care, when evaluating health states or use of heath services, the practical nature of using society's values may render this practice challenging because what would be required in order to establish the survey 'context' in terms of health-related descriptions, definitions, and meanings may be overly burdensome for the respondent. Further, the argument for using the status quo level of utility as a constant comparator may be difficult where health states were being valued that were not a common status quo in society.

12.8.3 Benefits transfer

Benefits transfer is an approach that makes use of previous welfare valuations of similar goods/services at a study site and, with any necessary adjustments, applies them to produce estimates for the same or similar good/service in a different context (known as the 'policy site) (79). In many situations, because of time and budget constraints, decision makers tasked with making decisions regarding the allocation of scarce resources are often required to extrapolate from existing data that were collected for a different purpose. Whilst similar exercises happen frequently in health care, in the form of meta-analyses and modelling exercises, the novelty of 'benefits transfer' is that preferences believed to be sensitive to changes in the *context* in which they were elicited, and subject to various uncertainties, are transferred to new settings and as such their validity is questionable (85).

In environmental economics, benefits transfer is increasingly being used by decision makers as a way of estimating environmental values suitable for use in CBA, however concerns have been raised over the validity of benefits transfer using contingent valuation methods (85). SPDCEs have been suggested as being particularly suitable for benefits transfer because it is possible to allow for differences in attributes and socio-economic characteristics when transferring benefit estimates. Namely, the flexibility of the data allow values to be obtained for different attribute level configurations, depending upon the new setting, as well as for different subgroups, depending upon the characteristics of the new population of interest. In health care SPDCE, marginal valuations could potentially be treated the same as standard 'outcomes' such as tariff values from the EQ-5D (86). Evidence in environmental economics to date suggests that transfers across different case study sites are likely to be subject to less error than those across different populations (87). However, particular attention should be paid to the specific challenges arising in *health care* 'sites' and the extent to which the benefits transfer approach is useful in a health care setting. It may be that alternative transfer methods are required for health care. In addition, alongside any benefits transfer will be 'cost transfer' and hence issues around the generalizability of costs in different settings/populations are equally as important as those around benefits transfer.

Whilst the use of SPDCEs in health care has increased markedly in recent years, this has not been matched with an equivalent increase in CBAs in health care using such SPDCE-derived valuations. The aim of this chapter was not to summarize the many challenges associated with deriving WTP using SPDCEs (19–23;25) but to treat these issues as 'work-in-progress', broaden the scope and outline some considerations for the development of SPDCE-deriven CBAs in health care. Indeed, topics including the aggregation of benefits, (88) and the validity of this practice, require further, in-depth insight and have not been covered within this chapter. Based upon the issues presented in this chapter, a suggested checklist is provided which outlines the key areas of consideration when devising a SPDCE-based CBA, see Appendix 12.2.

The aim of this chapter was to provide an impetus for this area to be explored in a more applied manner than previously, and to begin the task of providing a framework for such work. Whilst this chapter represents a type of 'wish list', further, more technical development of the individual topics arising is now required. A UK Health Technology Assessment (HTA) review carried out a systematic review of the effectiveness and cost-effectiveness of laparoscopic repair for inguinal hernia repair (89), this review was novel in that it is likely to be the first to include benefit evidence in the form of effectiveness, utility, *and* SPDCE-derived welfare estimates. Further, Markov modelling methods were used to generate incremental net benefit curves for the various alternatives using the SPDCE-derived data.

This chapter has shown that it is possible to develop a cost–benefit plane akin to the cost-effectiveness plane currently employed by many CEA practitioners. However, one advantage of the CBA plane approach would be that the outcomes would not be confined to a single measure of effectiveness or QALY, but would contain the full complement of benefits contained within the welfare estimate obtained and facilitate the answering of allocative efficiency questions. One practical way forward for researchers may be to include the use of 'shadow' CBA evaluations alongside CEAs and CUAs as a starting point within clinical trials and modelling exercises. This will allow policy makers to begin to not only see the usefulness of CBA results alongside more familiar CUA and CEA methods but also to use them to understand the implications of the CBA results more generally. However, it should be the ultimate goal to capture the preferences of the public as is the practice in areas such as environmental economics. The development of SPDCE methods in health care settings for use in formal CBAs should embrace appropriate methodology for 'context' setting so that the general public can be asked their preferences for health care scenarios/states they have no direct experience of. Finally, recognizing that it may not be possible to include everything in an economic evaluation, at the very least, CBA methods are transparent and as a minimum a balance sheet presentation of all the relevant costs and benefits provides the baseline estimates for policy makers (33).

Acknowledgement

Much of the material in this chapter is contained in: McIntosh, E. 2006. Using stated preference discrete choice experiments in cost–benefit analysis: some considerations. *Pharmacoeconomics* **24**(9): 855–869 and Petrou, S., and McIntosh, E. 2009. Women's preferences for attributes of first-trimester miscarriage management: A stated preference discrete-choice experiment. *Value in Health* **12**(4): 551–559.

References

1. Brent, R.J. 2003. *Cost-benefit analysis and health care evaluations.* Cheltenham: Edward Elgar Publishing.
2. Klose, T. 1999. The contingent valuation method in health care. *Health Policy* **47**: 97–123.
3. Borghi, J. 2008. Aggregation rules for cost-benefit analysis: A health economics perspective. *Health Economics* **17**(7): 863–875.
4. Drummond, M.F., Sculpher, M.J., Torrance, G.W., O'Brien, B., and Stoddart, G.L. 2005. *Methods for the economic evaluation of health care programmes.* 3rd ed. Oxford: Oxford University Press.
5. Bowling, A. 1991. *Measuring health: A review of quality of life measurement scales.* 4th ed. Buckingham: Open University Press.
6. Bowling, A. 1995. *Measuring disease.* 1st ed. Buckingham: Open University Press.
7. Sackett, D.L., and Torrance, G.W. 1978. The utility of different health states as perceived by the general public. *Journal of Chronic Disorders* **31**(11): 697–704.
8. Torrance, G.W., and Sackett, D.L. 1972. A utility maximising model for evaluation of health care programmes. *Health Services Research* **7**(2): 118–133.
9. Torrance, G.W. 1976. Social preferences for health states: An empirical evaluation of three measurement techniques. *Socioeconomic Planning Sciences* **10**(3): 128–136.
10. Torrance, G.W., Boyle, M.H., and Horwood, S.P. 1982. Application of multiattribute utility theory to measure social preferences for health states. *Operations Research* **30**(6): 1043–1069.
11. Culyer, A.J. 1989. The normative economics of health care finance and provision. *Oxford Review of Economic Policy* **5**: 34–58.
12. Williams, A. 1985. Economics of coronary artery bypass grafting. *British Medical Journal* **291**: 326–329.
13. Buckingham, K. 1993. A note on HYE (Healthy Years Equivalents). *Journal of Health Economics* **12**: 301–309.
14. Buckingham, K. 1995. Economics, health and health economics: HYEs versus QALYs. A response. *Journal of Health Economics* **14**: 397–398.
15. Richardson, J. 1994. Cost utility analysis – what should be measured? *Social Science and Medicine* **39**: 7–21.
16. Drummond, M.F., Stoddard, G.L., and Torrance, W. 1987. *Methods for the economic evaluation of health care programmes.* 1st ed. Oxford: Oxford University Press.
17. Drummond, M.F., Stoddard, G.L., and Torrance, W. 1987. *Methods for the economic evaluation of health care programmes.* 1st ed. Oxford: Oxford University Press.

18. McIntosh, E. 2006. Using stated preference discrete choice experiments in cost-benefit analysis: some considerations. *Pharmacoeconomics* **24**(9): 855–869.

19. Lancsar, E., and Savage, E. 2004. Deriving welfare measures from discrete choice experiments: inconsistency between current methods and random utility and welfare theory. *Health Economics Letters* **13**(9): 901–907.

20. Lancsar, E., and Savage, E. 2004. Deriving welfare measures from discrete choice experiments: a response to Ryan and Santos Silva. *Health Economics Letters* **13**(9): 919–924.

21. Ryan, M. 2004. Deriving welfare measures in discrete choice experiments: a comment to Lancsar and Savage (1). *Health Economics Letters* **13**(9): 909–912.

22. Ratcliffe, J. 2000. The use of conjoint analysis to elicit willingness-to-pay values. Proceed with caution? *International Journal of Technology Assess Health Care 2000* **16**: 270–275.

23. Slothuus, S.U., and Gyrd-Hansen, D. 2003. Conjoint analysis. The cost variable: An Achilles' heel? *Health Economics* **12**(6): 479–491.

24. McIntosh, E., and Ryan, M. 2002. Using discrete choice experiments to derive welfare estimates for the provision of elective surgery: impications of discontinuous preferences. *Journal of Economic Psychology* **23**(3): 367–382.

25. Santos Silva, J.M.C. 2004. Deriving welfare measures in discrete choice experiments: a comment to Lancsar and Savage (2). *Health Economics Letters* **13**(9): 913–918.

26. Clarke, P. 1998. Cost-benefit analysis and mammographic screening: a travel cost approach. *Journal of Health Economics* **17**: 767–787.

27. Haefeli, M., Elfering, A., McIntosh, E., Gray, A., Sukthankar, A., and Boos, N. 2008. A cost-benefit analysis using contingent valuation techniques: A feasibility study in spinal surgery. *Value in Health* **11**(4): 575–588.

28. Nocera, S., Bonato, D., and Telser, H. 2002. The contingency of contingent valuation: How much are people willing to pay against Alzheimer's Disease? *International Journal of Health Care Finance and Economics* **2**: 219–240.

29. Drummond, M.F., Sculpher, M.J., Torrance, G.W., O'Brien, B., and Stoddart, G.L. 2005. *Methods for the economic evaluation of health care programmes.* 3rd ed. Oxford University Press.

30. Cookson, R. 2003. Willingness to pay methods in health care: A sceptical view. *Health Economics* **12**: 891–894.

31. Oliver, A., Healey, A., and Donaldson, C. 2002. Choosing the method to match the perspective: economic assessment and its implications for health services efficiency. *The Lancet* **359**: 1771–1774.

32. Ryan, M. 2004. Discrete choice experiments in health care. *British Medical Journal* **328**: 360–361.

33. McIntosh, E., Donaldson, C., and Ryan, M. 1999. Recent advances in the methods of cost-benefit analysis in healthcare: Matching the art to the science. *Pharmacoeconomics* **15**: 357–367.

34. Louviere, J., Hensher, D.A., and Swait, J. 2000. *Stated choice methods: analysis and application.* 1st ed. Cambridge: Cambridge University Press.

35. Adamowicz, W.L., Louviere, J., and Swait, J. 1998. *Introduction to attribute based stated choice methods.* Washington, DC: NOAA Damage Assessment Centre.

36. Ryan, M. 1996. Using willingness to pay to assess the benefits of assisted reproductive techniques. *Health Economics* **5**: 543–558.

37. Kleinman, L., McIntosh, E., Ryan, M., Schmier, J., Crawley, J., Locke, G.R., *et al.* 2002. Willingness to pay for complete symptom relief of gastroesophogeal reflux disease. *Archives of Internal Medicine* **162**: 1361–1366.

38. Ryan, M., McIntosh, E., Dean,T., and Old, P. 2000. Trade-offs between location and waiting time in the provision of elective surgery. *Journal of Public Health Medicine* **22**(2): 202–210.

39. McIntosh, E. 2003. *Using discrete choice experiments to value the benefits of health care.* PhD Thesis University of Aberdeen.

40. Briggs, A.H., and O'Brien, B.J. 2001. The death of cost minimization analysis? *Health Economics* **10**: 179–184.

41. Briggs, A.H., and Fenn, P. 1998. Confidence intervals or surfaces? Uncertainty on the cost-effectiveness plane. *Health Economics* **7**: 723–740.

42. Fenwick, E., O'Brien, B.J., and Briggs, A.H. 2004. Cost-effectiveness Acceptability Curves - facts, fallacies and frequently asked questions. *Health Economics* **13**: 405–415.

43. Donaldson, C., Currie, G., and Mitton, C. 2002. Cost effectiveness analysis in health care: contradictions. *British Medical Journal* **325**(891): 894.

44. Briggs, A., and Fenn, P. 1998. Confidence intervals or surfaces? Uncertainty on the cost-effectiveness plane. *Health Economics* **7**: 723–740.

45. Louviere, J., Burgess, L., Street, D., and Marley, A. 2004. *Modeling the choices of single individuals by combining efficient choice experiment designs with extra preference information.* Sydney: University of Technology, Sydney; Report No.: Centre for the Study of Choice (CenSoC) Working Paper No. 04-005.

46. Stinnett, A.A., and Mullahy, J. 1998. Net health benefits: a new framework for the analysis of uncertainty in cost-effectiveness analysis. *Medical Decision Making* **18**: S65–S80.

47. Polsky, D., Glick, H., Willke, R., and Schulman, K. 1997. Confidence intervals for cost-effectivenss ratios: A comparison of four methods. *Health Economics* **6**: 243–252.

48. Risa Hole, A.A. 2007. A comparison of approaches to estimating confidence intervals for willingness to pay measures. *Health Economics* **16**: 827–840.

49. Fieller, E.C. 1954. Some problems on interval estimation with discussion. *Journal of the Royal Statistical Society* **16**: 175–188.

50. Kennedy, P. 1995. *A guide to econometrics.* 3rd ed. Oxford: Blackwell.

51. Efron, B. 1979. Bootstrap methods: Another look at the jackknife. *Annals of Statistics* **7**: 1–26.

52. McIntosh, E., and Ryan, M. 2002. Using discrete choice experiments to derive welfare estimates for the provision of elective surgery: implications of discontinuous preferences. *Journal of Economic Psychology* **23**(3): 367–382.

53. Claxton, K., Sculpher, M.J., McCabe, C., Briggs, A., Akehurst, R., Buxton, M., *et al.* 2005. Probabilistic sensitivity analysis for NICE technology assessment: not an optional extra. *Health Economics* **14**: 339–347.

54. Petrou, S., Trinder, J., Brocklehurst, P., and Smith, L. 2006. Economic evaluation of alternative management methods of first-trimester miscarriage based on results from the MIST Trial. *British Journal of Obstetrics and Gynaecology* **113**(8): 879–889.

55. Petrou, S., and McIntosh, E. 2009. Women's preferences for attributes of first-trimester miscarriage management: A stated preference discrete-choice experiment. *Value in Health* **12**(4): 551–559.

56. Bryan, S., Buxton, M., Sheldon, R., and Grant, A. 1998. Magnetic resonance imaging for the investigation of knee injuries: an investigation of preferences. *Health Economics* **7**: 595–604.

57. Johnson, F.R., Banzhaf, M.R., and Desvousges, W.H. 2000. Willingness to pay for improved respiratory and cardiovascular health: a multiple format stated-preference approach. *Health Economics* **9**: 295–317.

58. Johnson, F.R., Desvousges, W.H., Ruby, M., Stieb, D., and De Civita, P. 1998. Eliciting stated health preferences: an application to wilingness to pay for longevity. *Medical Decision Making* **18**: s57–s67.

59. Magat, W.A., Viscusi, W.K., and Huber, J. 1998. Paired comparison and contingent valuation approaches to morbidity risk valuation. *Journal of Environmental Economics and Management* **15**: 395–411.

60. van der Pol, M., and Cairns, J. 1998. Establishing patient preferences for blood transfusion support: an application of conjoint analysis. *Journal of Health Services Research Policy* **1998**3: 70–76.

61. Szeinbach, S.L., Barnes, J.H., McGhan, W.F., Murawski, M.M., and Corey, R. 1998. Using maximum difference conjoint and visual analogue scaling to measure patients utility for a particular health state. *Journal of Research in Pharmaceutical Economics* **9**(3): 83–100.

62. Freeman, J.K., Szeinbach, S.L., Barnes, J.H., Garner, D.D., and Gilbert, F.W. 1998. Assessing the need for student health services using maximum difference conjoint analysis. *Journal of Research in Pharmaceutical Economics* **9**(3): 35–49.

63. Anderson, N.H. 1971. An exchange on functional and conjoint measurement. *Psychological Review* **77**: 153–170.

64. Chakraborty, G., Ball, D., Gaeth, G.J., and Jun, S. 2002. The ability of ratings and choice conjoint to predict market shares: A monte carlo simulation. *Journal of Business Research* **55**: 237–249.

65. Reardon, G., and Pathak, D. 1990. Segmenting the antihistamine market: an investigation of consumer preferences. *Journal of Health Care Marketing* **10**(3): 23–33.

66. Boyle, K.J. 2001. A comparison of conjoint analysis response formats. *American Journal of Agricultural Economics* **83**(2): 441–454.

67. Huber, J., Wittink, D.R., Fiedler, J.A., and Miller, R. 1993. The effectiveness of alternative elicitation procedures in predicting choice. *Journal of Marketing Research* **30**: 105–114.

68. Elrod, T., Louviere, J.J., and Davey, K.S. 1992. An empirical comparison of ratings-based and choice-based conjoint models. *Journal of Market Research* **29**: 368–377.

69. Morey, E.R., Rowe, R.D., and Watson, M. 1993. A Repeated Nested-Logit Model of Atlantic Salmon Fishing. *American Journal of Agricultural Economics* **75**: 578–592.

70 . Mitchell, R.C., and Carson, R.T. 1989. *Using surveys to value public goods.* 3rd ed. Washington, DC: Resources for the Future.

71. Ryan, M., and Gerard, K. 2001. Using choice experiments to value ehalth care programmes: where are we and where should we go? Paper presented at the 3rd International Health Economics Association Conference, 22–25th July, 2001, University of York, UK.

72. Ruby, M.C., Johnson, F.R., and Mathews, K.E. 1999. Just say no: opt-out alternatives and anglers' stated-preferences. Technical working paper, No T-9801 R, Triangle Economic Research.

73. Ryan, M., and Skatun, D. 2004. Modelling non-demanders in choice experiments. *Health Economics* **13**(4): 397–402.

74. Small, K.A., and Rosen, H.S. 1981. Applied welfare economics with discrete choice models. *Econometrica* **49**: 105–130.

75. Hanemann, W.M. 1984. Welfare evaluations in contingent valuation experiments with discrete responses. *American Journal of Agricultural Economics* **66**: 332–341.

76. Freeman, A.M. 1993. *The measurement of environmental and resource values: theory and methods.* 3rd ed. Washington: Resources for the Future.

77. Hanson, K., McPake, B., Nakamba, P., and Archard, L. 2005. Preferences for hospital quality in Zambia: results from a discrete choice experiment. *Health Economics* **14**(7): 687–701.

78. Tversky, A., and Kahneman, D. 1991. Loss aversion in riskless choice: a reference dependent model. *Quarterly Journal of Economics* **106**: 1039–1061.

79. Bateman, I.J., Carson, R.T., Day, B., Hanemann, M., Hanley, N., Hett, T., *et al. Economic valuation with stated preference: A manual.* 1st ed. Cheltenham, UK: Edward Elgar.

80. Roe, B., Boyle, K.J., and Teisl, M.F. 1996. Using conjoint analysis to derive estimates of compensating variation. *Journal of Environmental Economics and Management* **31**: 145–159.

81. Pearmain, D., Swanson, J., Kroes, E., and Bradley, M. 1991. *Stated preference techniques: a guide to practice.* Hague: Steer Davis Gleave and Hague Consulting Group.

82. Johnson, F.R., Desvousges, W.H. 1997. Estimating stated preferences with rated-pair data: environmental, health, and employment effects of energy programs. *Journal of Environmental Economics and Management* **34**: 79–99.

83. Carson, R.T., Louviere, J., Anderson, P., Arabie, D., Bunch, D., Hensher, D.A., *et al.* Experimental analysis of choice. *Marketing Letters* **5**: 351–367.

84. Wathieu, L. 2004. Consumer habituation. *Management Science* **50**(5): 587–596.

85. Bergland, O., Magnussen, K., and Navrud, S. 1995. Benefit transfer: Testing for accuracy and reliability. 1995 Jun 20; Paper presented at the sixth Annual Conference of the European Association of Environmental and Resource Economists, Umea Sweden.

86. Dolan, P., Gudex, C., Kind, P., and Williams, A. 1995. *A social tariff for EuroQol: results from a UK general population survey. Discussion Paper no. 138.* York: University of York.

87. Morrison, M., Bennett, J., Blamey, R., and Louviere, J. 2002. Choice modeling and tests of benefit transfer. *American Journal of Agricultural Economics* **84**(1): 161–170.

88. Blackorby, C., and Donaldson, D. 1990. The case against the use of the sum of compensating variations in cost-benefit analysis. *Canadian Journal of Economics* **23**: 471–494.

89. McCormack, K., Wake, B., Perez, J., Fraser, C., Cook, J., and McIntosh, E., *et al.* 2005. Laparoscopic surgery for inguinal hernia repair: systematic review of effectiveness and economic evaluation. *Health Technology Assessment* **9**(14): 1–218.

Appendix 12.1

Pre-trial scenarios for surgical, medical, and expectant management miscarriage based on trial attributes and levels

Attributes	Surgical scenario	Medical scenario	Expectant scenario
• Time spent at hospital receiving treatment	1 day	0.5 day	0.5 day
• Level of pain experienced	Low	Moderate	Moderate
• Number of days bleeding following treatment	3 days	8 days	14 days
• Time taken to return to normal activities following treatment	3–4 days	3–4 days	3–4 days
• Chance of complications requiring more time or readmission to hospital	5%	10%	5%

Post-trial scenarios for surgical, medical, and expectant management of miscarriage based on actual MIST trial data

Attributes	Surgical scenario	Medical scenario	Expectant scenario
• Time spent at hospital receiving treatment	1 day	1.2 days	0 days
• Level of pain experienced	Low	Low	Low
• Number of days bleeding following treatment	8 days	11 days	12 days
• Time taken to return to normal activities following treatment	6.7 days	6.7 days	12 days
• Chance of complications requiring more time or readmission to hospital	3%	2%	3%

Appendix 12.2

Suggested checklist for developing a CBA using SPDCE methods for estimation of benefits

Elicitation method employed

◆ Consider requirement for modelling the participation decision as well as response scale (e.g. binary, graded) to ensure accurate welfare estimates (i.e. providing 'opt-out' so as not to overestimate welfare values)

◆ Consider whether inclusion of the status quo is feasible (and whether cost data are available for the status quo)

Form of and realism of payment vehicle

◆ Consider how to describe and present the cost attribute (e.g. cost to you, travel cost, donation, tax)

◆ Collect data on income of respondents to allow testing of theoretical validity of WTP responses

◆ Consider using equity weights in the final CBA within sensitivity analysis to explore impact on results

Timescale over which benefits and costs are elicited

◆ Consider period of discounting and extent to which the welfare values align with the costs required to achieve the welfare gain (loss)

◆ Consider whether preferences have a 'shelf life' (e.g. due to new developments) at which point they should be re-elicited for the purposes of updating the CBA

Resource use (cost) data required for CBA

◆ Ensure resource use data collected can be attributed to achieving the welfare gains i.e. improvements in attributes, from the SPDCE

◆ Consider the flexibility of the resource use data and the extent to which the cost data are as flexible as the SPDCE attributes and levels (e.g. consider economies of scale and issues around fixed costs; use marginal costs where possible)

Mapping attributes to alternative CBA scenarios

◆ Consider the nature of attributes and levels used (are they practical for extrapolating in a mapping exercise to estimate welfare values for alternative configurations of attributes and levels)

◆ Where trial data are available, consider designing attributes and levels in line with trial outcomes

◆ Consider realism of attributes and levels for mapping exercise (generalizability of scenarios)

◆ Carry out 'mock' welfare analysis with attributes and levels prior to finalization of design to ensure attributes and levels chosen in the design can be used post-analysis in the various CBA configurations of interest

Suggested checklist for developing a CBA using SPDCE methods for estimation of benefits *(continued)*

Accounting for uncertainty in the parameters/CBA ratio

♦ Explore alternative methods of estimating confidence intervals around the MRS (where applicable)

♦ Ensure resource use data estimated can be directly attributed to, and combined with, welfare gains (losses)

♦ Consider using the CBA plane to explore cost/benefit pairing variability where individual preference data are available

♦ Consider modelling SPDCE data along with cost data using Markov modelling methods to explore alternative CBA scenarios at the population/patient group level

♦ Consider using probabilistic sensitivity analysis methods where applicable (would need to consider the distribution of the data)

Generalizability: Habituation and context effects

♦ Consider whether habituation of preferences is likely in the respondents identified.

♦ Have preferences been explored for rationality and consistency? Are preferences well formed or are they susceptible to change depending upon context? Context dependency may affect the CBA ratio.

♦ Consideration of benefits transfer issues: Are CBA values to be transferred to another setting/population, etc.?

Chapter 13

The relevance of cost–benefit analysis in health care: Concluding comments

Emma McIntosh, W.L. (Vic) Adamowicz, and F. Reed Johnson

As outlined in Chapter 1, the purpose of this handbook was not to re-invent the theoretical wheel of CBA but to provide researchers with up-to-date methodological guidance and practical 'hands on' advice for carrying out applied CBA in health care and in doing so hopefully push forward this methodological area. The goal of the book was to provide readers with an understanding of the applied methods of CBA in health care as they stand to date as well as an insight to the ongoing methodological challenges in this area. Early chapters introduced important theoretical aspects such as key concepts in welfare economics and the relevance of market failure in health care to the development of economic evaluation methods (Chapter 1), the Household Production Model (HPM) and consumer preferences for own health and health care (Chapter 2). Key applied concepts related to the cost side of CBA including shadow pricing as well as a useful reference guide to key costing sources for economic evaluation were then provided (Chapters 3 and 4). Chapter 5 described the many parallels between environmental valuation and health valuation and the uses of CBA methods in both fields outlining the importance of strong economic conceptual frameworks. This comparison then set the scene for the subsequent chapters on measuring and valuing benefits for CBA. To this end, Chapters 6–8 explored the methodology of stated preference willingness to pay (WTP) methods in health care with the use of applied examples (including downloadable exercises) as well as provision of clear methodological guidance. Chapter 9 then outlined the use of revealed preference methods for valuing non-market and unpriced goods. An applied example of the travel cost method (as commonly used in environmental economics) in the area of mammographic screening was provided and this concluded with a formal CBA of this preventive programme. Recent years have seen a surge in the number of stated preference discrete choice experiments (SPDCEs) being carried out in health care hence Chapters 10–12 were dedicated to outlining the experimental design issues of this topic as well as how to estimate welfare using these techniques. Chapter 12 provided a practical guide to reporting and presenting SPDCE results within CBA.

This handbook has endeavored to provide a compilation of evidence in the areas of benefit assessment and costing specifically for use within a CBA framework in health care, in doing so this book hopefully provides some coherent guidance on applied methods of CBA in health care. The handbook has benefited from contributions from a number of emerging literatures most notably in the areas of costing methodology, WTP, and SPDCE research as well as other disciplines including environmental economics, accountancy, and marketing. One observation from these areas is the increasing reliance on statistical and econometric developments. Whilst these developments have aided the accuracy of measures, these advances have been developed independently of one another and as a consequence little attention has been paid to the science of CBA as an entity (1). The aim of this handbook was to attempt to rectify this somewhat and not only pull these developments together in a coherent fashion but to identify clear links between them with a view to providing some up-to-date guidance for carrying out applied CBA in health care.

As outlined, Chapter 5 described a number of parallels between environmental valuation and health valuation and the uses of valuation in CBA in environmental and health fields. The parallels are not surprising since both areas deal with decisions involving public goods, quasi-public goods, or publically provided goods that benefit from economic evaluation methods. Arrow and colleagues (2) recognized these similarities and argued for improved use of CBA and valuation in policy and management. What is perhaps surprising, however, is the somewhat divergent paths the two areas have taken – environmental economics following a more traditional welfare-economics orientation and health economics taking a 'cost-effectiveness' path. While there are clearly institutional reasons for the divergence, it is believed that both applications of economics and statistical analysis would benefit from a stronger economic conceptual framework and higher analytical standards in pursuit of good CBA practice.

In terms of research, there has been considerable effort in health economics to assess the extent to which findings in environmental economics apply to health care cases. Many of the same principles apply. The literatures would benefit, however, from collectively addressing problems in understanding revealed and stated choice behaviour, and identifying tools that can help in assessing tradeoffs. There are several areas where crossovers or hybridization can occur, including risk valuation, evaluation of public programmes and methodological, econometric, and experimental-design tool development.

Many advances in environmental economics occurred as a result of institutional arrangements that arose largely outside of the discipline such as Reagan's executive order and the Exxon Valdez incident. Recent debate in the USA over a greater public role in health care may or may not provide similar opportunities for exploring alternative valuation approaches. In any case, methodological advances in health care evaluation will require that health economists provide robust theoretical arguments from within the discipline of economics for adopting economic methods and techniques. In addition to this, a further skill required of health economists will be translating the theoretical core of such methods into 'applied' methodology for use in the complex health care setting. As Arrow *et al.* (2) state 'Because society has limited resources to spend on regulation, benefit–cost analysis can help illuminate the trade-offs involved in making different kinds of social investments. In this regard, it seems almost irresponsible to not conduct such analyses, because they can inform decisions about how scarce resources can be put to the greatest social good'.

References

1. McIntosh, E., Donaldson, C., and Ryan, M. 1999. Recent advances in the methods of cost-benefit analysis in healthcare: Matching the art to the science. *Pharmacoeconomics* **15**: 357–367.
2. Arrow, K.J., Cropper, M.L., Eads, G.C., Hahn, R.W., Lave, L.B., Noll, R.G., *et al.* 1996. Is there a role for benefit-cost analysis in environmental, health and safety regulation? *Science* **272**: 221–222.

Index